N. E. Brill

Mt. Sinai Hospital Reports

Vol. IV - For 1903 and 1904

N. E. Brill

Mt. Sinai Hospital Reports
Vol. IV - For 1903 and 1904

ISBN/EAN: 9783337173548

Printed in Europe, USA, Canada, Australia, Japan

Cover: Foto ©ninafisch / pixelio.de

More available books at **www.hansebooks.com**

MT. SINAI HOSPITAL REPORTS

VOLUME IV

For 1903 and 1904

EDITED FOR THE MEDICAL BOARD

BY

N. E. BRILL, A.M., M.D.

1905

CONTENTS.

	PAGE
Preface	5
Medical and Surgical Staff for 1903 and 1904	7
House Staff for 1903	9
House Staff for 1904	10
Statistics of Medical Service during 1903	11
Statistics of Medical Service during 1904	20
Some Further Observations on the Determination of Uric Acid and Xanthine Bodies in Urine. JULIUS RUDISCH, M.D.	27
Two Cases of Pernicious Anemia Due to the Dibothriocephalis Latus. ALFRED MEYER, M.D.	31
Primary Splenomegaly—Gaucher Type. N. E. BRILL, A.M., M.D., F. S. MANDLEBAUM, M.D., and E. LIBMAN, M.D.	35
The Diagnosis and Treatment of Perforation in Typhoid Fever. MORRIS MANGES, M.D.	53
The Present Limitations of Serum Therapy in the Treatment of Infectious Diseases. HENRY W. BERG, M.D.	78
Two Cases of Acute Yellow Atrophy of the Liver. ALBERT KOHN, M.D.	90
Statistical Report, Children's Service, 1903	98
Statistical Report, Children's Service, 1904	102
Posterior-Basic Meningitis. HENRY KOPLIK, M.D.	105
Bilateral Empyema in Children—A Report of Two Cases. HENRY HEIMAN, M.D.	125
Report of the Department of General Surgery—Introductory Remarks. ARPAD G. GERSTER, M.D.	129
Statistical Report of the First Surgical Division—1903	133
Statistical Report of the First Surgical Division—1904	148
Report on the Diseases of the Kidney and Ureter for 1903-1904. ARPAD G. GERSTER, M.D.	165
A Report of the Cases of Benign and Malign Diseases of the Stomach and Duodenum. A. A. BERG, M.D.	178
Dry Iodine Catgut. ALEXIS V. MOSCHCOWITZ, M.D.	206
Diseases Treated in the Second Surgical Division—1903	214
Diseases Treated in the Second Surgical Division—1904	229
Report of the Department of General Surgery—Second Surgical Division. HOWARD LILIENTHAL, M.D.	247
On the Treatment of Chronic Osteomyelitis and of Chronic Bone Cavities by the Iodoform Wax Filling. CHARLES A. ELSBERG, M.D.	322

	PAGE
Statistics of Gynecological Service	329
A Study of the Results of Abdominal Hysterectomy for Fibroid of the Uterus, With and Without Drainage. JOSEPH BRETTAUER, M.D.	340
Synopsis of Deaths—Service of JOSEPH BRETTAUER, M.D.	347
An Analytical and Clinical Study of Thirty Cases of Ectopic Pregnancy. SAMUEL M. BRICKNER, A.M., M.D.	358
Special Case. H. W. VINEBERG, M.D.	369
The Genito-Urinary Service. H. GOLDENBERG, M.D., and MARTIN M. WARE, M.D.	372
Poisoning by Wood Alcohol. CARL KOLLER, M.D.	376
Observations on the Thread Reaction; Its Occurrence in the Human Body. E. LIBMAN, M.D.	383
Notes on the Widal Reaction: (1) The Question of Dilution; (2) The Influence of Jaundice. E. LIBMAN, M.D.	389
A New Method for Staining the Capsules of Bacteria: Preliminary Communication. LEO BUERGER, M.D.	398
Investigations in Metabolism and Composition of the Urine in Disease. S. BOOKMAN, M.A., Ph.D., and EDWARD A. ARONSON, M.D.	401
A New X-Ray Tube Stand; A New X-Ray Table. WALTER M. BRICKNER, M.D.	413

PREFACE.

In presenting the fourth volume of the Medical and Surgical Reports of Mount Sinai Hospital the Editor expresses, on behalf of the Medical Board, its thanks to the Board of Directors of the hospital for the generous donation which made it possible to publish the following scientific contributions to medical literature.

This volume marks some of the work done in the new hospital which was opened for the reception of cases on March 19, 1904. Preparatory to the removal into the new buildings, it was deemed advisable to restrict the admission of patients to those suffering with conditions which required urgent treatment and to discharge those patients who remained in the hospital as soon as convalescence and improvement in their health justified such discharge. This method permitted a removal from the old to the new hospital with very little difficulty. The patients who were too sick to be removed were kept in the old hospital with an adequate medical and nursing staff until convalescence or improvement warranted their discharge or removal. Thus, for a time the two institutions were run simultaneously.

The various wards in the new hospital were opened, one after the other as soon as the resources of the institution permitted and the demand for beds became urgent. This explanation will make evident the apparent anomaly of a larger institution caring for a smaller number of patients. At the present writing the hospital is working at its full capacity. Future reports will show a much larger total number of cases treated.

In the Report of the First Surgical Division, Dr. A. G. Gerster has presented an outline of the general plan of the wards which obtains for both the surgical and medical wards of the hospital; he has shown the division of work between the two attending surgeons. For those who are interested in details as to the work in the Department of Internal Medicine, the Editor would say that there are four general medical wards, each of which is visited by an Attending Physician and Adjunct Attending Physician daily. There are two male wards and two female wards, comprising two medical divisions. At the end of each year, expiring on October 1, the Attending Physicians of each division change wards, so that the one having had the male service takes charge of the female service for the following year and *vice versa*. This plan gives each Attending Physician a continuous service which is deemed much more advantageous to the patient and the hospital. The neurologist and dermatologist have now small wards of their own instead of having their patients scattered throughout the various wards of the hospital.

In the equipment the minutest requirements have been supplied with a generous but judicious hand.

The work in no hospital could be done under better conditions than exist in the present magnificent institution, whose erection and equipment reflect the greatest honor upon the progressive and liberal minded spirit of those who had the work in charge.

N. E. BRILL, A.M., M.D.,
Editor for the Medical Board.

AUGUST 15, 1905.

MEDICAL AND SURGICAL STAFF FOR 1903 AND 1904.

CONSULTING PHYSICIANS.
A. JACOBI, M.D.,   E. G. JANEWAY, M.D.

CONSULTING SURGEONS.
DANIEL M. STIMSON, M.D.   WILLIAM F. FLUHRER, M.D.

ATTENDING PHYSICIANS.
JULIUS RUDISCH, M.D.   N. E. BRILL, M.D.
ALFRED MEYER, M.D.   MORRIS MANGES, M.D.
HENRY KOPLIK, M.D.
(*Diseases of Children.*)

ATTENDING SURGEONS.
A. G. GERSTER, M.D.   HOWARD LILIENTHAL, M.D.
HERMAN GOLDENBERG, M.D.
(*Genito-Urinary Service.*)

GYNECOLOGISTS.
JOSEPH BRETTAUER, M.D.   FLORIAN KRUG, M.D.

OPHTHALMIC AND AURAL SURGEON.
EMIL GRUENING, M.D.

ATTENDING NEUROLOGIST.
B. SACHS, M.D.

ATTENDING DERMATOLOGIST.
S. LUSTGARTEN, M.D.

ATTENDING LARYNGOLOGIST.
D. B. DELAVAN, M.D.

ADJUNCT ATTENDING PHYSICIANS.
D. H. DAVISON, M.D.   HENRY W. BERG, M.D.
E. LIBMAN, M.D.   ALBERT KOHN, M.D.
HENRY HEIMAN, M.D.
(*Diseases of Children.*)

ADJUNCT ATTENDING SURGEONS.
CHARLES A. ELSBERG, M.D.   A. V. MOSCHCOWITZ, M.D.
JOSEPH WIENER, M.D.   A. A. BERG, M.D.
MARTIN W. WARE, M.D.
(*Genito-Urinary Service.*)

MEDICAL AND SURGICAL STAFF FOR 1903 AND 1904.

(Continued.)

ADJUNCT OPHTHALMIC AND AURAL SURGEONS.

CHARLES H. MAY, M.D.   CARL KOLLER, M.D.

ADJUNCT GYNECOLOGISTS

HIRAM N. VINEBERG, M.D.   SAMUEL M. BRICKNER, M.D.*

ADJUNCT DERMATOLOGIST.

FRED. J. LEVISEUR, M.D.

ADJUNCT NEUROLOGIST.

WILLIAM HIRSCH, M.D.

ADJUNCT LARYNGOLOGIST.

EMIL MAYER, M.D.*

ADMITTING PHYSICIAN.

MAX ROSENBERG, M.D.

RADIOGRAPHIST.

WALTER M. BRICKNER, M.D.

ASSISTANT RADIOGRAPHIST.

EUGENE EISING, M.D.‡
ANDREW G. FOORD, M.D.*

ANESTHETISTS.

M. L. MADURO, M.D.†
MYRON P. DENTON, M.D.
THOMAS L. BENNETT, M.D.*

PATHOLOGICAL STAFF.

F. S. MANDLEBAUM, M.D., *Pathologist.*
E. LIBMAN, M.D., *Assistant Pathologist.*
E. P. BERNSTEIN, M.D., *Second Assistant Pathologist.*
HERBERT L. CELLER, M.D., *Laboratory Assistant.*
LEO BUERGER, M.D., *Pathological Interne.**

SAM. BOOKMAN, Ph.D., *Physiological Chemist.**
EDWARD A. ARONSON, M.D., *Assistant Physiological Chemist.**

*Appointed 1904.   †Deceased.   ‡Resigned 1904.

HOUSE STAFF.

From January 1 to June 30, 1903.

House Surgeon.
MEYER M. STARK, M.D.

House Physician.
HERBERT L. CELLER, M.D.

Senior Assistant Surgeons,
ROBERT T. FRANK, M.D.
ELI MOSCHCOWITZ, M.D.

Senior Assistant Physicians.
ALFRED FABIAN HESS, M.D.
DAVID KRAMER, M.D.

Junior Assistant Surgeons,
D. LEE HIRSCHLER, M.D.
FRED. H. McCARTHY, M.D.

Junior Assistant Physicians,
BERNH. OPPENHEIMER, M.D.
ARTHUR BOOKMAN, M.D.

First Externes,
C. F. JELLINGHAUS, M.D.
ALBERT G. SWIFT, M.D.

First Externes,
LOUIS BAUMAN, M.D.
FRANK B. MITCHELL, M.D.

Second Externes,
SOL. HYMAN, M.D.
ISADORE SEFF, M.D.

Second Externes,
SAMUEL FELDSTEIN, M.D.
GEORGE W. T. MILLS, M.D.

From July 1 to December 31, 1903.

House Surgeons,
ROBERT T. FRANK, M.D.
ELI MOSCHCOWITZ, M.D.

House Physicians,
ALFRED FABIAN HESS, M.D.
DAVID KRAMER, M.D.

Senior Assistant Surgeons,
D. LEE HIRSCHLER, M.D.
ALBERT G. SWIFT, M.D.

Senior Assistant Physicians,
BERNH. OPPENHEIMER, M.D.
ARTHUR BOOKMAN, M.D.

Junior Assistant Surgeons,
FRED. H. McCARTHY, M.D.
C. F. JELLINGHAUS, M.D.

Junior Assistant Physicians,
LOUIS BAUMAN, M.D.
H. F. L. ZIEGEL, M.D.

First Externes,
ISADORE SEFF, M.D.
SOL. HYMAN, M.D.

First Externes,
SAMUEL FELDSTEIN, M.D.
GEO. W. T. MILLS, M.D.

Second Externes,
LEO KESSEL, M.D.
G. A. FRIED, M.D.

Second Externes,
HORACE L. LEITER, M.D.
WILLIAM J. HABER, M.D.

HOUSE STAFF.
(Continued.)

From January 1 to June 30, 1904.

House Surgeons,
D. LEE HIRSCHLER, M.D.
ALBERT G. SWIFT, M.D.

Senior Assistant Surgeons,
FRED. H. McCARTHY, M.D.
C. F. JELLINGHAUS, M.D.

Junior Assistant Surgeons.
ISADORE SEFF, M.D.
SOL. HYMAN, M.D.

First Externes.
LEO KESSEL, M.D.
G. A. FRIED, M.D.

Second Externes.
MILTON BODENHEIMER, M.D.
CLARENCE M. HATHEWAY, M.D.

House Physicians,
BERNH. OPPENHEIMER, M.D
ARTHUR BOOKMAN, M.D.

Senior Assistant Physicians,
LOUIS BAUMAN, M.D.
H. F. L. ZIEGEL, M.D.

Junior Assistant Physicians,
SAMUEL FELDSTEIN, M.D.
GEO. W. T. MILLS, M.D.

First Externes,
HORACE L. LEITER, M.D.
WILLIAM J. HABER, M.D.

Second Externes,
JESSE G. M. BULLOWA, M.D.
JULIUS J. HERTZ, M.D.

From July 1 to December 31, 1904.

House Surgeons,
FRED. H. McCARTHY, M.D.
C. F. JELLINGHAUS, M.D.

Senior Assistant Surgeons,
SOL. HYMAN, M.D.
ISADORE SEFF, M.D.

Junior Assistant Surgeons.
WILLIAM J. HABER, M.D.
HORACE L. LEITER, M.D.

First Externes,
C. M. HATHEWAY, M.D.
MILTON BODENHEIMER, M.D.

Second Externes,
MAX TASHMAN, M.D.
JULIAN J. MEYER, M.D.

House Physicians,
LOUIS BAUMAN, M.D.
H. F. L. ZIEGEL, M.D.

Senior Assistant Physicians,
GEO. W. T. MILLS, M.D.
SAMUEL FELDSTEIN, M.D.

Junior Assistant Physicians,
G. A. FRIED, M.D.
LEO KESSEL, M.D.

First Externes,
JULIUS J. HERTZ, M.D.
JESSE G. M. BULLOWA, M.D.

Second Externes,
SOLOMON WIENER, M.D.
ERNST SACHS, M.D.

PRIVATE HOSPITAL STAFF.

Resident Physician,
ALBERT G. SWIFT, M.D.

Assistant Resident Physician,
EDWARD A. RIESENFELD, M.D.

PROVISIONALS.

From January 1, to December 31, 1904.

KAUFMAN SCHLIVEK, M.D.
ISIDORE GOLDSTEIN, M.D.

WILLIAM BRANOWER, M.D.
ISADORE KAUFMAN, M.D.

DEPARTMENT OF INTERNAL MEDICINE.

STATISTICS OF MEDICAL SERVICE DURING 1903.

ATTENDING PHYSICIANS.

JULIUS RUDISCH, M.D., NATHAN E. BRILL, M.D.,
ALFRED MEYER, M.D.,   MORRIS MANGES, M.D.

ADJUNCT ATTENDING PHYSICIANS.

D. H. DAVISON, M.D., E. LIBMAN, M.D.,
H. W. BERG, M.D.,   A. KOHN, M.D.

TOTAL OF ALL CASES IN DEPARTMENT OF INTERNAL MEDICINE FOR YEAR 1903.

Treated 1,012
Cured 338
Improved 431
Unimproved 87
Died 156

General Diseases.	Total.		Cured.		Improved.		Unimproved.		Died.	
	M	F	M	F	M	F	M	F	M	F
A. Diphtheria		1		1						
Influenza	19	2	17		2	2				
" with chr. sup. otitis media......	1		1							
" " " " " " exophthalmic goitre		1		1						
Malaria	5		5							
" æstivo-autumnal		1				1				
Measles		1		1						
Rötheln		2		2						
Mumps and orchitis...................	2			1			1			
Scarlet fever		2		1				1		
Typhoid fever	39	37	36	35			1	1	2	1
" " abortion		1		1						
" " nephritis	1		1							
" " periostitis	1						1			
" " intestinal perforation	2	1	1						1	1
" " phlebitis		1		1						
" " and post-typhoid sepsis.....		1		1						

General Diseases—Continued.	Total		Cured		Improved		Unimproved		Died	
	M	F	M	F	M	F	M	F	M	F
Para typhoid	8	1	8	1	..	..	..	..	..	..
Tuberculosis, acute general miliary	1	1	..	..	..	..	..	..	1	1
B. Arthritis, gonorrheal	5	5	4	3	1	2	..	..	..	..
" deformans	1	..	..	..	..	1	..	..	..	..
" peri	1	..	..	..	..	1	..	..	..	..
" chronic, of knee	1	2	1	..	..	1	..	1	..	..
" rheumatoid	..	2	..	..	..	2	..	..	..	..
Actinomycosis	1	..	..	..	1	..	..	..	..	..
Carcinomatosis, general	1	1	..	..	..	..	..	..	1	1
Cerebro-spinal meningitis	9	9	4	1	1	..	..	..	4	8
Diabetes mellitus	5	2	..	..	4	2	1	..	..	..
" " diphtheria	1	..	..	..	..	..	1	..	..	..
" coma, carcinoma of liver	..	1	..	..	..	..	..	..	..	1
" gangrene of lung	1	..	..	..	..	..	..	..	1	..
Filariasis	1	..	..	..	1	..	..	..	..	..
Hemophilia	1	..	..	..	..	..	1	..	..	..
Polyserositis, with abscess of leg	1	..	..	..	1	..	..	..	..	..
Rheumatism, acute articular	9	5	8	5	1	..	..	..	..	..
" " " pneumonia	1	..	1	..	..	..	..	..	..	..
" " " chr. endocarditis	7	4	4	2	3	2	..	..	..	..
" " " " and acute pericarditis	1	1	..	..	1	1	..	..	..	..
Rheumatism, acute articular, influenza	1	..	1	..	..	..	..	..	..	..
" subacute	10	4	7	2	3	1	..	1	..	..
" " chronic, endocarditis	1	..	1	..	..	..	..	..	..	..
" chronic articular	2	5	..	1	2	4	..	..	..	..
" " " insanity	..	1	..	..	..	1	..	..	..	..
" " " acute exacerbation	2	1	1	..	1	1	..	..	..	..
" muscular	1	..	1	..	..	..	..	..	..	..
Sarcomatosis, multiple	1	..	..	..	..	..	..	..	1	..
Sarcoma, lympho	3	..	..	..	3	..	..	..	..	..
" kidney and mediastinum	..	1	..	..	..	..	..	..	..	1
Sepsis	1	..	..	..	1	..	..	..	..	..
Staphylococcemia	..	1	..	..	..	..	..	..	..	1
Streptococcemia	..	2	..	..	..	..	..	..	..	2
" hemorrhagic nephritis and pneumonia	1	..	..	..	..	..	..	..	1	..
Syphilis, tertiary	..	1	..	..	..	1	..	..	..	..
" necrosis of nasal septum	1	1	1	1	..	..	..	..	..	..
Blood Diseases.										
Anemia, secondary	1	1	..	..	1	1	..	..	..	..
" " pernicious type	4	1	..	1	2	..	1	..	1	..
Chlorosis	..	3	..	..	..	3	..	..	..	..
Leukemia, splenic	1	..	..	..	..	..	..	..	1	..
" splenomyelogenous	1	1	..	..	1	1	..	..	..	..
Total	157	108	103	62	31	27	7	4	14	17

Diseases of Digestive Tract.	Total M	Total F	Cured M	Cured F	Improved M	Improved F	Unimproved M	Unimproved F	Died M	Died F
Alveolar abscess	..	1	..	1	..	..	..	..	..	..
Abdominal tumor	2	1	..	..	1	1	1	..	..	..
" carcinoma	..	1	..	..	..	..	..	..	..	1
Autointoxication	8	7	8	7	..	..	..	..	..	..
Biliary colic	..	1	..	..	..	1	..	..	..	..
Colitis, chronic, and ependymitis and chronic nephritis	1	..	..	..	..	..	..	..	1	..
Colitis, chronic, productive constipation	1	..	..	..	..	1	..	..	..	..
" "	3	..	1	..	2	..	..	..	..	..
" "	..	1	..	1	..	..	..	..	..	..
" and neurasthenia	1	..	..	..	..	1	..	..	..	..
" ulcerative	1	1	..	1	1	..	..	..	..	..
Constipation	3	2	2	2	1	..	..	..	..	..
Colic, intestinal	2	..	2	..	..	..	..	..	..	..
Cholecystitis	2	2	2	2	..	..	..	..	..	..
Cholelithiasis	4	1	1	..	3	..	..	1	..	..
" and multiple neuritis	1	..	..	..	1	..	..	..	..	..
Cholangitis, hemorrhagic pancreatitis and chronic nephritis	..	1	..	..	..	..	..	..	..	1
Diarrhea, nervous	..	2	..	2	..	..	..	..	..	..
Dyspepsia, intestinal	1	..	..	..	1	..	..	..	..	..
Duodenal ulcer with stenosis	1	..	1	..	..	..	..	..	..	..
Enteritis	1	..	1	..	..	..	..	..	..	..
" chronic	..	1	..	1	..	..	..	..	..	..
" tubercular	1	..	..	..	1	..	..	..	..	..
Esophagus, tumor	2	..	..	..	..	..	1	..	1	..
" (spasmodic stricture)	1	1	..	1	1	..	..	..	..	..
" carcinoma	2	..	..	..	..	..	..	..	2	..
Gastritis, alcoholic	1	..	1	..	..	..	..	..	..	..
" " with alcoholic neuritis	1	..	1	..	..	..	..	..	..	..
" acute	2	3	1	3	1	..	..	..	..	..
" chronic	1	7	..	2	1	5	..	..	..	..
" " and gastroptosis	1	..	..	..	1	..	..	..	..	..
" " " scoliosis	..	1	..	..	..	1	..	..	..	..
Gastric crises	1	..	..	..	1	..	..	..	..	..
Gastroptosis	1	..	..	..	1	..	..	..	..	..
Hyperchlorhydria	1	..	1	..	..	..	..	..	..	..
Hydrops vesicæ felleæ	..	1	..	..	..	1	..	..	..	..
Intestinal tumor	1	1	..	..	..	1	1	..	..	..
Jaundice, catarrhal	1	..	1	..	..	..	..	..	..	..
Liver, hypertrophic cirrhosis of	1	..	..	..	..	1	..	..	..	..
" cirrhosis of	3	1	..	..	1	..	..	..	2	1
" " and cholangitis	..	1	..	..	..	1	..	..	..	..
" carcinoma	..	3	..	..	..	..	..	2	..	1
" neoplasm	..	1	..	..	..	..	..	..	..	1
" fatty degeneration of, and sepsis	1	..	..	..	..	..	..	..	1	..
" biliary cirrhosis, jaundice, and stone in common duct	1	..	..	..	1	..	..	..	..	..
" biliary cirrhosis, stone in common duct	1	..	..	..	1	..	..	..	..	..

Diseases of Digestive Tract—Continued.	Total		Cured		Improved		Unimproved		Died	
	M	F	M	F	M	F	M	F	M	F
Liver, acute yellow atrophy	1	1	..	..	..	..	..	..	1	1
" cirrhosis and chronic endocarditis	1	..	..	..	..	1	..	..	..	..
Pyloric stenosis and gastrectasis	..	1	..	1	..	..	..	..	..	..
Pharyngitis, acute	1	..	1	..	..	..	..	..	..	..
Pancreas, tumor of	1	..	..	..	..	1	..	..	..	..
Peritonitis, tubercular	..	3	..	..	..	..	2	..	1	..
Pericholecystitis	..	1	..	..	..	..	..	..	1	..
Rectum, carcinoma of	1	..	..	..	..	..	..	..	..	1
Stomach "	10	2	..	..	..	..	..	5	2	5
" dilatation of	2	..	..	..	..	2	..	..	..	..
" ulcer of	2	8	..	8	..	1	..	..	..	1
" and omentum, carcinoma of	1	..	..	..	..	..	..	..	..	1
Stomatitis and abdominal pain	1	..	1	..	..	..	..	..	..	..
Tonsilitis, acute follicular	5	3	5	3	..	..	..	..	..	..
Visceroptosis	..	2	..	..	..	..	2	..	..	..
Total	82	63	30	35	28	15	8	7	16	6
Diseases of Respiratory Tract.										
Abscess of lung	1	..	..	..	..	..	..	..	1	..
Asthma	1	3	1	1	..	2	..	..	..	..
" and emphysema	1	1	..	..	1	1	..	..	..	..
Bronchitis, acute	..	2	..	2	..	..	..	..	..	..
" chronic	1	1	..	..	1	1	..	..	..	..
Cavity of lung	1	..	..	..	..	..	1	..	..	..
Endothelioma of lung	..	1	..	..	..	..	..	..	..	1
Empyema	2	..	..	..	..	..	1	..	1	..
" sacculated	..	1	..	..	..	..	..	..	..	1
" interlobar	1	..	1	..	..	..	..	..	..	..
Emphysema	4	1	..	..	4	1	..	..	..	..
" chronic, with chronic bronchitis	4	..	..	..	4	..	..	..	..	..
Gangrene of lung	1	..	..	..	..	..	..	..	1	..
Hydropneumothorax	1	..	..	..	1	..	..	..	..	..
Intrathoracic tumor	1	..	..	..	1	..	..	..	..	..
Neoplasm, mediastinal	..	2	..	..	..	1	..	1	..	..
Pleurisy, sicca	2	2	..	2	2	..	..	..	..	..
" with effusion	7	5	5	5	2	..	..	..	..	..
" tubercular	4	1	..	..	4	1	..	..	..	..
" with effusion and diabetes mellitus	1	..	..	..	1	..	..	..	..	..
" sicca, and emphysema	1	..	1	..	..	..	..	..	..	..
Pneumonia	3	1	2	..	..	..	..	..	1	1
" broncho	..	1	..	1	..	..	..	..	..	..
" acute lobar	21	10	14	6	..	1	..	..	7	3
" central	1	..	1	..	..	..	..	..	..	..
" interstitial	1	..	..	..	..	1	..	..	..	..
" resolvens	..	3	..	2	..	1	..	..	..	..
" tubercular	1	..	..	..	..	1	..	..	..	..
" and pleurisy with effusion	1	1	1	1	..	..	..	..	..	..
" " pulmonary edema	1	..	..	..	..	..	..	..	1	..

STATISTICS OF MEDICAL SERVICE FOR 1903.   15

Diseases of Respiratory Tract—Continued.	Total		Cured		Improved		Unimproved		Died	
	M	F	M	F	M	F	M	F	M	F
Pneumonia, lobar, with pericarditis	1	..	1	..	..	..	..	..	..	..
" " " empyema	1	..	1	..	..	..	..	..	..	..
Pneumothorax	1	..	..	..	1	..	..	..	..	..
Pyopneumothorax	..	1	..	..	..	..	..	..	..	1
Sarcoma of lung	1	..	..	..	..	..	..	..	1	..
Tuberculosis, incipient pulmonary	5	1	1	..	4	1	..	..	..	..
" pulmonary	30	7	..	..	24	5	5	1	1	1
" " and delirium tremens	1	..	..	..	..	..	1	..	..	..
" " " Pott's disease	1	..	..	..	1	..	..	..	..	..
" " " pyopneumothorax	1	..	..	..	1	..	..	..	..	..
" " " tubercular laryngitis	2	..	..	..	..	..	1	..	1	..
" " " pleurisy with effusion	1	..	..	..	1	..	..	..	..	..
Total	108	45	29	20	55	15	9	2	15	8

Diseases of the Circulatory System.

Diseases of the Heart.

	Total		Cured		Improved		Unimproved		Died	
	M	F	M	F	M	F	M	F	M	F
Cardiac neurosis	1	1	..	1	1	..	..	..	..	..
Chronic endocarditis	24	29	..	..	19	23	1	..	4	6
Chronic endocarditis with acute exacerbation	3	3	..	..	2	2	..	..	1	1
Chronic endocarditis with acute exacerbation and rheumatism	2	..	..	..	2	..	..	..	..	..
Chronic endocarditis with angina pectoris	1	..	..	..	1	..	..	..	..	..
Chronic endocarditis with asthma	..	2	..	..	..	2	..	..	..	..
Chronic endocarditis with femoral embolism	..	1	..	..	..	..	..	..	..	1
Chronic endocarditis with infarct of lung	3	3	..	..	2	2	..	..	1	1
Chronic endocarditis with lobar pneumonia	2	..	..	..	1	..	..	..	1	..
Chronic endocarditis with myocarditis	2	2	..	..	2	1	..	..	1	..
Chronic endocarditis with pneumonia	..	2	..	..	..	1	..	..	..	1
Chronic endocarditis, pleurisy with effusion	..	1	..	*1	..	*1	..	..	..	..
Chronic endocarditis, post-abortive sepsis and pulmonary infarct	..	1	..	..	..	..	..	..	..	1
Chronic endocarditis with pulmonary infarct, with thrombosis of internal jugular vein, with pulmonary edema	1	..	..	..	..	..	..	..	1	..
Chronic endocarditis with purpura	1	..	..	..	1	..	..	..	..	..
Chronic endocarditis with rheumatism	4	2	..	..	4	2	..	..	..	..
Endocarditis and myocarditis with erysipelas	..	1	..	..	..	..	..	..	..	1
Fatty heart	1	2	..	..	1	2	..	..	..	..
Malignant endocarditis	3	1	..	..	..	..	..	..	3	1
Myocarditis	4	9	..	..	2	7	1	2	1	..
Myocarditis with angina pectoris	1	..	..	..	..	..	..	..	1	..
Myocarditis with diabetes mellitus	..	1	..	..	..	..	..	..	..	1
Myocarditis with hepatic cirrhosis	1	..	..	..	..	..	..	..	1	..
Myocarditis with rheumatism	..	1	..	..	..	1	..	..	..	..
Pericarditis and endocarditis	..	2	..	..	..	2	..	..	..	..
Total	54	64	..	1	36	47	3	2	15	14

*One case.

Diseases of Circulatory System—*Continued.* Diseases of Vessels.	Total		Cured		Improved		Unimproved		Died	
	M	F	M	F	M	F	M	F	M	F
Aortitis	1	..	..	..	1	..	..	..	..	..
" chronic nephritis	1	..	..	..	..	..	1	..	..	..
" " endarteritis	..	1	..	..	..	1	..	..	..	..
Aneurism, arch of aorta	..	1	..	..	..	1	..	..	..	..
" descending aorta, rupture into left bronchus	1	..	..	..	..	..	..	..	1	..
Arterio-sclerosis, general	4	..	..	..	2	..	2	..	..	..
" " chronic endocarditis	1	..	..	..	1	..	..	..	..	..
" " diabetic gangrene	1	..	..	..	1	..	..	..	..	..
Obstruction of inferior vena cava (general peritonitis)	1	..	..	..	..	..	..	..	1	..
Total	10	2	..	..	5	2	3	..	2	..

Nervous Diseases.

	M	F	M	F	M	F	M	F	M	F
Alcoholic neuritis	2	..	1	..	1	..	..	..	..	..
Cerebral apoplexy	..	1	..	..	..	..	..	..	..	1
Cerebral embolism with hemiplegia	2	..	1	..	1	..	..	..	..	..
Cerebral gumma	..	1	..	1	..	..	..	..	..	..
Cerebral hemorrhage with nephritis	1	..	..	..	1	..	..	..	..	..
Cerebral syphilis	2	..	2	..	..	..	..	..	..	..
Cerebral thrombosis	5	3	..	..	2	1	..	..	3	2
Cerebral tumor	1	2	..	..	..	..	1	1	..	1
Cerebro-spinal syphilis	2	..	1	..	..	..	1	..	..	..
Chorea	2	1	1	..	1	1	..	..	..	..
Coccydinia	..	1	..	1	..	..	..	..	..	..
Dementia	..	1	..	..	..	..	..	1	..	..
Epilepsy	1	..	..	..	1	..	..	..	..	..
Erythromelalgia	2	2	1	..	2	..	1	..	..	..
Gastric neurosis	1	6	..	3	1	2	..	1	..	..
General paresis	1	..	..	..	1	..	..	..	..	..
Hemiplegia	4	4	..	..	2	2	2	..	..	2
Hemiplegia with nephritis	1	..	..	..	..	..	..	..	1	..
Hysteria	1	10	..	4	1	5	..	1	..	..
Hysterical hemianesthesia	1	..	..	..	1	..	..	..	..	..
Hysterical neurosis of spinal accessory nerve	..	1	..	..	..	1	..	..	..	..
Hysterical tic	..	1	..	..	..	1	..	..	..	..
Hysterical torticollis	1	1	1	..	..	1	..	..	..	..
Hystero-epilepsy	1	..	..	..	..	..	1	..	..	..
Insanity	1	1	..	..	1	..	..	1	..	..
Intercostal neuralgia	1	1	..	..	1	1	..	..	..	..
Lumbago	1	..	1	..	..	..	..	..	..	..
Lumbo-sacral neuralgia	..	1	..	..	..	1	..	..	..	..
Melancholia	..	2	..	..	..	..	..	2	..	..
Méniere's disease	1	..	..	..	1	..	..	..	..	..
Multiple neuritis	1	2	1	..	2	..	..	..	..	..
Multiple sclerosis	1	..	..	..	1	..	..	..	..	..
Neuralgia	..	1	..	..	..	1	..	..	..	..

STATISTICS OF MEDICAL SERVICE FOR 1903.   17

	Total		Cured		Improved		Unimproved		Died	
Nervous Diseases—*Continued.*	M	F	M	F	M	F	M	F	M	F
Neurasthenia	1	13	..	2	1	10	..	1	..	..
Occipital neuralgia	..	1	..	..	..	1	..	..	..	..
Occupation neurosis	1	..	1	..	..	..	..	..	..	..
Pachymeningitis cervicalis	1	..	..	..	1	..	..	..	..	..
Pachymeningitis, lumbar	1	..	..	..	..	..	1	..	..	..
Poliencephalitis and poliomyelitis	1	..	..	..	1	..	..	..	..	..
Poliencephalitis, superior and inferior	1	..	..	..	..	..	..	..	1	..
Psychosis	..	1	..	..	..	..	..	1	..	..
Sciatica	11	10	5	4	6	6	..	..	..	..
Senile dementia with chronic endocarditis	..	1	..	..	..	..	..	1	..	..
Spinal syphilis	1	..	1	..	..	..	..	..	..	..
Syphilitic neuritis	1	..	..	..	1	..	..	..	..	..
Tabes dorsalis	3	..	..	..	3	..	..	..	..	..
Tabes dorsalis, Charcot knee joint	..	1	..	..	..	1	..	..	..	..
Traumatic neuritis, brachial plexus	1	..	..	..	..	..	1	..	..	..
Trigeminal neuralgia	1	..	1	..	..	..	..	..	..	..
Typhoid spine	1	..	1	..	..	..	..	..	..	..
Total	62	70	19	15	34	35	8	10	5	6
Surgical Diseases.										
Abortion, retained secundines	..	1	..	..	..	1	..	..	..	..
Abscess, alveolar	1	..	1	..	..	..	..	..	..	..
" pelvic	..	1	..	1	..	..	..	..	..	..
" " with suppurative hepatitis	1	..	..	..	..	..	1	..	..	..
Appendicitis, subacute catarrhal with chronic endocarditis	1	..	..	..	1	..	..	..	..	..
Cellulitis, pelvic	..	1	..	..	..	1	..	..	..	..
Coxitis	..	1	..	..	..	..	..	1	..	..
" with otitis media	1	..	..	..	1	..	..	..	..	..
Fibroids, of uterus	..	2	..	..	..	2	..	..	..	..
Fracture, neck of femur, diabetes	..	1	..	..	..	..	..	..	..	1
Mastoiditis with sinus thrombosis and sepsis	1	..	1	..	..	..	..	..	..	..
Necrosis of rib	..	1	..	..	..	1	..	..	..	..
Oöphoritis, acute	..	1	..	1	..	..	..	..	..	..
Peritonitis, pelvic	..	1	..	..	..	1	..	..	..	..
Periostitis of femur with synovitis of knee	1	..	1	..	..	..	..	..	..	..
Pes planus	1	1	..	..	1	1	..	..	..	..
Phlebitis, multiple	1	..	..	..	1	..	..	..	..	..
Pyosalpinx with neurasthenia	..	1	..	..	..	..	..	1	..	..
Sarcoma of femur	..	1	..	..	..	..	..	1	..	..
Scoliosis	..	1	..	..	..	..	..	1	..	..
Sinusitis, frontal	..	1	..	1	..	..	..	..	..	..
Tuberculosis of epididymis and spine	1	..	..	..	..	..	1	..	..	..
" " kidney and testicle, uremia	1	..	..	..	..	..	..	..	1	..
" " knee	..	1	..	..	..	1	..	..	..	..
Tumor of breast	..	1	..	..	..	..	..	1	..	..
Varicose ulcer	..	1	..	..	..	1	..	..	..	..
" veins, emphysema	1	..	..	..	1	..	..	..	..	..
Total	11	18	3	3	5	9	2	5	1	1

Cutaneous Diseases.	Total		Cured		Improved		Unimproved		Died	
	M	F	M	F	M	F	M	F	M	F
Chronic eczema	1	1	1	1	..	..	..	..	..	..
Chronic eczema and lymphosarcomatosis	1	..	..	..	1	..	..	..	..	..
Darier's disease	1	..	..	..	1	..	..	..	..	..
Dermatitis chronica universalis	1	..	..	..	1	..	..	..	..	..
Diabetic eczema	1	1	..	..	1	1	..	..	..	..
Dysidrosis	1	..	..	..	..	..	1	..	..	..
Eczema parasitica	1	..	1	..	..	..	..	..	..	..
Erythema multiforme	1	..	1	..	..	..	..	..	..	..
Furunculosis	1	..	..	..	1	..	..	..	..	..
Herpes zoster	..	1	..	1	..	..	..	..	..	..
Pediculosis	1	..	1	..	..	..	..	..	..	..
Pemphigus foliaceus	..	1	..	..	..	..	..	..	..	1
Pityriasis rosea	..	1	..	1	..	..	..	..	..	..
Scleroderma	1	..	..	..	1	..	..	..	..	..
Seborrheal eczema	1	..	..	..	1	..	..	..	..	..
Total	12	5	4	3	7	1	1	..	..	1

Miscellaneous Diseases.

	M	F	M	F	M	F	M	F	M	F
Exophthalmic goitre	1	3	..	..	1	1	2	..	..	..
Exophthalmic goitre with chronic endocarditis	..	1	..	..	..	..	1	..	..	..
" " " glycosuria	1	..	..	..	1	..	..	..	..	..
Obesity	..	1	..	..	..	1	..	..	..	..
Total	2	5	..	..	2	2	3	..	..	..

Poisons.

	M	F	M	F	M	F	M	F	M	F
Acute alcoholism	1	..	1	..	..	..	..	..	..	..
Carbolic acid, suicide	1	..	..	..	..	..	..	..	1	..
Morphinism	1	..	..	..	1	..	..	..	..	..
Plumbism	3	..	3	..	..	..	..	..	..	..
Toxic amblyopia	1	..	1	..	..	..	..	..	..	..
Total	7	..	5	..	1	..	..	..	1	..

Genito-Urinary Diseases.

	M	F	M	F	M	F	M	F	M	F
Cystitis	..	1	..	..	..	1	..	..	..	..
" with stone left kidney	1	..	..	..	1	..	..	..	..	..
" urethritis and urinary sepsis	1	..	..	..	..	..	..	..	1	..
Chyluria	1	..	..	..	1	..	..	..	..	..
Hypernephroma of kidney	1	..	..	..	..	..	..	..	1	..
Nephritis, acute	2	1	1	..	1	..	1	..	..	..
" subacute	..	1	..	..	..	1	..	..	..	..
" chronic	23	19	..	..	21	16	..	2	2	1
" " with asthma	..	1	..	..	..	1	..	..	..	..
" " acute exacerbation of	4	..	..	..	4	..	..	..	..	..
" " with cirrhosis of liver	1	..	..	..	..	..	..	..	1	..

STATISTICS OF MEDICAL SERVICE FOR 1903.   19

Genito-Urinary Diseases—*Continued.*	Total		Cured		Improved		Unimproved		Died	
	M	F	M	F	M	F	M	F	M	F
Nephritis, chronic, with delirium tremens	1	..	..	..	..	..	1	..	..	..
" " " diabetes	..	1	..	..	..	1	..	..	..	..
" " " endocarditis	8	12	..	..	3	4	1	2	4	6
" " " chronic endocarditis and uremia	1	..	..	..	..	..	..	..	1	..
" " " emphysema	7	2	..	..	4	2	1	..	2	..
" " " cystitis	..	1	..	..	..	1	..	..	..	..
" " " hydropericardium	..	1	..	..	..	..	..	..	..	1
" " " myocarditis	2	1	..	..	..	1	..	..	2	..
" " " " and lobar pneumonia	1	1	..	..	..	..	..	..	1	1
" " " purpura	..	1	..	..	..	1	..	..	..	..
" " " sciatica	..	2	..	..	..	1	..	1	..	..
" " " tonsilitis	1	..	..	..	1	..	..	..	..	..
" " " pulmonary tuberculosis	1	..	..	..	..	..	..	..	1	..
" " " uremia	5	6	..	..	1	2	1	..	3	4
" " " " pericarditis and pleurisy	1	..	..	..	..	..	..	..	1	..
" " " chronic uremia, dysarthria	1	..	..	..	..	..	1	..	..	..
Nephrolithiasis	3	..	..	..	2	..	1	..	..	..
" with acute nephritis	1	..	..	..	..	..	..	..	1	..
" " hemicrania	..	1	..	..	..	1	..	..	..	..
Pyelitis	..	1	..	1	..	..	..	..	..	..
Ren mobilis	1	2	..	..	1	1	..	1	..	..
Renal colic	3	1	3	1	..	..	..	..	..	..
Total	71	56	4	2	40	34	6	7	21	13

DEPARTMENT OF INTERNAL MEDICINE.

STATISTICS OF THE MEDICAL SERVICE DURING 1904.

ATTENDING PHYSICIANS.

JULIUS RUDISCH, M.D.,   NATHAN E. BRILL, M.D.,
ALFRED MEYER, M.D.,   MORRIS MANGES, M.D.

ADJUNCT ATTENDING PHYSICIANS.

D. H. DAVISON, M.D.,   E. LIBMAN, M.D.,
H. W. BERG, M.D.,   A. KOHN, M.D.

Total of all cases in Department of Internal Medicine for year 1904:

```
Treated ............................................. 954
Cured ............................................... 391
Improved ............................................ 374
Unimproved .......................................... 74
Died ................................................ 115
```

General Diseases.	Total		Cured.		Improved.		Unimproved.		Died.	
	M	F	M	F	M	F	M	F	M	F
A. Tetanus, traumatic	1	..	..	..	..	..	..	..	1	..
Erysipelas	1	..	..	1	..	..	..	..	..	..
Erysipeloid	1	1	..	..	1	..	..	1	..	..
Influenza	18	13	18	13	..	..	..	..	..	..
Malaria	5	..	5	..	..	..	..	..	..	..
Scarlatina	..	1	..	1	..	..	..	..	..	..
Typhoid fever	43	27	39	26	..	..	..	..	4	1
" " with pneumonia	1	..	..	..	..	..	..	..	1	..
" " " hemorrhage	1	..	1	..	..	..	..	..	..	..
" " " phlebitis	1	..	1	..	..	..	..	..	..	..
" " " periostitis of tibia	1	..	1	..	..	..	..	..	..	..
" " " perforation, relapse and hemorrhage	1	..	1	..	..	..	..	..	..	..
Paratyphoid fever	3	..	3	..	..	..	..	..	..	..
B. Arthritis deformans	1	1	..	..	1	1	..	..	..	..
" gonorrheal	6	3	4	..	2	3	..	..	..	..
" tubercular	2	1	..	..	1	..	1	1	..	..

STATISTICS OF MEDICAL SERVICE FOR 1904.

General Diseases—Continued.	Total		Cured		Improved		Unimproved		Died	
	M	F	M	F	M	F	M	F	M	F
Sarcomatosis, acute	1	..	..	..	1	..	..	..	..	..
Carcinomatosis	..	3	..	..	..	..	..	1	..	2
Diabetes	5	1	..	..	2	1	..	..	3	..
Goitre	..	5	..	..	..	4	..	1	..	..
" with septic parotitis	..	1	..	..	..	..	..	..	..	1
Lumbago	11	2	7	2	4	..	..	..	..	..
Rheumatism, acute articular	14	9	14	7	..	2	..	..	..	..
" subacute	6	4	5	1	1	3	..	..	..	..
" chronic	3	7	1	..	2	7	..	..	..	..
" muscular	3	..	2	..	1	..	..	..	..	..
Costo-sternal arthritis	..	1	..	..	..	1	..	..	..	..
Syphilis, congenital	..	1	..	..	..	1	..	..	..	..
Septicemia, cryptogenetic	2	4	..	1	..	..	..	..	2	3
Sepsis, chronic	..	1	..	1	..	..	..	..	..	..
Scorbutus	1	..	1	..	..	..	..	..	..	..
Dermato-myositis	1	..	..	..	1	..	..	..	..	..
Meningitis, cerebro-spinal	3	2	1	2	..	..	..	..	2	..
" tubercular	2	..	..	..	1	..	..	..	1	..
Total	138	88	104	55	18	23	1	4	14	7
Diseases of the Digestive Tract.										
Abdominal tumor	1	1	..	..	..	1	1	..	..	..
" lymphosarcoma	..	1	..	..	..	..	..	..	..	1
Cholecystitis	6	1	4	1	..	..	2	..	..	..
Cholelithiasis	2	3	1	..	..	2	1	1	..	..
Colitis, acute	4	2	4	2	..	..	..	..	..	..
" chronic	3	1	3	..	1	..	..	..	..	..
" ulcerative	1	..	..	..	..	..	..	..	1	..
" amebic	..	1	..	..	..	1	..	..	..	..
Constipation	8	1	7	..	1	1	..	..	..	..
Diarrhea	..	2	..	2	..	..	..	..	..	..
Dysentery, acute	2	..	2	..	..	..	..	..	..	..
" " with septic peritonitis	..	1	..	..	..	..	..	..	..	1
Emesis of pregnancy	..	1	..	1	..	..	..	..	..	..
Enteralgia	1	..	1	..	..	..	..	..	..	..
Entero-colitis	2	2	1	1	..	1	..	..	1	..
Enteroptosis	1	3	..	..	1	3	..	..	..	..
Esophagus, carcinoma of	2	..	..	..	2	..	..	..	..	..
" spasmodic stricture of	2	..	..	..	2	..	..	..	..	..
Gastralgia	1	..	..	..	1	..	..	..	..	..
Gastritis, acute	1	1	1	1	..	..	..	..	..	..
" chronic	8	2	1	1	6	1	1	..	..	..
Gastroptosis	..	1	..	..	..	1	..	..	..	..
Hyperchlorhydria	2	..	..	..	1	..	1	..	..	..
Intestinal chronic atony	2	3	..	1	2	2	..	..	..	..
" auto-intoxication	26	7	24	7	1	..	1	..	..	..
" colic	4	..	3	..	1	..	..	..	..	..
Intestine, carcinoma of	1	..	..	..	..	..	..	..	1	..

Diseases of the Digestive Tract—*Continued.*	Total		Cured		Improved		Unimproved		Died	
	M	F	M	F	M	F	M	F	M	F
Intestine, sarcoma of	1	..	..	..	..	..	1	..	..	..
Jaundice, catarrhal	3	..	2	..	1	..	..	..	..	..
Liver, abscess of	1	..	..	..	..	..	..	..	1	..
" carcinoma of	3	..	..	..	..	..	..	..	3	..
" cirrhosis of	5	..	..	..	3	..	1	..	1	..
" with uremia	1	..	..	..	..	..	..	..	1	..
Pancreatitis, chronic, with cirrhosis of liver	1	..	..	..	..	..	..	..	1	..
Peritonitis, acute	2	..	..	..	..	..	1	..	1	..
" tuberculous	1	..	..	..	..	..	1	..	..	..
Peritonsilar abscess	..	1	..	1	..	..	..	..	..	..
Pharyngitis, acute	1	..	1	..	..	..	..	..	..	..
Rectum, carcinoma of	4	..	..	..	..	..	2	..	2	..
" " with metastases in peritoneum	1	..	..	..	1	..	..	..	..	..
" " and liver	1	..	..	..	..	..	1	..	..	..
Retroperitoneal sarcoma	1	..	..	..	..	..	1	..	..	..
Stomach, carcinoma of	7	2	..	..	4	..	3	..	..	2
" ulcer	3	4	3	3	..	1	..	..	..	..
Sigmoid flexure, carcinoma of	1	..	..	..	1	..	..	..	..	..
Tenia intestinalis	1	1	1	1	..	..	..	..	..	..
Throat, syphilis of	..	2	..	1	..	1	..	..	..	..
Tonsilitis, acute follicular	7	2	7	1	..	1	..	..	..	..
Intoxications: coal-gas poisoning	1	..	1	..	..	..	..	..	..	..
" lead arthropathy	1	..	1	..	..	..	..	..	..	..
" " colic	10	..	10	..	..	..	..	..	..	..
" " neuritis	2	..	1	..	1	..	..	..	..	..
Morphine poisoning	1	..	1	..	..	..	..	..	..	..
Total	140	46	80	24	30	16	18	1	13	4

Nervous Diseases.

	Total		Cured		Improved		Unimproved		Died	
	M	F	M	F	M	F	M	F	M	F
Amyotrophic lateral sclerosis	..	1	..	..	..	1	..	..	..	..
Brown-Sequard paralysis	..	1	..	..	..	1	..	..	..	..
Cerebral abscess	1	..	..	..	..	..	..	..	1	..
" hemorrhage	11	3	..	..	8	1	1	1	2	1
" syphilis	1	..	1	..	..	..	..	..	..	..
" tumor	2	1	..	..	1	1	..	..	1	..
" thrombus	1	1	..	..	1	..	..	..	..	1
Chorea	1	1	..	1	..	..	..	..	..	..
Dementia	2	..	..	..	..	..	2	..	..	..
" senile	1	..	..	..	..	..	1	..	..	..
Epilepsy	..	1	..	..	..	..	..	1	..	..
Functional tremor	1	..	..	..	..	..	1	..	..	..
Gumma of spinal cord	1	..	..	..	1	..	..	..	..	..
Hysteria	1	5	1	1	..	3	..	1	..	..
Malingering	1	..	1	..	..	..	..	..	..	..
Melancholia	1	..	..	..	..	..	1	..	..	..
Multiple sclerosis	1	..	..	..	..	1	..	..	..	..
Myelitis, specific	1	..	..	..	1	..	..	..	..	..

STATISTICS OF MEDICAL SERVICE FOR 1904.

Nervous Diseases—Continued.	Total		Cured.		Improved.		Unimproved.		Died.	
	M	F	M	F	M	F	M	F	M	F
Myelitis, transverse, traumatic	..	1	..	..	..	..	..	1	..	..
Neuralgia, facial	2	..	2	..	..	..	..	..	..	..
" intercostal	1	..	1	..	..	..	..	..	..	..
" supraorbital	1	..	1	..	..	..	..	..	..	..
Neurasthenia	11	16	3	9	8	6	..	1	..	..
Neuritis	1	..	..	..	1	..	..	..	..	..
" alcoholic	..	1	..	..	..	..	1	..	..	..
" brachial	1	1	..	1	..	..	1	..	..	..
Paramyoclonus, multiplex	..	1	..	1	..	..	..	..	..	..
Pachymeningitis, chronic	1	..	..	..	..	..	..	..	1	..
Sciatica	13	12	9	2	4	9	..	1	..	..
Spondylitis, cervical	1	..	..	..	1	..	..	..	..	..
Tumor spinal cord	1	..	..	..	..	..	..	..	1	..
Traumatic neurosis	1	1	1	..	..	1	..	..	..	..
Tabes dorsalis	4	..	..	..	4	..	..	..	..	..
Total	65	46	21	14	31	25	7	5	6	2
Cutaneous Diseases.										
Eczema	2	..	2	..	..	..	..	..	..	..
Scabies	1	..	..	..	1	..	..	..	..	..
Dermatitis exfoliativa	..	1	..	1	..	..	..	..	..	..
Chronic parasitic eczema	1	..	..	..	1	..	..	..	..	..
Total	4	1	2	1	2	..	..	..	..	..
Surgical Diseases.										
Post-operative adhesions	1	1	..	..	1	1	..	..	..	..
Periostitis of rib	1	..	1	..	..	..	..	..	..	..
Choroiditis	1	..	..	..	..	..	1	..	..	..
Fracture of femur	1	..	..	..	..	..	1	..	..	..
Contusion of back	1	..	1	..	..	..	..	..	..	..
Chronic appendicitis	..	2	..	1	..	1	..	..	..	..
Catarrhal "	1	..	1	..	..	..	..	..	..	..
Abscess of mamma	..	1	..	1	..	..	..	..	..	..
Osteomyelitis of maxilla	1	..	..	..	..	..	1	..	..	..
Specific iritis	1	1	1	..	..	..	1	..	..	..
" periostitis	..	1	..	1	..	..	..	..	..	..
Pes planus	..	1	..	..	..	..	1	..	..	..
Syphilitic osteomyelitis	1	..	..	..	..	..	1	..	..	..
Carcinoma of breast	..	1	..	..	..	..	..	1	..	..
Frontal synovitis	1	..	..	..	1	..	..	..	..	..
Vertebral scoliosis	..	1	..	..	..	..	1	..	..	..
Crutch paralysis	1	..	1	..	..	..	..	..	..	..
Sarcoma of fibula	1	..	..	..	..	..	1	..	..	..
Osteoma of femur, with sciatica	1	..	..	..	1	..	..	..	..	..
Total	13	9	5	3	3	5	5	1	..	..

Genito-Urinary Diseases.

	Total M	Total F	Cured M	Cured F	Improved M	Improved F	Unimproved M	Unimproved F	Died M	Died F
Neoplasm, kidney	2	1	..	..	..	..	1	..	1	1
Nephritis, chronic, with chronic endocarditis	1	1	..	..	1	1	..	..	..	..
" " uremia	5	1	..	..	..	..	1	..	4	1
" "	17	16	..	..	14	13	..	..	3	3
" " with myocarditis	4	1	..	..	3	..	..	..	1	1
" subacute	2	1	..	..	1	1	1	..	..	..
" acute	3	1	1	1	..	..	..	..	2	..
Renal calculus	2	..	..	..	1	..	1	..	..	..
Nephroptosis	1	3	..	..	1	3	..	..	..	..
Renal colic	3	..	3	..	..	..	..	..	..	..
Ren mobilis	..	5	..	1	..	2	..	2	..	..
Pyonephrosis	1	..	..	..	1	..	..	..	..	..
Hematuria	..	1	..	1	..	..	..	..	..	..
Hypertrophy of prostate	1	..	..	..	1	..	..	..	..	..
Tubercular testicle	1	..	..	..	..	..	1	..	..	..
Chronic cystitis	2	1	..	..	2	1	..	..	..	..
Subacute urethritis	1	..	..	..	1	..	..	..	..	..
Gonorrh. epidid. and orchitis	1	..	1	..	..	..	..	..	..	..
Sarcoma of ovary, with metastasis in lung	..	1	..	..	..	..	..	..	..	1
Pelvic tumor	..	1	..	..	..	..	..	1	..	..
" exudate	..	1	..	..	..	..	..	1	..	..
Total	47	35	5	3	26	21	5	4	11	7

Diseases of the Respiratory Tract.

	Total M	Total F	Cured M	Cured F	Improved M	Improved F	Unimproved M	Unimproved F	Died M	Died F
Asthma	5	1	1	..	4	1	..	..	..	..
Bronchiectasis	2	..	..	..	2	..	..	..	..	..
Bronchitis, acute	1	1	..	1	1	..	..	..	..	..
" chronic	1	6	1	4	..	2	..	..	..	..
Emphysema	3	1	..	..	3	1	..	..	..	..
" with asthma	2	1	1	..	1	1	..	..	..	..
" " bronchitis	7	7	2	..	5	6	..	1	..	..
" " endocarditis	1	..	..	..	..	..	..	..	1	..
" " pulmonary edema	1	..	..	..	..	..	..	..	1	..
Empyema with subphrenic abscess	..	1	..	..	..	..	..	1	..	..
Hydropneumothorax	1	..	1	..	..	..	..	..	..	..
Laryngitis, acute catarrhal	..	1	..	1	..	..	..	..	..	..
" tubercular	..	1	..	..	..	1	..	..	..	..
Lung, carcinoma of	1	3	..	..	1	1	..	2	..	..
" gangrene of	1	..	..	..	..	..	1	..	..	..
" metastatic carcinoma of	1	..	..	..	..	..	..	..	1	..
" " sarcoma of	..	1	..	..	..	..	..	..	..	1
Mediastinum, carcinoma of	..	1	..	..	..	..	..	..	..	1
Pleura, neoplasm of	1	..	..	..	..	..	1	..	..	..
Pleurisy, dry	3	2	2	1	..	1	1	..	..	..
" with effusion	6	1	5	1	1	..	..	..	..	..
Pneumonia, acute lobar	31	15	22	11	1	1	..	..	8	3
" " " with pleuritic effusion	1	..	1	..	..	..	..	..	..	..

STATISTICS OF MEDICAL SERVICE FOR 1904.

Diseases of the Respiratory Tract—*Continued.*	Total		Cured		Improved		Unimproved		Died	
	M	F	M	F	M	F	M	F	M	F
Pneumonia, influenza	5	2	5	1	..	1	..	..	..	..
" broncho	1	4	..	2	..	..	..	..	1	2
" lobar with chronic endocarditis	..	1	..	..	..	1	..	..	..	..
" " " abscess of lung	1	..	..	..	..	..	1	..	..	..
Pneumothorax	1	..	..	..	..	..	..	..	1	..
Pyopneumothorax	..	1	..	..	..	1	..	..	..	..
Tuberculosis, pulmonary	25	12	..	2	18	8	1	1	6	1
" " incipient	..	1	..	1	..	..	..	..	..	..
" " chronic	4	..	..	..	4	..	..	..	..	..
" general miliary	1	..	..	..	..	..	..	..	1	..
" lobar, with chronic endocarditis	..	1	..	..	..	1	..	..	..	..
Total	107	65	41	25	42	26	5	5	20	8

Diseases of Vessels.

	M	F	M	F	M	F	M	F	M	F
Aneurism of the arch of the aorta	2	..	..	..	2	..	..	..	..	..
Arterio-sclerosis specifica	1	..	..	..	1	..	..	..	..	..
" " with nephritis	1	..	..	..	1	..	..	..	..	..
Atresia of the superior and inferior vena cava and erysipelas	1	..	..	..	..	..	..	..	1	..
Erythromelalgia	..	1	..	..	..	1	..	..	..	..
Total	5	1	..	..	4	1	..	..	1	..

Diseases of the Heart.

	M	F	M	F	M	F	M	F	M	F
Endocarditis, acute	..	1	..	..	..	1	..	..	..	..
" chronic	41	34	..	..	33	25	5	2	3	7
" " with embolism	1	..	..	..	1	..	..	..	..	..
" " " nephritis	6	8	..	..	..	6	1	..	5	2
" " " rheumatism	11	5	2	2	9	3	..	..	..	..
" " " pericarditis	1	..	..	..	1	..	..	..	..	..
" " " pneumonia	1	..	..	..	..	..	..	..	1	..
" " " specific aortitis	1	..	..	..	1	..	..	..	..	..
Myocarditis	6	7	1	..	4	6	..	1	1	..
Pericarditis, with effusion	1	2	1	1	..	1	..	..	..	..
Total	69	57	4	3	49	42	6	3	10	9

Diseases of the Blood.

	M	F	M	F	M	F	M	F	M	F
Addison's disease with hemiplegia	1	..	..	..	1	..	..	..	..	..
Anemia, simple	1	1	..	1	1	..	..	..	..	..
" chlorotic	..	1	..	..	..	1	..	..	..	..
" secondary	1	..	..	..	1	..	..	..	..	..
" post-febrile	..	1	..	..	..	1	..	..	..	..

Diseases of the Blood—*Continued.*	Total		Cured		Improved		Unimproved		Died	
	M	F	M	F	M	F	M	F	M	F
Anemia, post-hemorrhagic	..	1	..	..	..	1	..	..	..	..
Leukemia, spleno-myelogenous	..	2	..	..	..	1	..	1	..	..
" acute lymphatic	1	2	..	..	..	..	..	..	1	2
" chronic	2	..	..	..	..	1	..	1	..	..
" pseudo	..	1	..	..	..	..	..	1	..	..
Lympho-sarcoma, general	1	..	..	..	..	..	..	1	..	..
Splenomegaly	..	2	..	..	..	2	..	..	..	..
Total	7	11	..	1	4	6	2	2	1	2

SOME FURTHER OBSERVATIONS ON THE DETERMINATION OF URIC ACID AND XANTHINE BODIES IN URINE.

By Julius Rudisch, M.D.,
ATTENDING PHYSICIAN.

As will be remembered by those who are interested in this important subject, the principal points in the paper written by myself and Dr. Kleeberg, of this city,[*] were as follows:

"All the more exact methods are founded upon the property of uric acid and the purin bases of forming definite compounds with silver in ammoniacal solution of the latter in the presence of a neutral salt of the alkaline and alkaline earth group, preferably chloride of magnesium, chloride of lithium, or chloride of ammonium. Under the above conditions, uric acid combines with silver in the proportion of one molecule of the former to one atom of the latter; the purin bases in the proportion of two molecules of xanthine to one of silver. The compound of silver urate formed under the above conditions is insoluble in both weak and strong ammonia up to 1:200,000 parts. The compounds of silver and purin bases are soluble in strong ammonia, insoluble in weak ammonia.

"Our method is founded upon the titration of the excess of silver added. For titration, we use a solution of potassium iodide, the titre of which is unchangeable; and, having by experiments found that silver urate in strong ammonia solutions is insoluble, and that silver compounds which the purin bases form in the same menstruum are soluble, we are enabled to determine both these bodies by the same procedure.

"METHOD: *To Determine Uric Acid.*—To 110 c.c. of urine add 55 c.c. N/50 Ag. solution, and dilute with NH$_4$OH (sp. gr. 0.90) to 220 c.c. All these measurements can be conveniently made in flasks of the Giles pattern. Mix and filter through a dry folded filter, either

[*] J. Rudisch and F. Kleeberg, American Journal of the Medical Sciences, November, 1904.

at once or after standing a few minutes. Two portions of 100 c.c., each of which corresponds to 50 c.c. of urine, are collected.

"In the meantime a half-dozen small test-tubes (about 6 cm. long and 1 cm. in diameter) are filled for about 1 cm. with a mixture of, roughly, two parts of the nitrous-sulphuric acid (the nitrous-sulphuric acid mixture is prepared by adding 25 c.c. concentrated H_2SO_4 to 75 c.c. of H_2O, and then adding 1 c.c. fuming nitric acid) and one part starch solution.

"To one of the above portions of 100 c.c., N/50 KI is rapidly added, and after each addition of 2 c.c. a small portion, not exceeding 0.5 c.c., is removed by means of a pipette, which also answers as a stirring rod, and carefully introduced down the side of one of the test-tubes in such a manner that two absolutely distinct layers are formed. The end reaction manifests itself sharply by the formation of a blue ring (iodide of starch) at the point of juncture. Having now found the end point approximately with the first 100 c.c., the exact end point is determined with the second 100 c.c.—e.g., say that more than 10 c.c. and less than 12 c.c. are required with the first 100 c.c. The second 100 c.c. are then taken, and 10 c.c. N/50 KI run into the solution at once; then a few drops at a time are carefully added, until the exact end point is reached. With a little practice the exact end point can be obtained without having removed more than 1 c.c. from the solution being tested. The entire analysis need not require more than from twenty to twenty-five minutes."

The principal difficulty for those who are not thoroughly conversant with this method, is the inability to perceive the end reaction, the sometimes very faint blue ring at the junction of the two liquids, but only a very little perseverance and practice will soon enable one to be absolutely accurate. A few hints will be of great use to the experimenter.

1. I find it of advantage to have two solutions of silver ready. (a) The N/50 of silver diluted with an equal amount of strong (36%) ammonia water for the determination of uric acid alone. (b) The N/50 silver solution diluted with an equal amount of distilled water to determine all the purin bodies. Thus for the determination, *equal amounts* of the urine and either one of the above solutions are used, and some time is hereby saved.

2. To shorten the time of filtering, I find Carl Scheicher & Schull's No. 588 filter, diameter $18\frac{1}{2}$ cm. (to be had, in New York, at Eimer

& Amend's) of great value. The time of filtration is shortened considerably.

3. It is advisable to make the nitrous-sulphuric acid fresh every two weeks at least.

4. I find it better to put in the test-tubes at least 2½ cm. of the mixture of the nitrous-sulphuric acid and starch, instead of the 1 cm., as described in the quoted paper.

5. In case of necessity, the same amount of urine may be used both for the preliminary and for the accurate determination, in the following manner. For example, if, at the preliminary determination, at 10 c.c. there is no blue ring, and at 12 c.c. the ring is present, pour back the contents of all of the test-tubes into the urine, taking care that there is more than enough ammonia to neutralize the nitrous-sulphuric acid, and add 2 c.c of the $N/50$ silver solution. Then proceed by titrating with the KI, drop by drop, until the blue ring shows. Supposing the reaction has shown itself at $13\frac{1}{4}$ c.c. Deduct 2 c.c. for the silver added, and ¾ of 1 c.c. for the correction. The true value will be $10\frac{1}{2}$ c.c.

To test the correctness of the ring method, three controls were occasionally used. As all are of some interest, I will describe them.

1. The aliquot portion of the filtrate was acidified, preferably by acetic acid, the resulting precipitate of silver chloride filtered through a Carl Scheicher & Schull's No. 589 filter. The precipitate was dissolved in a large excess of a saturated solution of muriate of ammonia. An excess of acetic acid and some hydrogen peroxide and starch were added, and titrated with the $N/50KI$, until the blue color remained permanent.

2. The precipitate of the mixture of the urine and silver chloride was filtered off, and washed out until free from chlorine; then dissolved in nitric acid, and titrated by the Vollhard method. Both methods agreed absolutely with the ring method.

3. In a paper of ours ("A New Method for the Approximate Determination of Uric Acid in Urine," by Julius Rudisch and Leopold Boroscheck, *Journal of American Chemical Society*, vol. xxiv., 6, June, 1902), we describe the way for precipitation of uric acid in a strongly alkaline urine by a solution of chloride of silver in a concentrated solution of sulphite of soda. The results obtained were always slightly lower than those by the Salkowski method. In going lately over the work done, I found that the loss was due to the washing

of the precipitate with a solution of carbonate of soda. When I used instead the concentrated solution of the sulphite of soda, the result agreed fully with the iodine ring method. Since in the precipitation with chloride of silver and sulphite of soda no ammonia is used, the determination of nitrogen is very much facilitated, and as there is no darkening of the uric acid and xanthine silver, I think this method will be used with great advantage for the demonstration of these bodies in a pure form.

The ideal way of determining the silver, either suspended as an insoluble chloride, or in solution, by means of iodine is as follows:

The solution to be titrated is acidified by acetic acid. Hydrogen peroxide and starch are added, and titrated with iodine until a permanent blue color results. This is one of the most delicate volumetric methods; but, unfortunately, this procedure is not applicable to urine, because a great many of the constituents of the urine combine with the iodine, and the acetic acid and peroxide are not able to break the combination. The use of inorganic acids is not admissible, as they in combination with the hydrogen peroxide evolve chlorine, which combines with the iodine and materially interferes with the end reaction.

In the last few weeks, though, I believe I have found a way to overcome this difficulty, and if further experiments confirm me in my expectation, there will be a way to determine uric acid and xanthine bodies in the urine as rapid and much more accurate than the determination of glucose.

TWO CASES OF PERNICIOUS ANEMIA DUE TO THE DIBOTHRIOCEPHALUS LATUS.

By Alfred Meyer, M.D.

There is perhaps no pathological state so commonly met with in private or in hospital practice, whether by the general practitioner or the specialist, as that of secondary anemia. In many cases the cause is readily ascertained: a hemorrhage, convalescence from a long febrile disease, a carcinoma, a chronic nephritis, a malarial toxemia, a tuberculosis, a leukemia; and the success of the treatment instituted depends more or less upon the success with which we can reach the etiological factor. Other secondary anemias—as for instance those accompanying chronic cystic degeneration of the kidneys—are in most cases not even diagnosed and their causative treatment therefore not even discussed. But there is a type of severe secondary anemia due to the presence of certain parasites in the intestines, notably the *Anchylostomum duodenale* and the *Dibothriocephalus latus* which, when recognized, are not only amenable to treatment by anthelmintics, but so prompt and striking is the cure at times that almost the whole field of medicine may be searched in vain for similar illustrations of its beneficent power. It ought to be both a warning and a stimulus to medical men not to be satisfied with the routine administration of iron and arsenic, especially in progressive anemia of obscure origin or long duration, but to examine the stools for links and ova, for upon their discovery may depend absolutely the issue of the case. The temptation to use iron is particularly great, for have we not a very large list of iron preparations to choose from? And is not the enterprise of chemists and pharmaceutical houses continually adding to the number? And may we not, varying the poet's language a bit, say with perfect truth that the medical profession is "Dragging a lengthening chain of iron behind it"?

It has often been observed and commented upon by medical men having large hospital services that if a rare disease occurs in the service, or a rare complication of a common disease, the same is not infrequently met with again after a short interval. Within the present year I have had confirmation of this "law of chances," if you choose, in the wards of Mt. Sinai Hospital. For many years the stools of every patient suffering from a high grade of anemia, for which no cause could be found, have been systematically searched for intestinal parasites and their ova; never, so far as I know, was there found a single case of *Dibothriocephalus latus* anemia, and then, curiously enough, two cases followed each other within about a year—both of them anemias of the severest kind, clinically and microscopically. I shall only give extracts from the complete histories of the cases as taken by the house staff.

CASE 1.—Edith H., twenty-two years old, domestic, born in Finland; admitted November 6, 1903; marked tuberculous history on mother's side, but no subjective tuberculous history. Ill one year with weakness and increasing pallor with occasional vomiting. On admission the pallor was marked with a yellowish hue, the conjunctivæ fatty looking, loud systolic murmurs at the apex and in the aortic area. Slight edema of extremities. No petechiæ.

Blood.—Red blood corpuscles, 780,000; white blood corpuscles, 5,000; hemoglobin, 15 per cent.; poikilocytosis, microcytes, macrocytes, cells showing polychromatophilic degeneration, some normoblasts.

Differential count 100 cells: Polynuclears, 37 per cent.; mononuclears, 8 per cent.; lymphocytes, large and small, 54 per cent.; mastzellen, 1 per cent.

Numerous ecchymoses upon arms and about ankles and trochanter. Large retinal hemorrhages, especially in the right eye. Temperature 100° to 102°F. for first twenty days in the hospital. The first few days no ova were found in the stools. On the eighth day after admission ova were found, but not recognized as those of any known parasite. A few days later 30 grains of thymol were given in two doses and four hours later a tapeworm was passed which proved to be a *Dibothriocephalus latus*, measuring 8 feet and 8 inches in length. Ova were still found in the stools from time to time, until nine days after the expulsion of the worm, when they disappeared for a period of three weeks and then were found again on one day only. For fear that there might be a second *Dibothriocephalus latus*, thymol and male fern were given successively without the expulsion of another parasite, and after that no ova were found during the remaining five weeks of the patient's stay in the hospital. The improvement of the patient was immediate and truly marvelous. The mucous membranes steadily and rapidly improved in color, she gained thirteen pounds in weight, the hemoglobin rose from 15 to 63 per cent. and the red blood cells from 780,000 to 3,460,000.

CASE II.—The history of this patient was as follows: Is still in the Mt. Sinai Hospital. Jennie L., twenty-five years old, married, born in Russian Poland; admitted December 7, 1904. First child born four months ago. Her illness began about two months before birth of baby with swelling of feet and legs. Pallor began about the same time and progressively increased. Says that she saw segments of worm in stools about one year before. Marked pallor of body and mucous membranes with an icteric tinge; edema of lids and of extremities; systolic blowing murmur at apex and pulmonic area. Temperature, 101.2°F.

Blood.—Red blood corpuscles, 660,000; white blood corpuscles, 5,400; hemoglobin, 10 per cent.

Differential count, 200 cells: polynuclears, 53½ per cent.; eosinophiles, ½ per cent.; large mononuclears, 15 per cent.; large lymphocytes, 6 per cent.; small lymphocytes, 25 per cent. Marked poikilocytosis and basophile degeneration; one normoblast, 6 megaloblasts.

Dr. Grüning, who made the fundus examination, reported numerous hemorrhages along the veins, also hemorrhages where there are no veins. When I first saw this patient and before the report of the stool examination was handed in, I was inclined to regard the case as one of progressive pernicious anemia of the pregnant, of which seven fatal cases were originally reported by Gusserow of Zurich, Switzerland, in 1871, and of which type I have reported one case without autopsy in the Mt. Sinai Hospital reports of 1898. I might very reasonably omit this reference to my first erroneous impression of the case, because it was not a final diagnosis and necessarily was subject to revision after the stool examination which I immediately ordered, and which examination had actually been begun by the house staff before the order was given. But I mention it deliberately in order to show the very grave condition of the patient that would have justified such an opinion—an opinion which, if verified, would have meant death in a few weeks. The following day a large number of ova of the *Dibothriocephalus latus* were found in the stools. Thymol was given in half-dram doses with the same precautions as in the first case in regard to withholding the food and the administration of castor oil the day before and two hours after the remedy, but the worm was not expelled. The same negative result with 2½ drams of the ethereal extract of filix mas.

December 19: Red blood corpuscles, 556,000 (a loss in eleven days of 100,000).

January 3: Red blood corpuscles, 468,000 (another loss of about 90,000).

January 7: Some segments of *Dibothriocephalus latus* passed and ova were found for the first and only time since the administration of anthelmintics was begun. Many and varied doses of thymol, filix mas and pelletierine sulphate were employed but without expelling the parasite (so far as known).

January 16: Red blood corpuscles, 1,176,000 (nearly trebled in thirteen days); white blood corpuscles, 5,800; hemoglobin, 21 per cent. (doubled in the same period).

It is hard to determine why in some cases the *Dibothriocephalus latus* develops only slight gastric or nervous symptoms and in others the severest grades of anemia. Braun (Thier. Parasiten des Menschen, p. 202) believes the latter due to the absorption by the hosts of poisonous material excreted by the parasite. In this connection it is interesting to note that in the second case reported by me the improvement in the anemia followed soon after the use of anthelmintics and the disappearance of eggs from the stools.

The worm had not been discovered in the stools up to the date of discharge, April 4, 1905, but the persistent absence of ova for a period of sixty-one days made it certain that the same had been expelled and escaped the observation of the nurse.

The patient steadily improved. The blood examination showed, on January 27: Red corpuscles, 1,648,000 (nearly quadrupled in twenty-four days); hemoglobin, 36 per cent. (nearly quadrupled in twenty-four days). Only a faint systolic murmur was still present in the pulmonic area.

In view of the claim that has been made in some quarters "that healing may occur without removal of the worm or before the worm has passed, and that possibly the improvement is only a temporary improvement of a primary pernicious anemia," the patient was kept under observation for some months at the hospital in order to continue the search for ova, but none were found.

On March 14, the blood showed: Red corpuscles, 3,928,000; hemoglobin, 72 per cent.; differential count, 100 cells: polynuclear neutrophiles, 61 per cent.; large mononuclears, 12 per cent.; lymphocytes, 21 per cent.; eosinophiles, 6 per cent.; no nucleated reds, no mastzellen, some poikilocytosis.

One week after discharge patient reappeared for examination (April 12, 1905), and the hemoglobin and blood count were practically the same.

PRIMARY SPLENOMEGALY—GAUCHER TYPE.*

REPORT ON ONE OF FOUR CASES OCCURRING IN A SINGLE GENERATION OF ONE FAMILY.

By N. E. BRILL, A.M., M.D.,
ATTENDING PHYSICIAN TO MOUNT SINAI HOSPITAL,

F. S. MANDLEBAUM, M.D.,
PATHOLOGIST TO MOUNT SINAI HOSPITAL,

AND

E. LIBMAN, M.D.,
ASSISTANT PATHOLOGIST TO MOUNT SINAI HOSPITAL.

CLINICAL (DR. N. E. BRILL). Under the caption of primary splenomegaly have been heaped together indiscriminately a large variety of non-leukemic enlargements of the spleen developing with or without anemia. Osler, in an attempt to establish order out of chaos, suggested calling the cases of enlarged spleen associated with an anemia of the chlorotic type and with hemorrhages, but unaccompanied by a leukocytosis, splenic anemia, adopting as the cognomen the term first used by Griesinger for the splenic variety of Hodgkin's disease. He insists that these cases in their evolution present a terminal stage characterized by secondary cirrhosis of the liver associated with jaundice and ascites, which Banti described as constituting a disease *sui generis*, and which cases have been known as those of Banti's disease. But even with Osler's limitation, under the term of splenic anemia, there have been associated diverse splenic enlargements, differing both in their clinical and pathological conditions, such as the cases described by Sippy,[1] Osler,[2] Rolleston,[3] Taylor,[4] Gilbert and Fournier,[5] Stengel,[6] and others. Much more work will

*An abstract of this report was presented at a meeting of the New York Pathological Society on December 14, 1904; the article was reported in the American Journal of the Medical Sciences, March, 1905.

have to be done, many more clinical and pathological investigations will have to be made, before a satisfactory classification of the varieties of types of so-called splenic anemia can be agreed upon.

The writer insists that the type of splenomegaly first described in 1882 by Gaucher[7] as "Splenomegalie Primitive—Primary Epithelioma of the Spleen," and after him by Picou and Raymond,[8] Collier,[9] and Bovaird,[10] ought not to be included in the category of splenic anemia, because its pathology is unique and typical and the clinical picture so distinctive that it can be recognized during life. It was from the clinical picture presented by the patients whose histories I reported in *The American Journal of the Medical Sciences* for April, 1901, that I was able to predict that my cases* belonged only to the class described by Gaucher as splenomegalie primitive. Indeed, one of the distinctive features of this class, which alone might separate it from all the cases belonging to the category of splenic anemia, is the enormous increase in the size of the liver, which almost equals the colossal size of the spleen.

For the benefit of those who have not access to the original article, a *resumé* of the clinical data of the case which forms the topic of this report is herewith given; for full details the reader is referred to the original publication. It is the first male case ever reported in literature:

Maximilian R., born in 1870, had suffered from the common infections diseases of childhood, but never had malaria, rheumatism, or tuberculosis. He had not been rachitic and never contracted gonorrhea or syphilis. After his ninth year he was a sturdy, muscular, healthy chap, and never was ill outside of an occasional attack of bronchitis. The only features of an abnormal nature which the patient himself observed was a tendency to sweat easily, the frequent presence of sudamina, even in winter, and a persistent patch of erythematous papules which extended from the malar prominence of one side across the skin covering the nasal bone to the same prominence on the other side, most intense, however, on the bridge of the nose. The latter developed about his fourteenth year, and, notwithstanding treatment by skin specialists, was persistent. In 1885, when he came under my observation, this patch was prominent. No signs of splenic enlargement appeared until 1889. Patient felt in perfect health all

---

*The disease has since been discovered by me in another sister, who constitutes the fourth member of the one generation of the family thus afflicted.

the years since his ninth. There were no pains in the splenic region at any time up to the date of the detection of an enlarged spleen. Since 1889, after an apparent initial slight reduction in the size of the spleen, there had been a steady, slow, progressive increase in size of that organ, with occasional attacks of epistaxis. In 1899 the first absolute signs of liver enlargement became demonstrable, and about this time was noticed a peculiar *hard, pale, ochre-colored*, wedge-shaped infiltration of the sclerotic of the nasal side of each eye, the base being limited by the cornea, the apex extending toward the nasal angle, thus differing from the ordinary pinguecula.

While feeling in perfect health the patient was losing weight very slowly but progressively. Between 1899 and 1900 the skin of the face, neck, and hands began to assume a dusky, light yellowish-brown tint. Wherever the skin was not exposed to the light and air it was perfectly normal in color. There was an entire absence of jaundice; examination of the blood and urine showed no bile.

Frequent blood examinations were made, blood counts dating from 1893, and showing a normal red and white count, and normal proportions of polynuclear neutrophiles, small and large mononuclears and eosinophiles. The hemoglobin up to 1900 was never lower than 80 per cent. by Gowers' instrument.

The progress of the disease became rapid from August, 1900, when the patient was seized by an attack of acute colitis, starting with a chill, and followed by hyperpyrexia and diarrhea, the movements finally becoming bloody and composed then of mucus and sanguineous fluid. Immediately after convalescence hemorrhagic furuncles appeared on the legs, thighs, trunk, arms, and forehead, leaving behind them, when healed, permanent pigmented spots at the site of each furuncle. Excepting these spots and the peculiar change in color of the face and hands, there was no pigmentation anywhere of the skin or of the mucous membranes accessible to inspection. Later in the year the first signs of petechiae appeared, three on the thorax.

From January, 1902, to May, 1902, there was very little if any change in the condition of the patient. In May he began to complain of pain in the lower end of the left tibia. Physical examination at the seat of pain revealed nothing, there being no swelling, redness, or tenderness.

On June 6, 1902, he was seized by an attack of malarial infection, with the usual signs of the tertian type; plasmodia were found in the blood. A course of quinine dissipated the organisms. Epistaxis, which had not been frequent in the past, now became more so, and the blood examinations revealed a steady decrease in hemoglobin to 45 per cent., and a slight increase in leukocytes, 8,240; the red cells being diminished, 3,420,000. The red cells showed a few normoblasts (August 1, 1902). He complained less of pain in the lower part of the tibia; occasionally this pain disappeared entirely, even for a month at a time. During the attack of malarial infection there was no demonstrable increase in the size of the spleen.

In September the patient was so well that he again attended actively to business. He remained in a condition of relative well-being throughout the rest of the year and the first half of the following year, 1903. During these nine months he had but four attacks of epistaxis. In April, 1903, he began to complain again of the pain in the neighborhood of the ankle and also about the left knee. There were no local signs of swelling, etc., and no indications of a hemarthrosis. A blood examination at this date revealed the following: red cells, 4,400,000; white, 5,240; Hemoglobin, 55 per cent.; polynuclear neutrophiles, 65 per cent.; small mononuclear, 26.5 per cent.; large mononuclear, 6.5 per cent.; transitional forms, 1 per cent.; eosinophiles, 0.5 per cent.

In June, 1903, in the warm spell, his sudaminia became pronounced, a few miliaria becoming hemorrhagic; the erythematous patch on the nose became more livid. The pain in the left knee and ankle, however, disappeared. The heated term weakened him considerably, and he left town, spending the next three months in the mountains, where he felt very well.

On his return examination revealed a slight increase in the size of the spleen, its anterior border extending 3 cm. beyond the middle line; the upper border (dullness) was at the fifth rib in the midaxillary line; the posterior border could be felt in a line with the angle of the scapula about 4 cm. from the lumbar spines, and became lost to the touch behind the iliac crest. The liver had relatively increased more in size. Liver flatness was elicited at the fourth rib, lower border palpable 4 cm. below the level of the umbilicus, extending below the iliac crest in the midaxillary and postaxillary lines. His chest and abdomen were more bulging than ever.

September 27, 1903.—Red cells, 4,200,000; white cells, 6,200; polynuclears, 70 per cent.; small lymphocytes, 22 per cent.; large lymphocytes and transitionals, 7 per cent.; eosinophiles, 0.5 per cent.

Heart.—Loud systolic murmur at apex and over pulmonary area; upper border of cardiac dullness at lower border of second rib; right border at right sternal line; apex in third interspace.

November 17th.—A moderately severe epistaxis.

November 27th.—A few petechiae are noted in the dorsum of each hand; none on conjunctivae. Hemoglobin, 50 per cent. Patient has a ravenous appetite. Again complains of pain in left knee and ankle. He, however, has been taking long walks daily. No demonstrable increase in size of spleen or liver.

January 6, 1904.—First appearance of ecchymosis—one ecchymotic spot on left lower leg near the end of the fibula and one on dorsum of left foot, each about 2 cm. in diameter. Emaciation much more marked since last note. Hemic murmur increased in intensity. Hemoglobin, 45 per cent. No epistaxis since November 17, 1903.

yet a gradual hemoglobin reduction. No ascites. Has had dyspeptic symptoms, perhaps partly due to the excessive amount of food he has been taking.

March 12th.—Patient began to complain of dyspnea and fever, with great weakness. Temperature, 101°. Limit of cardiac dullness considerably to right of sternum; left border not definable, owing to interference of spleen; apex beat feeble and in third interspace. Same hemic murmur. No recognizable increase in spleen and liver.

March 13th.—Patient feeling better. Temperature, 100°; two ecchymotic (fresh) spots over right tibia; another on dorsum of left foot. Dyspnea; respirations, 34. Says he feels comfortable.

March 20th.—Since last note normal temperature until yesterday. To-day increased difficulty in breathing, pain behind sternum, sticking and rubbing in character; chills; respiration, 38 and labored; pulse, 116; temperature, 103°. Apex beat cannot be felt; to-and-fro superficial friction at junction of third right rib with sternum. Diagnosis of pericarditis, with probable bloody effusion. From this day on fever persisted, weakness became extreme, the patient became irritable, objected to further blood examinations. Signs of fluid in peritoneal cavity. Dyspnea more extreme, the pericardial friction more rough and superficial, the pulse became weaker; exitus, with mental faculties preserved to final moment, on March 30, 1904.

Negative Symptoms.—Urine never contained bile; negative examination for pathological urobilin (Jaffé); never any casts; never albumin; urea never much above normal limits; highest 3.4 per cent. Ascites never present, except two days before death. Edema absent. Jaundice absent throughout. Superficial lymph nodes never enlarged.

Blood.—Never contained bile; coagulation time gradually increased in length toward terminal stage of disease to fourteen minutes, first examination in 1899 being three minutes.

Hemorrhages.—Epistaxis was the only form. The attack of colitis associated with bloody stools cannot be considered as a melena. Toward the last two years of life petechiæ and ecchymosis, few, however, in number.

Discoloration of Skin.—Limited to face and neck, wrist and hands. Skin of body not discolored. Discoloration not that of Addison's disease; color, yellowish-brown. It would appear as if the light and air had some influence in changing the tint of the exposed parts. The color is not one due to ordinary exposure; it remained permanent. Bovaird mentions bronzing of the face and hands of his patient. Bronzing is not applicable to this case.

Local pain over spleen and liver absent, though such could be elicited by pressure.

No bone tenderness; pressure over lower end of femur and tibia relieved the pain when present in those regions.

No feeling of being sick except during an intercurrent affection—

colitis, malarial disease, terminal pericarditis—on the contrary, a feeling of well-being.

Owing to the unusual importance of this case, I have been happy to call into its collaboration the aid of Dr. Mandlebaum, who made the histological examination and who prepared the photomicrographs, and of Dr. Libman, who made the autopsy.

REPORT ON POST-MORTEM EXAMINATION MADE MARCH 31, 1904, 11.45 P. M.—No rigor mortis; body emaciated; pupils large; yellowish-brown discoloration of face and hands. A few small lymph nodes in both axillæ the size of peas; in supraclavicular regions a few half the size; the same in the epitrochlear and inguinal regions. Panniculus adiposus atrophic; muscles of the abdominal wall succulent. In the abdomen 1,000 c.c. of hemorrhagic fluid, chocolate in color. The body musculature is atrophic, pale.

Old and recent adhesions over liver; omentum adherent to anterior surface of the spleen; the spleen at its upper pole is adherent to the surrounding tissues.

Diaphragm on the right side at the third rib and on the left at the fourth rib. Lower part of the chest markedly expanded. All the intra-abdominal veins are distended.

Anterior mediastinal nodes enlarged the size of peas, yellowish-brown in color; on section there are pinpoint hemorrhagic areas.

Lungs.—No fluid in pleural sacs; both lungs congested, lower lobes compressed. Lingula emphysematous. Bronchial nodes moderately enlarged and anthracotic.

Pericardium.—Very markedly distended by 2 litres of very bloody fluid. Microscopic examination of the fluid reveals altered erythrocytes only. The visceral pericardium is coated by a layer of shaggy fibrin, which is easily removed.

Heart.—Small, old thickening of posterior visceral pericardium; right auricle dilated. Tricuspid orifice admits three fingers; the valve is slightly thickened. The wall of the right ventricle is thin. The pulmonary valves are negative. The left ventricle is small; the auricle dilated. The heart muscle is firm, brownish. The coronaries and aorta show no lesions. There are no congenital defects.

Esophagus and Stomach.—Marked congestion. Stomach is dilated.

Spleen.—Immensely enlarged, filling the larger part of the abdominal cavity. The weight is 5,280 gm. (11 pounds). It measures 40 x 20 x 14 cm. The organ is of an elongated ovoid form. The surface as a whole is of a reddish-brown color and shows marked recent and old perisplenitis. There are irregular depressed areas on the surface, evidently the result of infarctions. The organ is very firm. On section the color is that of chocolate, but here and there are lighter areas of a grayish-red color. The pulp is moderately swollen. There is a large number of old and recent infarctions, mostly peripheral. In some sections the whole periphery is made up of infarcted tissue; some of these infarcts are surrounded by hemorrhagic zones; most are anemic and look cheesy. In the lower pole there is a white area about 1.5 cm. wide, crossing the entire width of the spleen. Where the pulp is less swollen the connective tissue is seen to be decidedly increased. In the pulp are a number of small hemorrhages. The splenic vessels show no changes. At the lower part there is a globular mass of splenic tissue attached by a flat pedicle to the main organ; it measures 4 x 6 cm. On section it is dark brown in color, with grayish markings.

Liver.—Weight 4.8 k. (10 pounds). It measures 35 cm. in width; both lobes are 27 cm. in length; thickness of the organ is 13 cm. There is marked old and recent perihepatitis. The surface is pale reddish-brown, with irregular white and dark-brown markings. The right lobe is oblong; the left ovoid; the free border is rounded. On section the organ is quite firm. As a whole it is chocolate-colored; the cut surface is rather granular. Throughout the liver are irregular white markings, varying in diameter from 0.5 cm. to 2 or 3 cm., which, for the most part, are ramifying. They do not seem to bear any definite relation to the lobular markings. In both lobes, but especially in the right, there is a number of fine hemorrhages. The portal vein and the gall-ducts show no changes. The gall-bladder is distended by a large amount of very dark bile. The wall appears to be normal.

Kidneys.—Left: weight, 150 gm., capsule markedly adherent; moderate lobulation; surface slightly granular; veins injected. On section the organ is quite firm. The cortex is narrow, but swollen; the markings are poor. There is a hemorrhagic area in the labyrinth. There are uric acid deposits in the cortex and in the papillæ; also lime infarctions in the latter. In the pelvis there are petechiæ and one large hemorrhage. Right: weight, 120 gm.; surface the same as that of the left kidney; cortex, yellow in color. The organ is succulent; there are hemorrhages in the pelvis. Just external to the pelvis there is a border of very succulent, reddish tissue, varying in width from 0.5 cm. to 1 cm. There are uric acid and lime deposits as in the left kidney.

Ureters.—Negative.

Adrenals.—Negative.

Pancreas.—Negative.

Small Intestine.—The walls of the jejunum and duodenum show blood injection; the contents are tarry. The mucosa of the ileum is swollen, and there are hemorrhages in the wall.

Colon.—Small effusion of blood in and under the mucosa of the ileocecal valve and the cecum. The contents of the large intestine are hemorrhagic. No evidences of lymphatic hyperplasia. The wall of the rectum is injected.

Bladder.—Marked injection of the vessels of the trigone. Prostate normal in size; color, yellowish.

Lymph Nodes.—The mesenteric nodes moderately enlarged; they look like the prevertebral nodes. The latter vary in size, the largest being about the size of a large bean. They are fairly soft, ochre in color, and show some hemorrhagic markings.

Bone-marrow of Femur.—Uniformly dark red in color; quite firm; no changes in bone.

Thoracic duct is formed by two separate channels, which coalesce just below the diaphragm.

Bacteriological Examination.—Cultures made from the heart blood remain sterile. Those made from the spleen show the staphylococcus albus.

MICROSCOPIC FINDINGS.—Pieces of tissue from various parts of the organs were fixed in Zenker's solution, saturated sublimate, formaline, alcohol, Müller's fluid, and Orth's solution, and were embedded both in celloidin and paraffin. The ordinary histological stains were employed, also iron hemotoxylin, Biondi-Heidenhain, Pappenheim's methyl-green pyronin, Mallory's connective-tissue stain, Unna's polychrome methylene blue, Weigert's modified Van Gieson's stain, and others.

Spleen.—Certain peculiarities are found in sections from different parts of the organ. Many dense bands of fibrous connective tissue are seen surrounding certain parts of the splenic tissue. In places where these bands are less dense, the individual connective-tissue fibres are seen to be slightly separated from one another by a faintly staining homogeneous substance containing a few mononuclear cells and giving the usual appearances of edema. Occasionally an area is found near the margin of a band of connective tissue, where the fibres are more widely separated, giving rise to small, irregularly-shaped spaces or meshes. As a rule, these spaces contain a few normal pulp cells, though here and there an endothelial cell of the type described below is seen, entirely surrounded by delicate connective-tissue fibres. The capsule and the trabecular arrangement are quite normal, with the exception of certain pigment, which will be mentioned below, and a slight increase in the amount of connective tissue. The infarcts are of the usual anemic variety. Some of these contain areas of necrosis, with many slit-like openings, due, in all probability, to the presence of cholesterin crystals. In some of the necrotic areas the remnants of alveolar spaces filled with endothelial cells, as described below, can be seen.

Scattered throughout all the sections are large masses of cells which require further description and which seem to be the principal and characteristic feature of the disease. The cells are found mainly in large, irregularly shaped, alveolar spaces, whose walls are composed of delicate connective tissue lined by endothelium. Fine capillaries are seen in the walls in places where the latter are somewhat thickened. These alveolar spaces measure from 130μ by 269μ to 9.5μ by 108μ, respectively. Many variations in size occur between these extremes. The alveolar spaces or pulp spaces may be looked upon, according to Weidenreich,[11] as the venous capillaries of the spleen. In some places a direct connection between adjacent alveoli is found to exist.

The endothelial cells which line these spaces can readily be seen.

In some places they are of normal appearance; in other places they are distinctly swollen. Occasionally a few very delicate connective-tissue fibres may be found within the alveoli. The endothelial cells filling these spaces are so abundant in number that in many places it is impossible to distinguish any of the normal splenic tissue. Only here and there can a single Malpighian body be seen. These bodies have no degenerative changes, but the central artery shows a slight thickening of its walls. Here and there a few connective-tissue fibres can be found in the Malpighian bodies themselves, principally at the periphery. The cells are found both lying free and attached to the wall of the spaces, and their size and shape correspond to the amount of pressure exerted upon them. For the most part, the cells resemble swollen endothelial cells. They are, as a rule, quite large in size, round, oval, or polygonal in shape, depending upon the number in a given space (Fig. 1). The cell bodies stain faintly, but distinctly, with eosin or picric acid, and show a slightly granular appearance of the cytoplasm, but no degenerative changes. The outline of the cell body is usually well preserved. In thin paraffin sections a distinct network of fine linear markings can be seen in some of the cells; with the high power these fine lines seem to be composed of minute dots. In other cells very delicate wavy lines are distinguished, arranged in a more or less concentric form, giving a streaked or wrinkled appearance to the cell. This appearance of the cytoplasm is well brought out by Mallory's phosphomolybdic acid hematoxylin stain. Fig. 2 shows the general granular and streaked appearance of the cells under high amplification. Vacuoles are not uncommon, as many as four or five being present in some of the larger cells. In favorable parts of the sections the cells can be seen arising directly from the endothelial lining of the pulp spaces, or, more properly, venous capillaries. In size the cells vary from 17.4μ by 21.75μ, to 34.8μ by 47.85μ, respectively. Nuclei of a relatively small size are seen in the cells. The average measurement is 5.43μ by 8.7μ. These are found either centrally placed or near the periphery. Some of the cells contain three or four nuclei, but the number of nuclei found in a single cell does not correspond always to the size of the latter, for some of the very largest cells contain but a single nucleus. The nuclei vary considerably in size, from small, round, deeply staining bodies rich in chromatin, to larger, irregular forms staining rather freely. Some of the nuclei show atypical mitotic changes, and a few contain distinct nucleoli. No typical giant cells are seen in any of the sections. Here and there the pulp spaces are seen well distended with red blood cells and normal adenoid tissues. Some of these spaces contain but a few endothelial cells; others show a relatively large number. Many of the bloodvessels throughout the sections are surrounded by a slight increase of connective tissue. A few veins, however, are noted whose walls appear quite normal. These are filled with blood.

Light, brownish-colored pigment particles are scattered here and there in the pulp spaces and also in some of the pulp cells. Throughout the trabeculæ fine granules of brownish-yellow pigment are seen, in long spindle-form arrangement, corresponding to the capillaries and also lying free between the connective-tissue fibres. Sections treated with potassium ferrocyanide and hydrochloric acid give the characteristic iron reaction. Sections were stained for bacteria, but none could be discovered. Neither could any bodies be found resembling protozoa.

Liver.—The capsule is much thickened and contains many pigment granules. A striking feature in all the sections is the enormous increase in the amount of interlobular connective tissue throughout the organ, without any apparent influence upon the liver cells themselves. This interlobular structure is composed of very delicate connective-tissue fibres containing numerous capillaries and some pigment. With Mallory's aniline-blue stain a few very fine fibrillæ can be seen extending into the lobules here and there. The bile-ducts are not increased in number and appear quite normal. Under the low power the general picture is that of a diffuse hepatic cirrhosis (Fig. 3). The liver cells, for the most part, are normal, though occasionally a cell is seen containing minute fat-droplets, and a few nuclei show the usual appearance of degeneration.

The peculiar endothelial cells described in the spleen are also found in abundance in this organ. A few are seen in the lobule proper, but the majority are situated in interlobular connective-tissue spaces. In the lobules these cells are, for the most part, situated in the capillaries at the periphery, though now and then single cells can be found in the deeper parts of the lobule surrounded by liver cells. The individual endothelial cells can be made out quite readily, though they are not so clearly defined as in the spleen. In the interlobular connective-tissue spaces the cells are so intimately fused together that their recognition is somewhat more difficult, but sections treated by Weigert's modified Van Gieson's stain show the cell bodies quite distinctly. In every other respect the cells are identical in appearance with those found in the spleen. In a few places there seems to be a tendency for these cells to invade the lobule itself, but, for the most part, the cells seem to be confined to these spaces and in intimate union with the connective-tissue fibres. The pigment in this organ responds also to the test for hemosiderin. The bloodvessels appear quite normal, as a rule. Some of the arteries have slightly thickened walls.

Mesenteric Lymph Nodes.—The capsule and trabeculæ are sharply defined by the large amount of pigment which outlines their course. Throughout the nodes the trabeculæ are deeply pigmented, but not otherwise affected (Fig. 4). The pigment is dark brown in color, and in the thinnest sections can be seen either as elongated whetstone-shaped crystals or as fine amorphous particles. Smaller masses of pigment are also seen distributed in the cortical and medullary portions of the node. The lymph sinuses are all filled with pigment. Iron reaction is present. The nodes are so changed in general appearance and structure that the usual characteristics have entirely disappeared. A section through the central portion of a somewhat enlarged node shows less than ten follicles. The germinal centres are not well marked, but otherwise the follicles are quite normal, excepting that occasionally a few delicate connective-tissue fibres may be seen in the follicle near its periphery. Only here and there are small remnants of normal lymphoid tissue seen (Fig. 5). The medullary portion of the node is somewhat less affected than the cortical substance. The reticulum of the organ is well preserved.

The entire node is practically transformed by the presence of endothelial cells, such as were described in the spleen and liver. With the exception of the connective-tissue structures, follicles, and small remnants of lymphoid tissue, the whole section is but one mass of these cells. Notwithstanding this fact, the individual cells are most distinctly outlined and clearly seen and show but a slight tendency to fuse together. The cells can be seen arising from the walls of the lymph sinuses (Fig. 6), and from the reticulum throughout the node (Fig. 7). In size, shape, structure, and staining properties, the cells are identical with those described above. A few very large cells, measuring 39.15μ by 56.55μ, are present. Some contain as many as nine nuclei. These are not arranged in any particular form, and no cells are found presenting any of the usual appearances of giant cells. The bloodvessels are surrounded by a slightly increased amount of connective tissue, but show no other changes.

Bronchial Lymph Nodes.—These nodes are affected in a like manner. The endothelial cells are of the same general structure and appearance as in the mesenteric lymph nodes and distributed in a similar manner, but they are not present in such great numbers. Here and there small areas of quite normal adenoid tissue are seen, with fairly well-preserved follicles. Pigment is also present and is identical in color, distribution, and reaction with that found in the mesenteric nodes. Besides this, a moderate amount of anthracosis is present. The capsule and trabeculæ show a rather marked increase in amount of connective tissue. The bloodvessels are prominent throughout and well distended with blood. Their walls are somewhat thickened, but show no degenerative changes.

Retroperitoneal Lymph Nodes.—The same process is also found here. The general picture is identical, but a few slight differences may be noted. The capsule is more markedly thickened than in the other nodes, but the pigment, particularly in the lymph sinuses, is not as prominent. Surrounding the follicles are quite a number of small capillaries, and the margins of the follicles show the presence of young connective-tissue fibres. Numerous small bloodvessels, mostly arteries, are seen. These vessels show hyaline changes. In parts of the section degenerative processes have occurred, so that many of the endothelial cells, as well as the adenoid tissue, do not stain distinctly. The entire process in these nodes seems somewhat older than in those described above.

Bone-marrow.—Cells identical with those in the above-described organs are found in abundance in the bone-marrow. There is considerable variation in the size of the cells in the bone-marrow as compared with those found in the other organs, but the general characteristics are preserved. Vacuoles are common in these cells. No forms are found with an excessive number of nuclei, neither are any of the very large types, such as were described in the lymph nodes, to be seen. Occasionally a large mass of these cells is noted, but for the greater part they are found either singly or in groups of from four to ten cells (Fig. 8). In the latter instance the cells are always found in intimate relationship with the walls of the capillaries or attached to the connective-tissue reticulum. The larger masses cannot always be seen to have such a relationship, and occasionally they are found surrounded by a considerable number of red blood cells. In a few places the cells are distinctly seen within the lumen of dilated capillaries.

A large number of stains were employed in the examination of these sections, but the Biondi-Heidenhain method gave the best results, bringing out the connective-tissue reticulum with much clearness. A few polynuclear leukocytes, some of which show eosinophile granulations, are present, also normoblasts and giant cells in considerable numbers. The larger bloodvessels appear normal. No pigment is present.

Spreads made from the bone-marrow by Dr. Libman, and stained with eosin-hematoxylin, Ehrlich's triacid stain, Jenner's stain, and Wright's stain, show the following: There are present many erythrocytes; these are of about the normal size or larger (macrocytes). Slight poikilocytosis is also noted. Normoblasts are very abundant, showing karyokinetic and karyolytic changes. Small and large lymphocytes and mononuclears are present; also polynuclear neutrophilic and eosinophilic leukocytes, but the main bulk of leukocytes is made up by neutrophilic and eosinophilic myelocytes. Some of these are quite large, as are also some of the polynuclear leukocytes. With the Wright stain azurophile granules are seen in a few lymphocytes. Mastzellen are not to be found. The large endothelial cells have basophilic nuclei; their cytoplasm stains slightly basophilic and faintly acidophilic. Giant cells are abundant.

The spreads of the spleen and liver show no nucleated erythrocytes, no giant cells of the type seen in the marrow, and no myelocytes. The cytoplasm of a few of the endothelial cells is granular-looking, the granules taking on an appearance resembling neutrophilic granulations, but they do not impress one as possessing true granulations.

Lung.—The vessels are all distended with blood. The vesicles are compressed in a great measure and show evidences of edema. A moderate amount of fibroid induration is present. The sections show a moderate degree of anthracosis, and some hematogenous pigment is seen scattered through the organ.

Heart.—The pericardium shows a recent serofibrinous exudate with the production of young connective-tissue fibres. In the meshes of this exudate are a large number of small round cells and some red blood cells. Many newly-formed capillaries are also noted. The muscle fibres of the heart show considerable parenchymatous degeneration; also a moderate amount of brown atrophy. No changes are seen in the bloodvessels.

Kidney.—Sections show the usual picture of a chronic interstitial nephritis. Bowman's capsule is much thickened, and here and there the glomeruli are entirely replaced by fibrous tissue. The tubular epithelium is coarsely granular, and the nuclei are occasionally missing. The epithelium shows vacuoles in places. There is also some increase in connective tissue between the tubules, and a few areas of infiltration by small round cells are seen. The vessels are the seat of endarteritis, and the sections also show a slight amount of congestion. Small deposits of lime salts are present. The right kidney shows rather more congestion than the left, and in the medulla is a large hemorrhagic area containing blood pigment and surrounded by a zone of chronic inflammatory tissue.

Pancreas.—This organ shows no lesion.

Andrenal.—The sections are normal.

Colon.—The mucosa is somewhat congested. In the submucosa are many dilated veins filled with blood. Otherwise the sections are quite normal.

While the study of this case was nearing completion, the sister of this patient met with a fatal accident. Her organs are now being studied. Owing to the fact that these may give additional information, we shall reserve our full discussion of the features of these cases to a subsequent publication.

We may state, however, that our findings enable us to place this case in the group described by Gaucher, Picou and Raymond, Collier, and Bovaird. The spleen and liver show the same changes as described by Gaucher, but he has not reported fully in regard to the lymph nodes. Picou and Raymond report simply on the spleen and lymph nodes, as in their case the spleen was removed at operation. Our findings correspond with theirs in nearly every respect. The spleen in Collier's case is also identical. Bovaird's case and ours are also similar, but our case is the first one in which the bone-marrow was examined and the endothelial hyperplasia discovered.

REFERENCES.

[1] SIPPY: The American Journal of the Medical Sciences, November, 1899, p. 445; and December, 1899, p. 570.

[2] OSLER: Edinburgh Medical Journal, May, 1899; The American Journal of the Medical Sciences, January, 1900; and ibid., November, 1902.

[3] ROLLESTON: Clinical Journal, 1902.

[4] FREDERICK TAYLOR: Guy's Hospital Reports, 1895, vol. lii.; and 1897, vol. liv.

[5] GILBERT AND FOURNIER: Rev. mens. des malad. de l'enfance, 1895, p. 309.

[6] STENGEL: The American Journal of the Medical Sciences, September, 1904.

[7] GAUCHER: Thèse de doctorat, 1882; Splenomegalie primitive, Epithelioma primitif de la rate.

[8] PICOU ET RAYMOND: Arch. de méd. exp. et anat. path., 1896, p. 168.

[9] WILLIAM COLLIER: Transactions of the London Pathological Society, 1895, p. 148.

[10] BOVAIRD: The American Journal of the Medical Sciences, 1900, vol. cxx. p. 377.

[11] WEIDENREICH: Arch. f. mikrosk. Anat. und Entwick, 1901, Bd. lviii.

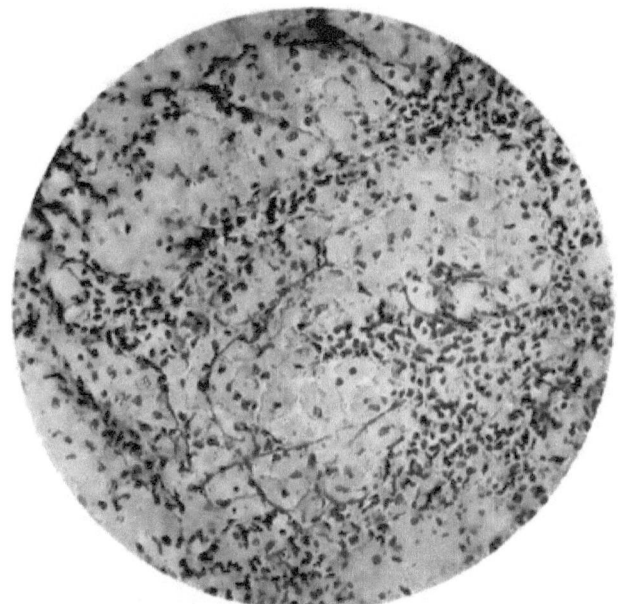

Fig. 1.—Photomicrograph of spleen, showing the alveoli filled with endothelial cells. × 250.

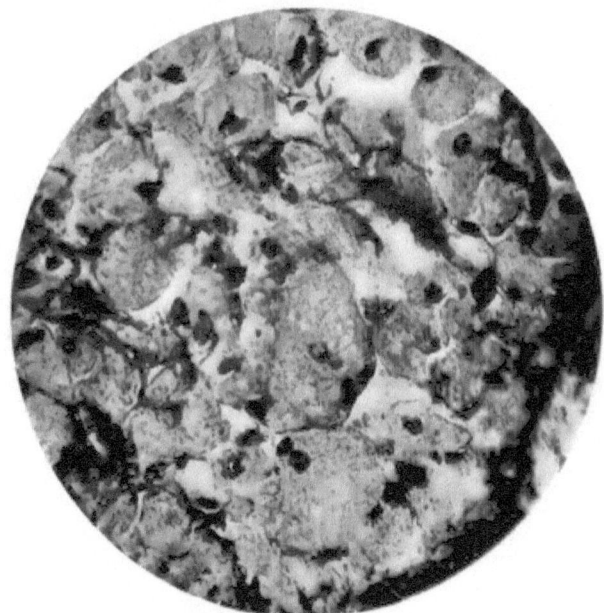

Fig. 2.—Photomicrograph, showing the general granular and streaked appearance of the endothelial cells. × 500.

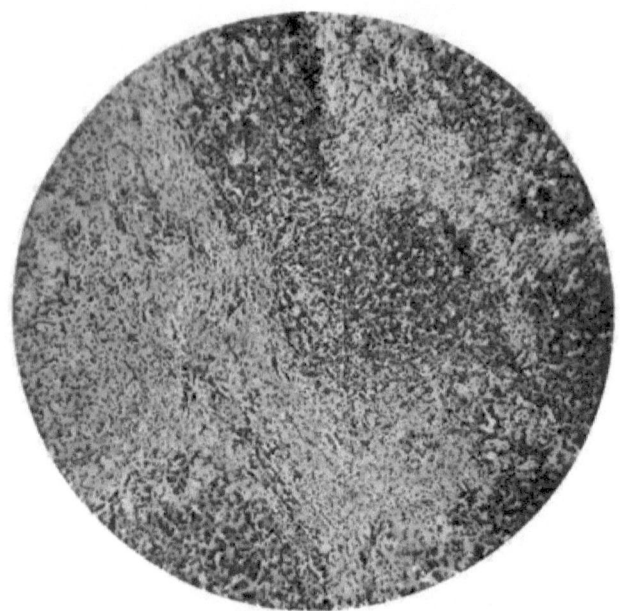

FIG. 3.—Photomicrograph of liver, low power, showing the increase in connective tissue and the general appearance of diffuse cirrhosis.

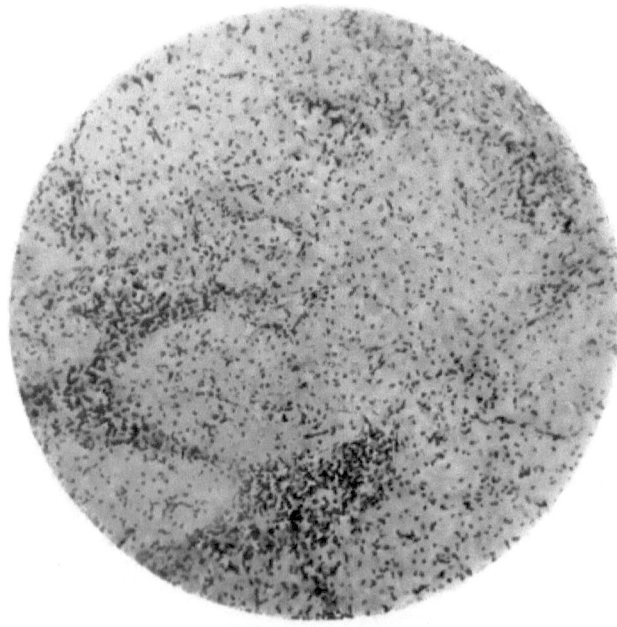

FIG. 4.—Photomicrograph of lymph node, showing the pigment distribution and the endothelial hyperplasia. × 125.

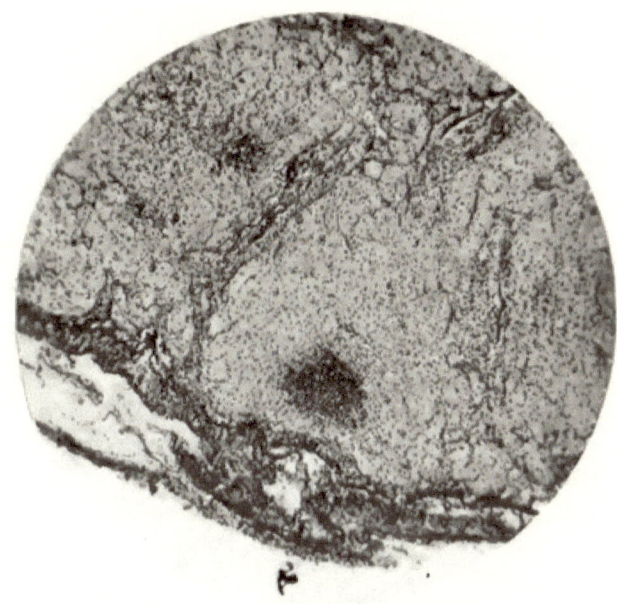

FIG. 5.—Photomicrograph of lymph node, low power, showing remnants of two follicles and absence of normal lymphoid tissue.

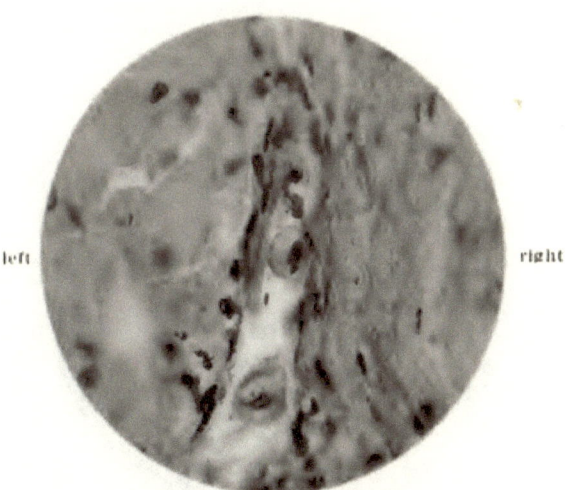

FIG. 6.—Photomicrograph of lymph sinus containing pigment granules and endothelial cells in its lumen. On the right is the connective tissue of the capsule; on the left are endothelial cells arising from the wall. × 500.

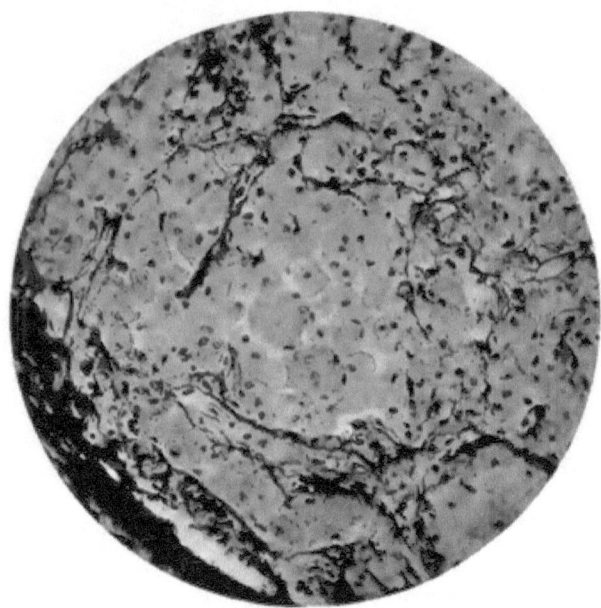

FIG. 7.—Photomicrograph of lymph node, showing the endothelial cells arising from the reticulum, and the general type of the multinuclear endothelial cells. × 250.

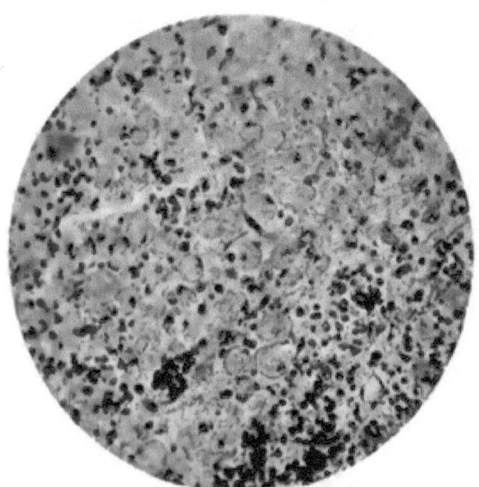

FIG. 8.—Photomicrograph of bone-marrow, showing a small group of endothelial cells. × 250.

THE DIAGNOSIS AND TREATMENT OF PERFORATION IN TYPHOID FEVER.

WITH A REPORT OF 19 CASES, OF WHICH 16 WERE OPERATED ON, WITH 5 RECOVERIES.

MORRIS MANGES, M.D.,

VISITING PHYSICIAN.

The diagnosis and treatment of acute appendicitis are now so clearly defined and so generally recognized that it hardly seems credible that about twenty-five years ago bitter controversies were being waged in New York City as to the propriety of the use of the aspirating needle in the diagnosis of this condition, and an occasional recovery after the opening of an appendicular abscess attracted great attention.

It was at about this time, in 1884, that Leyden first made the suggestion that perforation occurring during the course of typhoid fever should be treated surgically. Contrast the fact that thousands of cases of appendicitis are now successfully operated on annually and that a paltry 362 cases constitute the whole literature of surgically treated typhoid perforation! And this for a condition which, according to the well-known statistics of Taylor, costs from 20,000 to 25,000 lives yearly in the United States alone.

The surprise, which at first glance seems inevitable, yields on a more careful consideration of the situation. While there are many things in which the two conditions have a close resemblance, there are other important points of difference. The first is that the majority of practitioners see relatively few cases of typhoid fever, and the clinical picture is one which is, unfortunately, only well known in all its various forms to those who have had the opportunity of hospital practice. Appendicitis is a disease of every-day occurrence, and the practitioner whose field of work is even limited has a more or less extensive opportunity for knowing the disease. Then, too, appendicitis strikes in health or after a previous attack, and the differential diagnosis is between unassociated conditions. Perforation, on the other hand, occurs during the course of a disease, the progress of which presents an infinite number of variations, which irregularities may be due to a great variety of causes. The typhoid stupor is not conducive to affording much aid from the patient, and hence we must depend on the intelligent observation of nurses rather than on the subjective complaint of the patient; so that, while the diagnosis of perforation may in some cases be exceedingly easy, in other cases it may be very difficult, and in still others absolutely impossible.

Advances have been made, it is true; yet, when compared with what has been accomplished in appendicitis, much remains to be done to popularize the diagnostic features of perforation, in spite of the fact that not a few excellent papers have been published which present the clinical aspect of this condition in the clearest possible way and leave nothing to be desired. Yet, look at the majority of the text-books now in the hands of students and practitioners and judge whether anyone, from reading even the latest editions of some of them, could recognize the occurrence of perforation early enough to render surgical interference possible. This is all the more unpardonable, since this subject has been so actively and ably studied during the past few years. The lore which lies buried in society reports, hospital bulletins and medical journals is not the working stuff which reaches the general practitioner and guides him in the darkness and despair which envelop these gloomy hours.

A review of the recent experiences at Mt. Sinai Hospital may possibly be of some value in showing some of the varied clinical aspects of perforation.

This series of 19 cases of perforation, out of a total of 216 cases (8.8 per cent.) of typhoid fever occurring at one hospital, may possibly now subserve a better purpose than a collection of cases in different parts of the country, observed by different men under different conditions. Indeed, there is no excuse for this since the statistical side has been so ably treated by Keen, the Johns Hopkins School, Hare, Hays, Elsberg, Harte and Ashhurst, and other writers.

I have restricted myself to the cases which have occurred during the past two years, since those before that time have not been reported in sufficient detail to make them of special value for this purpose.

I am indebted to my colleages, Drs. Meyer, Rudisch, Berg, Davison and Koplik for their courtesy in allowing me to report the cases which occurred in their services.

It will at once strike one that this is a very large number of cases to report for so short a period. It must remain an open question whether there may not be some seasonable variations which are peculiar to typhoid fever—that is, whether the typhoid bacilli which are responsible for the present epidemic have more ulcerating qualities, if one may be allowed to use this expression, or whether the large number may not be due to peculiarities of treatment; or, again, whether the question may not be explained by the better training and constant watch for the possibility of the occurrence of perforation.

As regards the first point, it has been frequently noted that there have been variations in the frequency of perforation. Curschman and Osler also refer to the great variations in the frequency of perforation in different epidemics, both from the clinical and from the autopsy records, the variations being from 4 per cent. to 33 per cent. There is also a difference in the statistics as to mortality from perforation, the German being much lower, Curschman giving 9 per cent. to 10 per cent. as the average mortality rate, while Osler's figures give 30 per cent. of all deaths as being due to perforation.

As regards the influence of treatment in this series, this can be dismissed in the present instance, since the cases occurred in various services and were not subject to any particular plan of treatment.

The third point probably affords the correct solution, namely, our better training and the ability to correctly interpret symptoms which formerly would have escaped notice. I have gone over many hospital reports and series of cases which have been published, and without exception I have noted that, whereas the first few cases occurred scattered at long intervals, the latter part of the series consisted of cases which occurred within a comparatively short time, thus showing that, as each observer's knowledge of the symptoms had improved, so had his diagnostic skill.

That a diagnosis is possible in the majority of cases is shown by the fact that of the 16 cases of this series which were operated on, the diagnosis was verified at the time of operation, and the 3 cases which were not operated on leave no room for doubt, either in the case which recovered or in the two which died.

To attempt any classification of these cases from a diagnostic standpoint is at present both impossible and futile. Thus, it is idle to divide them into the appendicular, the intestinal, and so forth, and it is useless to conjecture what pathologic changes might be present, since there is, unfortunately, no relation between the latter and the patient's symptoms. It is this lack of relation which often makes the diagnostic problem so difficult, and the confusion which has resulted from confounding perforation with a resulting peritonitis must be cleared up if early diagnoses are to be made. No more striking proof of the great extent to which this confusion still prevails can be offered than that which is afforded by the most recent and certainly the most elaborate and best work on typhoid fever in the German and English languages, i.e., Curschman's treatise and its American edition by Osler. In neither is there any index reference for perforation, and it is only referred to under perforative peritonitis.

A much more practical classification is that which is based on the mode of onset, whether abrupt or gradual. This is a useful grouping; it aids greatly in making a prognosis as well as a diagnosis, since a careful examination which I have made of a large number of published cases has demonstrated the fact that cases with an abrupt onset are much more favorable than the other group, because not only is early operative interference possible, but also, as a rule, the general course is more favorable.

In the present series the onset was gradual in 4, all of whom died, 2 having been operated on. In the other 15 cases the onset was abrupt, with 6 recoveries, 5 of which were operative cases. The mortality in the cases of gradual onset was 100 per cent., while in those of abrupt onset it was but 60 per cent.

It is not my purpose to present a wearisome recital of the details of the 19 cases of perforation, since those who are interested will find these data in the report of the cases. Instead, I will give, as briefly as possible, the important features which may be serviceable from a diagnostic standpoint.

As usual, males predominated, there being 15 males to 4 females. The ages ranged between 6½ years and 42; 3 were under 10 years, 5 between 10 and 20, 6 between 20 and 30, 3 between 30 and 40, and 2 were 42 years old.

Plunges were used in 5 cases; not used in 14.

Bowels were constipated in 7; diarrhea in 4; variable in 8.

The day of perforation varied from the ninth to the fifty-eighth day of the disease.

	CASES		CASES
First week	0	Sixth week	1
Second week	5	Seventh week	1
Third week	5	Eighth week	0
Fourth week	3	Ninth week	1
Fifth week	3		

The onset was gradual in 4, and sudden in 15 cases.

FIRST SYMPTOM: CASES
- Abdominal pain 10
- Pain and chill................s........................ 2
- Pain and vomiting 2
- Vomiting 1
- Chill 2
- Changes in condition and rise in pulse and respiration.... 1
- Changes in condition and abdominal tenderness............. 1

Of all the symptoms, pain will always remain the most important. It was present in 17 of the 19 cases of the series, being absent only in the 2 delirious and comatose cases, and in 14 it was the first symptom or onset. As this symptom deserves special attention it will be considered in detail later on.

Of the conditions of the abdomen, tenderness is a very varying symptoms as regards extent, locality and severity. A far better guide is abdominal rigidity, which was present in 16 cases, was variable in 2 and absent in 1.

Distension is also an uncertain guide, as it was marked in only 6, was slight in 8 and absent in 3; in some of the latter the abdomen was even retracted.

Movable dullness in the flanks forms quite an important symptom, and was present in 8 cases, absent in 8, and not stated in 3.

As to the obliteration of liver dullness, much more would be gained from this symptom if physicians would make it a rule to note the variations in the size of the liver dullness throughout the disease. The time which is now wasted in examining the spleen during the course of the disease would be far better spent if devoted to the percussion of the liver and abdomen. The obliteration of the liver dullness is best noted in the axillary line, since this area is less subject to disturbing factors from undue distension of the colon and small intestine. The time of the occurrence of the obliteration of liver dullness is variable, and may even be absent in cases of perforation where free gas is localized in the peritoneal cavity by pre-formed adhesions. It was present in 11 cases, and was either absent or of doubtful value in 8 cases.

Posture: All children had flexed thighs.

Temperature: Fell, 3; rose, 9; unchanged, 4; could not be ascertained, 3.

Pulse: Fell, 0; rose, 12; unchanged, 4; could not be ascertained, 3.

Respirations: Fell, 0; rose, 10; unchanged, 6; could not be ascertained, 3.

Number of leucocytes: Rose, 7; fell, 3; no marked change, 6; could not be learned, 3.

Collapse was present only once; sweating, twice.

No observations on changes in blood pressure, to which some observers (Elsner and Crile[1]) have called attention, were made. For obvious reasons this will never be an important guiding symptom in this condition.

Results: Died, 13 (68.4 per cent.); recovered, 6 (31.6 per cent.).

Operated on, 16; died, 11 (68.75 per cent.); recovered, 5 (31.25 per cent.).

Not operated on, 3; died, 2 (66+ per cent.); recovered, 1 (33+ per cent.).

In 1902, out of 107 cases of typhoid fever treated at the hospital, there were 9 cases of perforation, with 1 operative recovery and 1 non-operative recovery, giving an operative recovery of 11+ per cent. In 1903, out of 109 cases of typhoid fever, there were 10 cases of perforation, 8 of which were operated on and 2 were not operated on; both of the latter died. Of the 8 operated on, there were 4 recoveries (50 per cent.). If objection be made to including the 2 cases of recovery where fecal abscesses were opened, there would still remain 2 operative recoveries out of 6 cases of perforation operated on, namely, 33+ per cent. of recoveries.

Time of operation (reservation being always made as regards the exactness of such estimation):

	CASES		CASES
5 hours	1	21 hours	1
6 hours	3	43 hours	1
8 hours	1	48 hours	1
11 hours	2	72 hours	1
12 hours	2	Unknown	6[2]

[1] Journal American Medical Association, 1903, vol. xl. p. 1292.
[2] Further details will be found in the reports of the cases.

I wish to draw especial attention to the diagnostic significance of pain. As already stated, it occurred in 17 of the cases of this series, and in 14 was the very first symptom of onset. It varies in degree and in location. It also varies in its character, but is usually more or less paroxysmal. Its severity may be so marked that the more or less comatose patient may cry out with pain; on the other hand, it may be very mild, indeed. It may remain more or less constant or it may gradually disappear; it may even be concealed, as occurred in Case No. 6, to avoid operation. It may be referred to any part of the abdomen, and even to other parts, like the penis, the umbilicus, or to the left iliac fossa. In the latter, which occurred in Case No. 6, an omental abscess was found near the tender area.

It is the constancy of the early occurrence of pain in cases of perforation which renders the proper interpretation a matter of very great importance. The correct appreciation of the exact significance of attacks of pain during the course of typhoid fever is by no means an easy task, and we are greatly indebted to McCrae[3] for his instructive analysis of the relation of pain in 500 cases of typhoid fever. Of this series the most important were the 161 cases (32 per cent.) in which there was more or less marked pain during the course of the disease. In these 161 cases of pain the pain was referred to perforation in 13 cases, to hemorrhage in 13, to some known cause in 65, but in 70 cases no explanation could be found.

This subject is so important that I may be pardoned if I name the various conditions to which the pain was referred in the 65 cases where the cause was discoverable. They were, first, hysteria, pleurisy, pneumonia, distended bladder, abortion, labor and menstruation; second, gastrointestinal conditions apart from complications, i. e., taking solid food, vomiting, constipation, fecal impaction and diarrhea; third, various abdominal conditions, i. e., appendicitis, peritonitis, cholecystitis, rupture of the gall bladder, liver abscess, painful spleen (rupture or infarction), phlebitis and thrombosis of iliac vessels.

Among the 70 cases in which no cause was discoverable were included several cases in which the pain was very severe and accompanied by rigidity, tenderness, leucocytosis and diminished liver dull-

[3] New York Med. Jour., May 4, 1901; see also Martin, de la Douleur Abdominale dans la Fievre Typhoide, These de Paris, 1901, which corroborates McCrae's statements.

ness. Two of these cases were operated on; in one only the angry bases of inflamed Peyer's patches could be found; in the other nothing was discoverable. In others of these cases it was surmised that enlarged mesenteric glands might have caused the pain.

McCrae states that of the various conditions in which pain occurred, the association of perforation and hemorrhage was most puzzling. The two cases in my series corroborate this statement. The possibility of the two conditions occurring together should always be borne in mind, and McCrae very properly warns against the danger of opium in such cases, since the symptoms may be masked by it. Every case of hemorrhage with marked symptoms should be regarded as being possibly associated with perforation.

It is unfortunate that the space at my disposal does not permit a more careful discussion of these two conditions, for the further consideration of which and the other associated conditions I would refer to the paper above cited, and also to a most careful analysis by McCrae and Mitchell on the "Surgical Features of Typhoid Fever."[4]

The solution of some of these problems of the real significance of pain will be found when we know more about the exact relation of non-perforative peritonitis in typhoid fever. A recent paper by Yates[5] contains a very full bibliography and presents a number of most instructive facts as to its varied relations. Non-perforative peritonitis is one-third as frequent as perforation, since it was found present in 73 out of 4,300 cases (1.7 per cent.) collected by Horton Smith and Hoelscher and Liebermeister.

The symptoms of peritonitis as given by Yates are exactly those of perforative peritonitis, and in the 20 cases which he has collected were so regarded, as will be detailed later on in the discussion of the treatment.

These cases of localized peritonitis without perforation, like the case of Murphy,[6] the 5 cases of Gairdner,[7] the 2 of Shattuck, Warren and Cobb,[8] and others, may be cited as showing how exceedingly important it is to always bear in mind the relation of non-perforative peritonitis in the differential diagnosis of pain.

[4]Johns Hopkins Hospital Reports, vol. x.
[5]American Medicine, May 2, 1903.
[6]KEEN: Surgical Complications and Sequels of Typhoid Fever, Philadelphia, 1898, p. 238.
[7]Glasgow Medical Journal, vol. xlvi. p. 114.
[8]Boston Medical and Surgical Journal, June 28, 1900.

In drawing practical conclusions from this analysis of the varied clinical features of perforation as it occurred in this series, it will at once be seen that there is no one symptom or group of symptoms which is pathognomonic. Its recognition demands intelligent watchfulness and judgment on the part of the physician, and especially the nurses.

Osler's[9] schema for the observation of symptoms in suspected perforation is a useful guide which should be both studied and used by the physician, and especially for the instruction of nurses.

To my mind the first important fact to note is that there is a more or less marked change in the condition of the patient; associated with this, there is usually some form of abdominal pain which is very variable. The condition of the abdomen as regards tenderness, rigidity, distension, respiratory excursions and the liver dullness which have been routinely observed, now afford valuable aid. Movable dullness in the flanks gives distinct evidence of peritoneal exudate. In the meantime the anxious facies and sweating are significant guides. Changes in the rate and character of the pulse mean much more than do changes in the temperature and respiration. The leucocyte count is of so little value that the general practitioner may very well disregard it in private work. Probably more will be gained from a simple hemoglobin test to exclude a concealed or misleading hemorrhage.

Finally, it is the combination of the symptoms, their progressive character and development which must enable one to make a presumptive diagnosis.[10] It is far safer to assume that the symptoms point to the occurrence of perforation and to prepare for possibilities and rapid action than to take the opposite standpoint and wait for the fully developed symptoms of peritonitis.

If these facts be borne in mind it becomes much easier to understand the statements made by all writers that the marked symptoms are not those of perforation, but of the complicating peritonitis. It also becomes easy of comprehension that most physicians expect too many and too pronounced symptoms for an early diagnosis of perforation, for the appearance of which they often sacrifice the golden time for successful operative interference, since the fact is so often

[9]Philadelphia Medical Journal, Jan. 19, 1901.
[10]See also McCrae and Mitchell's summing up of the various symptoms on pp. 410-411, Amer. Med., Sept. 13, 1902.

overlooked and so seldom understood that the perforation itself causes little shock and may even afford temporary relief.

It is absurd to state definitely in many cases that the perforation occurred at this or that time, and that the operation was performed a certain number of hours after perforation. Such estimates are only approximate and are liable to great errors. We are really only entitled to say that the operation was performed at such an interval after the occurrence of certain symptoms. However, as no other guides are given, this is often the best that can be done, and in what follows I would have such statements as to the time of operation so understood.

The reason for this statement is that the occurrence of acute symptoms does not necessarily mean that this coincides with the time of perforation. Anyone who has seen a number of cases of perforation must have been struck by the difficulty of estimating the exact time of the occurrence of the accident. Corroboration of this will be found in the statement made by Shattuck, Warren and Cobb, that early warning pains, earlier by a definite number of hours than the severe symptoms, occurred in 14 out of the 21 cases of perforation reported by them.

Before considering the question of treatment, a few words may be said as to the possibility of the spontaneous cure of perforation. Most authorities deny this positively. The views of Fitz[11] and Curschman and Osler[12] leave little room for doubt as to the certainty of their convictions. The cases in which spontaneous cures have occurred are supposed to have been either appendicular perforations in the course of typhoid, or cases of peritonitis which have simulated perforation. My own belief, from what I have seen, is that spontaneous cure is possible and probably occurs more often than we think, if the perforation is a small one and is immediately shut off by adhesions or omentum. I may refer to Case No. 8 as one of spontaneous cure, and to Case No. 18, in which a small perforation was found at the autopsy well sealed by adhesion of omentum.

Cases have been reported by Bucquoy, Trousseau, Cruveilhier, Reunert, Bühl, Widal, Dieulafoy, Chantemesse and Remlinger[13] in

---

[11]Trans. of the Assn. of Amer. Physicians, vol. vi, 1891, p. 207.

[12]Typhoid and Typhus Fever, Nothnagel's Encyclopedia, American translation, p. 233.

[13]Bull. de la Soc. Imp. de Constantinople, Seance du 15 March, 1901.

which recovery has been due to protective adhesions, fibrinous deposits and by the agglutination of intestines, omentum or mesentery. Furthermore, Haegle-Pasavant, Villemin and Walther have reported recoveries with intestinal fistulæ. The cases of Bucquoy and Widal are especially interesting, since the patients having died from other conditions, the evidences of the healed perforations and adhesions were found at autopsy.

Granting the possibility of spontaneous cure, the best results ever claimed for nature's method have been 5 per cent., and even the recoveries with fecal abscesses can hardly be called ideal recoveries. Contrast this with the latest statistics published by Hare and Ashhurst of 362 cases which they collected from the literature, with a recovery of 26 per cent. Granting that these statistics represent in the main successful cases and may not include many unreported unsuccessful cases, yet the contrast is sufficiently striking as to leave no doubt as to the best plan for treatment.

This consists in making as early a diagnosis as possible, and this, or a strongly probable diagnosis having been made, an immediate operation is indicated.

It is a matter of great regret that in private practice the patients are under a great disadvantage in regard to what constitutes an early operation, for reasons which are obvious, unless the possibility of surgical complications receive that prompt consideration and action which is afforded to patients in the hospital. No time should be lost by the attending physician in making suitable preparations for the surgeon while he is stimulating the patient and awaiting the final decision as to the course of action. No harm will be done by making needless preparations; much will be gained by making timely preparation for prompt action.

The only exception to the rule of early operation is that moribund patients should not be operated on.

In making the prognosis it must not be forgotten that the patient must still run the gauntlet of the balance of his attack of typhoid fever, in passing through which, however, he will have been made none the worse by the operation. This also holds for those cases in which no perforation has been found, unless, of course, the underlying condition which produced the misleading symptoms should cause a fatal issue. The wonderful endurance and resistance of typhoid patients enable us to hold out a much more hopeful prognosis than would be deemed advisable under other conditions. The operation in skillful hands, with local or general anesthesia, is infinitely less dangerous than the possibilities of the complications of the disease. Furthermore, I have observed that in some of the patients who have survived the operation for perforation, the balance of the disease seems to have been cut short by the operation. McCrae and Mitchell have also observed this. Lenander, quoted by Cushing[14] discourages delay, and even goes so far as to regard the narcosis and operation as a means for combating the shock due to perforation.[15]

The cases in which a perforation has not been found are often by no means needless interferences, since an impending perforation may be prevented or undue distension may be relieved by low ileostomy, as done by Cushing and Esher. Furthermore, Yates' statistics show that of 20 cases of peritonitis in typhoid fever which he collected, 11 were operated on with 4 recoveries; 9 were not operated on, and all died. Of the 11 cases operated on, one was a case which was operated on for appendicitis, but proved to be a walking case of typhoid fever with peritonitis. All of the others were cases of typhoid fever which were operated on for supposed perforation, but in which only peritonitis was found. Finally, Cushing has reported a case which was under his care in 1889, and was operated on for symptoms of supposed perforation. No intestinal lesion was found except a chronic adherent appendicitis. The removal of the appendix under cocain anesthesia gave immediate relief from the abdominal symptoms, and the patient recovered from his typhoid fever.

If, however, an early diagnosis has not been made, the indications for immediate operation are not so clear and the cases must be individualized as to the advantage of waiting or of operating, since nature does cure some of these cases. But who can surely pick them out and what means have we at our disposal to know whether the opening has been closed by the adhesion of omentum or by a thick layer of fibrin?

Cases 17 and 19, in which successful operations were performed many hours after perforation, enormous fecal abscesses being found

[14] Studies in Typhoid Fever, Johns Hopkins Hospital Reports, Series 3, pp. 229-230.

[15] In the cases reported general anesthesia was always used in preference to local anesthesia, unless there was some special contraindication.

notwithstanding the fact that the patient's general condition was good, show that even a late operation has its indications.

These 2 cases (17 and 19) deserve a few words. No one looking at Case 17 would have suspected that he had nearly two quarts of fecal fluid in his peritoneal cavity—nothing in his condition on his admission to the hospital, even after his transportation, would have warranted this assumption, except a careful consideration of the history and the proper interpretation of the physical signs. To have relied on the clinical text-book description would have been absolutely misleading.

Even more striking is the last case (No. 19). This was a walking case where perforation occurred on the fifteenth day. He was admitted to the hospital twenty-four hours later. A leucocytosis of 14,000 was found; the local rigidity and tenderness in the abdomen lessened; his temperature dropped from 105.2°F. to 101.8°F.; pulse and respiration improved decidedly, and his whole appearance was better. On the following day the only disturbing features were that there was a little more distension, the liver dullness had decreased, and he had vomited twice during the night. The operation was then performed, and an enormous fecal abscess was found. The patient has recovered in spite of a complicating pneumonia. An additional feature of interest is the fact that the Widal reaction was repeatedly negative until the forty-second day; the positive diagnosis of typhoid fever had, however, been made on the twenty-sixth day by the finding of typhoid bacilli in the blood culture.

Wilson, of Philadelphia, the earliest advocate of operative interference in this country, wrote as follows in 1886:[15]

"Granted that the chance of a successful issue is heavily against you; that the patient is in the midst, or at the end, of a long sickness; that the tissues are in the worst state to stand the injuries of the surgeon's knife; that the lesions of the gut may be very extensive; that the vital forces are at the lowest ebb; no one has yet for these reasons refused to perform tracheotomy in the laryngeal complications of typhoid fever, which requires it to save life. The operative treatment of purulent peritonitis has been performed successfully many times by gynecologists in conditions scarcely less promising. In point of fact, the objections which may be urged against laparotomy in intestinal perforation in enteric fever are no more forcible than those which would

[15]Quoted from Finney, Johns Hopkins Hospital Reports, vol. viii. p. 56.

have been made use of at first against the same operation in gunshot wounds of the abdomen.

". . . . The courage to perform it will come of the knowledge that the only alternative is the patient's death."

Mikulicz[17] stated in 1884:

"If suspicious of a perforation, one should not wait for an exact diagnosis and for peritonitis to reach a pronounced degree; but, on the contrary, one should immediately proceed to an exploratory operation which in many cases is free from danger."

It is hard to believe that these views were written in 1886 and 1884, respectively; it is still more difficult to modify or change in any respect these terse and telling sentences which so truthfully represent the experience and opinions of all physicians who have had practical experience with this most trying complication of typhoid fever.

Cases 1 to 7 and 9 have already been published in Mount Sinai Hospital Reports, 1903, vol. iii, pp. 104, 75, 383, 207, 208, 384, and hence the histories are omitted.

CASE 8.—*Typhoid fever; moderately severe course of long duration; symptoms of perforation on forty-third day; spontaneous recovery.*

Patient.—Hyman B., aged 12, was admitted October 2, 1902, to the service of Dr. Koplik, with a history of typhoid of ten days' duration. Among the early symptoms was abdominal pain, which was present at the time of admission. He had also vomited at different times.

Examination.—White blood count on the day after admission, 10,200. Widal positive in 1 to 50. The liver enlarged three finger breadths below the costal border.

October 8: Temperature approaching normal. General abdominal tympany, but lax. Leucocytes, 5,000.

October 11: Slight abdominal pain on pressure in the right iliac fossa; soon passed off. Lower border of the liver at the free border of the ribs.

October 27: (thirty-fifth day). A sudden short rise of temperature to 104°F.; pulse, 110 to 120; leucocytes, 7,000.

The following week the temperature gradually fell, reaching 99°F. on November 2. General condition good. Pulse 90 to 104; respiration, 24.

November 4: (forty-third day). Morning temperature, 99.1°F. At 4 p. m. he complained of sudden severe abdominal pain at the um-

[17]Curschman and Osler, op. cit., p. 235.

bilious; abdomen rigid and general tenderness, especially in the right iliac fossa. Temperature, 100.2°F.; pulse, 104; respiration, 24; leucocytes, 14,000. At 4:30 p. m. vomited. At 6 p. m. temperature, 102°; pulse, 116 to 128. Expression anxious; condition of the abdomen unchanged. Rectal examination showed tenderness in Douglas' pouch. At 8 p. m. the temperature had fallen to 99.8°; pulse and respiration remain 104 and 24. At 9 p. m. temperature rose to 104°; pulse, 124; respiration, 32. Condition of the abdomen the same. Liver dullness unchanged.

November 5: Midnight temperature, 103.8°; respiration, 32; pulse, 128. Abdominal pain was the same; no vomiting. Liver dullness reached from the sixth rib to just above the free border. Abdomen was slightly distended, rigid, and with a tender area in the right iliac fossa. Temperature during the day ranged between 103° and 104.4°; pulse kept about 120; respiration varied from 26 to 38, superficial. Leucocyte count at 10 a. m. 12,200. At 3 p. m. he still had abdominal pain. Liver dullness was half gone in the middle line. Abdomen rigid; slight dullness in both flanks.

November 6: Temperature, which had reached 104.4° at 6 a. m., gradually fell during the day, being 103° at 3 p. m., 101° at 9 p. m., and 99.8° at midnight. The pulse rose to 148 at 6 p. m., and then rapidly fell to 100 at midnight. Respiration, 26 at 6 a. m., 36 at noon, 38 at 6 p. m., and fell to 28 at midnight. The abdomen became more distended and was very tender. Liver dullness remained the same; no friction sounds could be heard. Throughout the day the patient's condition remained unchanged, the face being very anxious and the general impression being made that of a child who was desperately ill.

November 7: Both pulse and respiration gradually fell during the course of the day, temperature dropping from 101° at 3 a. m. to 98.6° at 6 p. m. Pulse from 110 at 3 a. m. to 72 at 6 p. m. Respiration ranged from 26 to 24. Blood count at noon was 5,800. General condition better; quality of the pulse decidedly improved. Abdomen, especially the right iliac fossa, being less tender. Dullness in both flanks still persisted; liver dullness remained unchanged. He passed a stool voluntarily.

November 8: Temperature normal. Abdomen less distended; very little tenderness of the right iliac fossa; liver percusses to the free border; leucocytes, 7,000.

Subsequent course of the disease was uneventful; discharged on December 10.

The case attracted a great deal of attention, owing to the fact that the parents refused to have an operation performed, and I am indebted to Dr. Koplik for the privilege of observing the course of this spontaneous cure of a perforation.

As to the occurrence of a perforation on the afternoon of the forty-third day there can be absolutely no doubt, since the presence of pain, rise in temperature, pulse and respiration range, the increase in the number of leucocytes, the occurrence of abdominal distension, the characteristic pain in the right iliac fossa, the tenderness and doughiness of the pouch in the rectum, the partial obliteration of the liver dullness, the dullness in both flanks and the change in the patient's condition, constitute a group of clinical phenomena for which no other explanation than that of perforation with peritoneal effusion can be found. This diagnosis is strengthened by the subsequent disappearance of all these signs.

CASE 10.—*Typhoid fever; severe course; perforation on eighteenth day; operation; death.*

Patient.—Samuel H., aged 38, Russian, was admitted on January 28, 1903, on the fifteenth day of his disease. Markedly alcoholic history.

History.—He had been in bed a few days at a time until three days ago, when he remained in bed constantly. There was obstinate constipation.

Examination.—On admission his condition was apathetic. Abdomen tympanitic, somewhat distended, moderate rigidity, no tenderness, no roseola. The liver dullness extended to the free border. Bronchitis. General condition poor. Temperature, 104.4°F.; pulse, 118; respiration, 28. At 3 p. m. temperature rose to 106°, but dropped to 104°F. at midnight. Leucocyte count, 8,400.

January 29: Temperature ranged from 104° to 105.4°F.; pulse between 90 and 104; respiration between 24 and 34.

January 30: Patient decidedly worse, temperature suddenly rising at noon at 107°; pulse, 120; respiration, 38. Widal remained negative. At 6 p. m., temperature 106°; at midnight, 105.4°; pulse, 120; respiration, 40.

January 31: At 4.30 a. m. he complained of severe generalized abdominal pain with marked rigidity and tenderness, both being more marked on the right side and especially in the iliac fossa. Complete obliteration of liver dullness anteriorly; dullness of upper border of liver in axilla became tympanitic when the patient was turned on his left side. Respiration thoracic and had fallen to 34, but soon rose to 48. Temperature fell to 104°, pulse to 112. At 9 a. m. temperature, 105°; pulse, 148 and very weak; respiration, 48. Leucocyte count, 5,800. The abdominal signs unchanged.

Operation.—Consent for an operation having been obtained, patient was transferred to Dr. Lilienthal's service for operation. Free fecal fluid in peritoneal cavity; perforation found in lower ileum and sutured.

Patient died eight hours after the operation. No autopsy.

CASE 11.—*Typhoid fever; moderate course; perforation on tenth day; no operation; death.*

Patient.—Joseph C., aged 13, American, was admitted to the children's service July 17, 1903, with a history of typhoid fever of one week's duration. Bowels normal; has had slight pain in the abdomen since onset.

Examination.—The attack was of moderate severity. Positive Widal, 1 to 50. White blood cells, 5,200; hemoglobin, 75 per cent. Abdomen retracted and tympanitic, except in the rigid area over the right upper rectus, where there was some dullness; rigidity of right upper rectus, tenderness in the right iliac fossa. The liver extended from the fifth space to the free border in the mammillary line, and in the anterior axillary line from the sixth space to one finger's breadth below the free border. Spleen palpable; a few roseola. Temperature, 103.8°F.; pulse, 120; respiration, 30.

Treatment.—Plunge on the first day was badly borne and only one given, sponges being used thereafter.

July 19: At 9 a.m. temperature dropped to 100.4°, pulse remaining stationary at 110; respiration, 24. At noon, white blood cells, 9,400. In the evening the temperature rose to 103.4°, respiration to 52, pulse to 144, fair quality. No vomiting. Liver dullness not obliterated; abdomen tympanitic except dullness in the left iliac fossa. Flexion of the left thigh caused pain. The breathing is thoracic and superficial.

July 20: General condition unchanged and physical signs as last noted. The temperature at noon had dropped to 100.8°, pulse to 128; respiration remained stationary at 48. White blood count, 10,600. At 9 p.m. the temperature rose to 102.4°, pulse to 140, respiration to 56.

July 21: General condition the same; abdomen still tense, slightly distended and tender, especially in the left iliac fossa. General tympany, except dullness in the left iliac fossa. Liver dullness in the mammillary line obliterated up to two finger breadths above the free border of the ribs. In the axillary line dullness from the eighth space to the free border. Lies with thighs flexed. Thoracic breathing; vomits occasionally; bowels respond slightly to enemata; rectal feeding begun. The temperature dropped to 100.6° at 9 a.m., but rose to 102.8° in the afternoon. Pulse kept between 130 and 140. Respiration, which had fallen to 36 in the morning, in the afternoon and evening kept at 52. White blood count at noon, 11,200.

July 22: General condition worse. Extreme thirst; tongue dry and coated; vomits everything. Lies with flexed thighs. Abdomen is tense, slightly distended, especially in the lower half; dullness in the left iliac fossa. Tympany over the liver is one finger breadth higher than noted yesterday.

July 23: Grew progressively worse. The vomiting was incessant; the abdomen was less rigid but still tender. The liver dullness remained as last noted. The temperature, which had remained at about 100.5° on July 22, fell to 98° at 9 a. m. on July 23, and rapidly rose to 104.8° at midnight; pulse oscillated between 150 and 160; respiration between 36 and 48. Died July 24, at 2 a. m. No autopsy.

Comments.—The clinical picture of this case was that of perforation, which probably occurred on July 19. Operation was proposed on that day, but consent could never be obtained.

CASE 12.—*Typhoid fever; mild course; perforation on fifteenth day. Admitted with perforation; operation thirty hours (?) after perforation. Recovery.*

Patient.—Harry R., aged 7, American, admitted to the surgical service on August 6, 1903, with a history of typhoid fever of two weeks' duration.

History.—He had really been very ill only for twenty-eight hours before admission, the history being that of an acute onset of severe burning pain in the abdomen, then general cramplike pains, which were most marked on the right side of the abdomen. Vomited once after eating; bowels moved slightly after an enema. Two chills, one at onset and one four hours after the enema. Eighteen hours before admission the child's temperature was 104°. These were the only details that could be obtained from the physician who had attended the child before admission to the hospital.

Examination.—On admission the child's general condition was poor. He was somnolent, but when aroused the expression was anxious. Heart and lungs negative. Abdomen was generally distended, rigid, tense and tender, the tenderness being most marked in the right iliac fossa; movable dullness in the flanks; no mass palpable. The liver and splenic dullness was obscured by tympany and rigidity. Rectal examination negative. Temperature on admission was 100.4°; pulse, 120; respiration, 22.

Operation.—Patient was admitted at noon and operated on at 2 p. m. by Dr. Elsberg; cloudy fluid was found in the peritoneal cavity. A perforation was found twelve inches from the cecum; the neighboring intestines were covered with fibrin for from three to four inches above the perforation. The perforation was sutured. The appendix was removed but found normal. The peritoneal cavity was irrigated with normal saline solution and the wound saturated.

Shortly after the operation temperature rose to 103.4°, pulse to 146, respiration to 44. The subsequent history was that of a rapid convalescence, temperature reaching normal on August 8, the third day after the operation and the seventeenth day of the disease. A positive Widal was obtained on the day after admission, on which day the leucocytes were 10,900.

He was discharged cured October 3, 1903.

CASE 13.—*Typhoid fever; moderate course; perforation on twenty-seventh day; operation five hours later; death from perforation of another ulcer.*

Patient.—Becky B., aged 9 years, American, was admitted on September 11, 1903, to the children's service with a history of typhoid fever of eight days' duration. Constipated. The disease ran a course of moderate severity. Leucocyte count between 6,000 and 7,000; hemoglobin between 75 per cent. and 65 per cent. Temperature began to fall on September 28, the twenty-fifth day of the disease.

September 30: Child takes nourishment poorly; slight distension; vomiting. Liver dullness extends from the fifth space to the free border. 6.20 p. m., complained of pain when position was changed; nauseated one hour ago; legs flexed on abdomen; abdomen more rigid and tender, especially on the right side, being most marked in the iliac fossa, where there is dullness, the rest of the abdomen being tympanitic. Dullness in the right flank which is not movable. Liver percusses to the costal border. The temperature, which had been 104° at 1 a. m., and had dropped to 100.8° at 11 a. m., was 102.2° at 3 p. m., 102.6° at 6 p. m., and 105° at midnight. Pulse at 1 a. m., 134; at 3 p. m. and 6 p. m., 108. Leucocytes, 10,600. At 7:30 p. m. the patient went into collapse.

Operation.—At 10:45 the patient, having responded to stimulation, was sent to the operating room, where laparotomy was performed by Dr. Elsberg and a large quantity of yellowish fluid found. Four inches above the ileocecal junction a perforation was found and sutured. There were three other suspicious ulcers within the foot of gut above the ileocecal valve. Irrigation with normal saline solution. Dr. Libman reported bacterium coli in the peritoneal fluid.

Result.—Death occurred twenty-four hours later with marked abdominal distension and rise of temperature, which had fallen after the operation. Twelve hours after the operation the patient seemed to have rallied, but this change was only temporary.

Autopsy.—An ulcer was found through which feces and gas escaped; general peritonitis; fibrinous exudate on coils of bowels; moderate amount of purulent peritoneal fluid; sutured perforation intact; other organs showed the usual lesions of typhoid fever.

CASE 14.—*Typhoid fever; walking case; perforation on thirty-first day; operation six hours later; recovery; normal temperature in nine days; long and severe relapse with hemorrhages, severe myo-endocarditis; recovery.*

Patient.—Jacob F., aged 19, Austrian, admitted on September 18, 1903, to male ward I, with a history of typhoid fever of four weeks' duration, but he had only gone to bed six days before. Diarrhea, four or five stools a day.

Examination.—On admission, temperature, 104°; pulse, 132; respiration, 26. Positive Widal; white blood count, 8,200. Abdomen lax, tympanitic; roseolæ on chest and back. Hemorrhagic eruption over the right tibia. Liver extends from the sixth rib to one finger breadth below the free border. General condition good.

September 21, 4 a. m.: Complains of sudden, sharp, sticking cramp-like pain in the lower abdomen, most marked in the right iliac fossa. Temperature rose from 102.2° to 105°. Slight chill. Temperature 105° at 5 a. m. Pulse rose from 90 to 120. Looks somewhat worse, being distinctly sicker, crying out with pain, which is continuous with exacerbations. Rigidity and tenderness in the right iliac region; nothing palpable; no other rigidity. Some tenderness in the left iliac fossa. Whole abdomen tympanitic. Liver dullness extends from the fourth space to two finger breadths above the free border, where there is tympany. No obliteration of liver dullness in axilla. Slight abdominal distension, most marked in epigastrium. Respiratory movements present in abdomen. Respiration causes pain. Resists flexion of legs. No sweat. 7 a. m., general condition the same. Tongue dry; no change in temperature or pulse rate. Quality of pulse very good. Rigidity very much increased in right iliac fossa and extends upward to free border of ribs. Rigidity in left iliac fossa as high as umbilicus. Liver flatness obliterated anteriorly as high as tenth rib (tympany). Flat and dull area in axilla over liver became tympanitic with patient on left side. No signs of fluid. Pain somewhat diminished. 9.30 a. m., condition the same. Temperature, 105.6°. Transferred to second surgical service and operated on by Dr. Elsberg.

Operation.—Laparotomy disclosed a moderate amount of cloudy serous fluid. About eight inches from the ileocecal valve a perforation was found and sutured. About a foot further on there was a suspicious ulcer which was also sutured. The abdominal cavity was flushed with normal saline solution and closed. The peritoneal fluid contained the bacterium coli.

The patient made an uninterrupted recovery from the operation except for some vomiting and distension, the typhoid fever running its course and the temperature coming down to normal on September 29. On September 30 began a relapse.

Relapse.—October 5, patient had a hemorrhage and was sent back to the medical service with a sinus due to infection of the abdominal wall. No further hemorrhages. Relapse exceedingly severe owing to the fact that he suffered from a severe myocarditis superadded to an old endocarditis. For eight days (up to October 13) patient was *in extremis*, the pulse being exceedingly poor in quality and very irregular, both in rate and force, at times being imperceptible for hours. After eight days the cardiac condition improved and the temperature fell to 98.8°, immediately shooting up again to 103°, where it remained until October 17, when it became normal. The patient was discharged cured November 4, 1903.

CASE 15.—*Typhoid fever; very severe course; profuse hemorrhages; perforation on twenty-fifth day; no operation; death.*

Patient.—Abram L., aged 30, Austrian, admitted on September 26, 1903, to male ward I, with a history of typhoid fever of two weeks' duration.

Examination.—His general condition on admission to the hospital was poor. Temperature, 105.6°; pulse, 120°; respiration, 30. Liver extends to the free border. Abdomen somewhat distended and tympanitic; no rigidity. Positive Widal, 1 to 50. White blood cells, 8,600. The case ran an extremely severe, septic course with marked delirium, subsultus, etc. Moderate diarrhea; fairly marked distension of abdomen but no tenderness.

This severe toxemia continued until October 5 (twenty-fourth day) when, at 9 a. m., he had an intestinal hemorrhage of about four ounces. Temperature dropped from 104.4° to 101°. Pulse rose from 94 to 114. White cells, 4,900. Abdomen soft; no tenderness, no rigidity. Liver percusses to the free border. At 8 p. m., temperature, 103.4°; pulse, 110; white cells, 4,500. In the afternoon a subcutaneous gelatin injection was given and a gelatin enema was also used.

October 6: During the night had two hemorrhages, about a pint altogether. Temperature fell from 104.4° at 3 a. m. to 99.2° at 3 p. m. The pulse dropped from 110 to 82, respiration the same as yesterday, 32. White cells, 5,800 at noon; 5,400 at 6 p. m. During the day the patient's condition became worse; abdomen somewhat distended but not tender; liver dullness obliterated for three finger breadths above the free border; flatness beginning at the sixth rib; dullness not obscured in the axilla. 6 p. m., abdomen not distended, but somewhat rigid, especially in the right iliac fossa. Respiratory movements absent in the upper part of the abdomen, with general tenderness, especially in the lower half. Liver dullness decreasing in the mammillary line, reaching to fifth rib, but not obscured in axilla. No nausea, vomiting, chill nor leucocytosis, the count at 6 p. m. being 5,400. Temperature between 99.2° and 102°; respiration, 38; pulse between 90 and 100. The symptoms gradually increasing, a perforative peritonitis was diagnosed, but operation was not permitted.

October 7: 8 a. m., condition worse; hippocratic facies; marked sul-saltus; cold sweats; pulse, 120; respiration, 35; temperature, 100.6°; white blood cells, 5,000. Vomited for the first time, the vomitus being brownish. Abdomen is more distended, with greater tenderness in the lower half; liver tympany reaches fifth space in the mammillary line, being two finger breadths higher than yesterday. Spleen entirely obscured. Respiration thoracic. Much flatus expelled through rectal tube. At 9 p. m. temperature fell to 98.6°; respiration, 38. This improvement was of temporary duration only, for the pulse, respiration and temperature rapidly rose and the patient died at 1 a. m. on October 9. No autopsy.

CASE 16.—*Typhoid fever; severe course; perforation on twenty-third day; operation; death.*

Patient.—Jacob C., aged 16, Austrian, was admitted to the male ward I, October 27, 1903, with a history of typhoid fever of insidious onset and of twenty days' duration. He took to bed twelve days previously on account of chill, severe headache, fever and abdominal pain; he also had profuse sweats and from five to six diarrheal movements daily.

Examination.—On admission general condition only fair; delirious; abdomen generally tympanitic; slight tenderness, but no rigidity. Liver flatness in the mammillary line extends from the seventh space to the free border edge, being just palpable. Spleen palpable. Temperature, 105°; pulse, 100; respiration, 26; white blood count, 11,600. Widal positive, 1 to 50.

October 29: 6 a. m., general condition not so good. Abdomen slightly distended and tender, especially in the right iliac fossa. General tympany, liver dullness obliterated in the axillary line, in the axilla flatness to the free border. The temperature, which had fallen from 104° at 3 a. m. to 101.8° at 6 a. m., rose to 104° at noon; pulse, which had remained at 88, rose to 100 at noon, and respiration rose from 23 at 6 a. m. to 37 at noon. 6 p. m., no special change in the patient's condition, but it is noted that there is increased abdominal rigidity; no distension; no pain, but slight general tenderness; no vomiting; no chill. Liver dullness at the fourth space in the mammillary line; in the axilla sixth space. Temperature remained steady at 104.5°, but the pulse rose at 6 p. m. to 130°, dropped to 102° at 9 p. m., and rose to 124° at midnight. Respiration, which had fallen to 28, rose to 37 at midnight. No special character about the breathing. Leucocyte count at 9.30 p. m., 11,700.

October 30: Signs the same with the exception that there was a little more distension and there was dullness in the left flank. Diarrhea.

Operation.—Diagnosis of perforation having been made, he was transferred to the service of Dr. Lilienthal, who operated at noon and found a perforation low down in the ileum, covered with omentum; fibrinous adhesions; no free gas nor feces in the peritoneal cavity, only some cloudy serum. The perforation was sutured, but the patient never rallied after the operation. There was continuous vomiting and in spite of vigorous stimulation he died on November 3.

Note.—The exact time of perforation could not be determined in this case owing to the patient being delirious and to the vagueness of the onset of the symptoms.

CASE 17.—*Perforation at the end of the fifth week of typhoid fever; operation two days after perforation; evacuation of large fecal abscess; artificial anus; drainage; recovery.*

Patient.—X., aged 21, Russian, was admitted on November 13, 1903,

He had been ill with typhoid fever for five weeks, having been referred to the hospital by Dr. Alfred Meyer, who had seen him in consulation. The details of the history of his illness are very vague.

History.—Two days previously he had had an attack of severe general crampy abdominal pain; since then there had been severe general abdominal tenderness. No chill at onset; did not vomit and has not vomited since; has had no movement of the bowels even after an enema; no gas has passed.

Examination.—On admission his general condition was fair and he certainly did not give one the impression of a patient who had a large quantity of purulent fluid in his abdomen, as was afterward found at the operation. The abdomen was generally tympanitic, tender and distended; the lower border of the liver and spleen obscured by tympany; there was movable dullness in both flanks. Temperature on admission, 100.2°; pulse, 12; respiration, 26; white blood count, 9,000.

Operation.—He was immediately operated on by Dr. Moschcowitz. There were adhesions of the coils of gut to the abdominal wall, collections of foul, yellow pus being found between the coils; there was a large abscess in the pelvis and a perforation the size of a quarter of a dollar was found in the ileum and sutured. The edge of the perforation was sutured to the peritoneum, the abscess was drained with a tube, and the rest of the wound closed in layers.

Result.—November 14. The temperature, which had arisen to 104° nine hours after the operation, fell to 99° in twenty-six hours. His convalescence was uninterrupted. The artificial anus was subsequently closed and the patient left the hospital cured in the middle of December.

CASE 18.—*Typhoid fever; walking case; perforation on thirty-fifth day while on bed-pan; operation six hours later; death.*

Patient.—Samuel L., aged 24, was admitted December 14, 1903, to male ward I, with typhoid fever of three weeks' duration. For two weeks he had taken cathartics for the constipation a number of times, the last cathartic being taken two days before admission. Has been in bed for only two days. Fever has only been marked since the day before admission. Has complained of abdominal pain for two days.

Examination.—On admission, temperature, 102°, shortly after that he had a severe chill, after which the temperature rose to 105°. Abdomen is lax, no distension, no tenderness. Liver dullness to the free border, not palpable. Widal positive, 1 to 50.

The course of the disease was severe. Various blood counts between 5,000 and 6,000. Abdomen was scaphoid; no tenderness.

December 26: Patient improving; temperature beginning to fall, ranging between 102° and 103°; leucocyte count, 6,000; abdomen negative.

December 27: At 4:30 a. m., while the patient was on the bed-pan, he suddenly experienced a severe abdominal pain which caused him to cry out. This lasted only a short time and when seen fifteen minutes later he was quiet. Pulse, 100. Abdomen somewhat scaphoid and soft, but with slight rigidity over the lower part of the right rectus muscle. Patient lies with thighs flexed; tenderness in the lower half of the abdomen, especially on the right side. General tympany; tympany over the liver two finger breadths above the free border in the mammillary line; no axillary tympany. Breathing thoracic and upper abdominal. Temperature at this time, 102.8°; pulse, 100; white blood count, 6,600. At 6:30 he had another attack of pain. Pulse rose to 116. At 9 a. m. patient's general condition was the same; had one stool which contained no blood. No nausea, vomiting, chill nor collapse. Pulse of fair quality; temperature has fallen to 101.6°. Rectal examination negative.

Operation.—At 10.45 a. m. he was operated on by Dr. Gerster; duration of operation, 45 minutes. Free fluid was found in the peritoneal cavity, but no free gas or fecal material; no peritonitis; no injection of intestine. A small perforation was found in the lower ileum surrounded by a necrotic area and was closed by Lembert suture. No other perforation was looked for on account of the poor condition of the patient at this time, pulse being 160 and of poor quality.

Following the operation the temperature rose to 105.6°, then fell rapidly. Pulse after the operation, 132, and respiration, 32.

December 28: Temperature has fallen to 96.2°; pulse, 82; respiration, 22. No nausea nor vomiting, but complains of some abdominal pain, with slight distension and tenderness in the epigastrium. Liver flatness obliterated from the sixth space downward in the mammillary line. In the afternoon there was hiccough; vomited once in the evening; bowels moved during the day. In the evening pulse grew more rapid and feeble. Patient died at midnight.

Wound Examination.—A sutured perforation with sutures intact was found in the ileum ten inches above the cecum and a second perforation beyond this, this being protected by the adherence of the omentum. No peritonitis present.

CASE 19.—*Typhoid fever; walking case; admitted with perforation, which had occurred on fifteenth day; operation forty-eight hours later; fecal abscess drained; recovery.*

Patient.—Jacob M., aged 25, Russian, admitted to male ward II, December 10, 1903, with a history of walking typhoid of two weeks' duration.

History.—Stopped work two days before admission because he felt "sleepy," but did not go to bed. Had one watery, yellow stool each day. No abdominal pain until the day before admission, when he had severe, sudden sticking pain in the lower abdomen on both sides, which caused him to go to bed. Was chilly, vomited some watery fluid at the onset of the pain. The vomiting persisted every fifteen minutes.

That night he was seen by a physician, who found a temperature of 106°; pulse, 120. At 5 a. m. on the day of his admission the pain and vomiting had abated.

Examination.—On admission to the hospital at 9 a. m. his general condition was good. Temperature, 105.2°; pulse, 110; respiration, 26; white blood count, 14,200; negative Widal. Abdomen retracted and tender, especially on the left side; walls rigid and tympanitic. Dullness in the left flank; dull tympany in the right flank, but no change with change of posture. Liver dullness begins at the fourth space; no flatness; tympany begins three finger breadths above the free costal border in the mammillary line, the same in the axillary line. Spleen, in axillary line, dullness at the sixth rib, becomes tympanitic four finger breadths above the free border. Rectal examination: On the left side, high up, a small, irregular mass which was not hard nor tender, could be felt.

Urine: Trace of albumin, hyaline casts, a few blood cells.

After admission he twice vomited bile-stained fluid and the abdomen became more distended. There was an elliptical area of tenderness the size of an orange in the left iliac fossa, midway between the symphisis and the umbilicus. The tympany over the liver had risen two finger breadths above the line first noted.

Operation.—There was delay in obtaining consent for operation, which was not performed until 6 p. m., by Dr. Lilienthal. A median incision was made below the umbilicus, two and one-half inches long. To the left of the median line, corresponding to the area of tenderness above noted, a large fecal abscess was evacuated. No further exploration was made. Tube drainage.

The further course of his disease was that of a severe typhoid.

December 11: Condition of the patient worse; temperature ranged between 102° and 103°. Frequent vomiting, but no abdominal tenderness except over the wound. Slight icterus. Leucocytes, 13,600; negative Widal. Hypostasis at both bases.

December 14: Leucocytes, 7,400. Vomiting has ceased. He now takes nourishment by mouth. Temperature range, 102°; general condition better.

December 15: Temperature still high. No rectal mass to be felt.

December 21: Still running continuous temperature between 102° and 103°; general condition fair. Fecal fistula persists; granulations healthy. Repeated Widal tests having been negative, a blood culture was made by Dr. Libman, who reported the presence of typhoid bacilli in the blood. The first positive Widal, 1 to 50, was reported five days later, December 26, the thirty-first day of the disease. It remained positive thereafter.

The further course of his disease was complicated by a pneumonia and a right otitis which required perforation.

Temperature reached normal on January 12. The fecal sinus closed at the end of January, when he was discharged cured.

THE PRESENT LIMITATIONS OF SERUM THERAPY IN THE TREATMENT OF THE INFECTIOUS DISEASES.

By Henry W. Berg, M.D.,
ADJUNCT ATTENDING PHYSICIAN.

One of the earliest practical results of the studies concerning acquired immunity was the wonderfully successful antitoxin serum therapy in diphtheria. This practical application of the principles upon which acquired immunity depends was in reality premature, evolved by the genius of Behring and his confreres some years before the principles themselves were more than vaguely understood. But while, thanks to the work of Metschnikoff, Ehrlich, and a host of others, the knowledge concerning immunity, antitoxic and bacteriolytic sera has been rapidly developed and amplified, serum therapy has not advanced with anything like equal rapidity. While the logical clinician is now able to understand the *raison d'être* of the success of serum therapy in diphtheria, the broader knowledge of the laws upon which immunity depends has not yet increased the number of infectious diseases which are amenable to curative and prophylactic treatment by antitoxic or antimicrobic sera.

To understand the reasons for this it is necessary to recall some essential facts. The pathogenic bacteria which have been hitherto identified with specific infectious diseases naturally fall into three groups, as far as the production or non-production of toxins is concerned.

First, those bacteria which produce in living cultures outside of the body, best shown in fluid media, as a free secretion, a virulent toxin. The chief members of this group are the diphtheria and tetanus bacillus. A subsidiary member is the bacillus pyocyaneus.

Second, those bacteria which secrete little or no free toxin in living cultures, but do contain a powerful toxin, known as an endotoxin, in the living bacterial cell, which is partly set free only upon the death and disorganization of the bacterial cells. To this class belong by far the largest number of known pathogenic bacteria; good examples are the pneumococcus, the typhoid bacillus, the various streptococci, etc.

Third, those bacteria that produce no free toxins, nor have the bacterial cells endotoxins of any power, but in which the cell plasma contains other poisons in addition to the protein poisons, which all bacterial cells in common contain. For our purposes the most important member of this group is the tubercle baccillus.

The importance of such a classification will be evident when it is recalled that in the diseases with the causation of which the bacteria belonging to the first group have been identified, there is present a local growth of the specific bacteria at some favorite site, together with a more or less general toxemia, to which are due the constitutional manifestations of the disease. The toxic products are absorbed by the lymphatics and bloodvessels and carried throughout the system. This does not preclude the spread to new centres of bacterial growth either by direct extension or by a limited dissemination of the bacteria themselves by means of the circulation. But the toxin and its dissemination are the important factors. On the other hand, in those numerous diseases in which bacteria belonging to the second group are the pathogenetic factor, there is practically no free toxin produced, to be absorbed and carried through the circulating and lymphatic vessels. The pathological changes in the cells, tissues and organs are due to the bacteria themselves, and while endotoxins are set free on the destruction of the bacteria, and their absorption does give rise to toxic symptoms, it is evident that its quantity depends upon the quantity of bacterial growth. Furthermore, these endotoxins are not as toxic as the real toxins produced by the bacteria belonging to the first group. In a word, in this group the microbes are the important and direct pathogenic element, as are the free toxins in the first group.

In the third group the symptoms of the disease are due to the bacterial growth, poisons in the cell plasma and protein contents of the bacteria, and the pathological changes which result from their influence. There are no toxins or endotoxins. It is unnecessary to say here that all three groups of these infections may be complicated by mixed infections in which organisms of various kinds may take part.

Studies of the methods by which an acquired immunity can be induced in the living body which has become the seat of an infectious disease, have shown that the diseases due to the bacteria of the first group can be logically treated by antagonizing the free toxin, by the injection of the blood serum of an animal which has been immunized to that toxin. Such immunization is accomplished by repeated injections of the toxin, until the animal no longer reacts to the largest and most virulent possible doses. The serum of such an animal contains antitoxins which enter into chemical combination with the toxins in the blood of the diseased animal and neutralize it. Diseases due to the bacteria of the second group can *not* be treated by such antitoxic sera, because the bacteria belonging to this group do not secrete a free toxin in the course of their growth, or practically do not, or at least no toxin of sufficient virulence for the purpose of immunizing animals—apart from that in the diseases produced by this group the pathogenetic factors are the bacteria, and antitoxic sera would not antagonize them nor inhibit their growth. For example, even the diphtheria baccillus grows excellently in diphtheria antitoxic serum. So that in these diseases we are logically forced to rely upon antimicrobic sera, which produce immunity in an infected animal by producing a bacteriolytic or destructive action upon the bacteria in the tissues and fluids of the body. Such a curative serum is produced by immunizing animals to repeated injections of virulent sterilized or pure cultures of the bacteria, against which it is sought to immunize the animal. The blood serum of such an animal contains a comparatively stable body, known as the immune body, which is bacteriolytic, however, only in the presence of an unstable body present in the blood serum in the living body, and in freshly drawn serum this is called the alexin or complement. This alexin or complement, so necessary to the bacteriolytic action of the antimicrobic serum, is present in very small quantity only in the blood serum of the living body, hence one of the reasons for the inefficiency of the antimicrobic sera. For the alexin is rapidly destroyed when the blood serum has left the living body, so that the antiserum contains none of it, while that present in the body of the patient is insufficient to enable the antimicrobic serum to neutralize more than a limited quantity of the bacteria. Wassermann has advised that the necessary alexin be supplied by injecting with the antisera *fresh* normal ox or horse serum—surely a difficult thing to accomplish.

As to the diseases dependent upon bacteria belonging to the third group, medicine has as yet received so little encouragement in the treatment of such diseases, as tuberculosis, by a therapeutic serum, that so limited a paper as this may well leave this portion of the subject to more minute and special investigation.

In the case of both the antitoxic and antimicrobic sera the therapeutic action, both curative and prophylactic, is only potential and not positive in any individual case.

It is true that, for instance, in the laboratory experiment a given fixed quantity of diphtheria antitoxin will safely antagonize and neutralize the effect of a fatal dose of diphtheria toxin when both are injected simultaneously into an animal, or when the injection of the antitoxin immediately follows the injection of the toxin. Yet it is apparent that the conditions present in the laboratory experiment are not duplicated in sickroom. First and foremost is the element of time. The injection of the antitoxin does not immediately follow the infection of the patient. Even were the antitoxin injected on the first appearance of pseudo membrane in the throat, the antitoxic injection would still be as many days behind the laboratory experiment as is indicated by the duration of the incubation period of the infection in the given patient. Indeed, when this fact is taken into consideration, it is marvelous that such magnificent results from the antitoxin treatment of diphtheria are obtained. For it is essential that the antitoxin of the injected serum come in contact with the toxin in such a condition that it can enter into chemical combination with it. In other words, it can only bind the free toxin which it finds in the blood and tissues. That which has already entered into firm combination with the body cells, for some of which it has a selective action, is no longer amenable to neutralization with antitoxin. Hence, one of the important practical limitations to the efficacy of the antitoxic sera in therapy is the length of time that has elapsed since the infection has occurred. The Ehrlich side chain theory enables us to comprehend why it is that, in spite of considerable lapse of time, the antitoxic sera are effective. The toxin molecule becomes anchored to the body cell by a certain atomic group or side chain, which Ehrlich terms the haptophore group; but its toxic action upon the cell does not take place until after some time (the incubation period), when it is further attached to the body cell by another atomic group, the toxophore group. The body cell, on the other hand, possesses corresponding side chains to unite with those of the toxin molecule; these chains are termed the haptophile and toxophile groups. If the antitoxin enters the circulation before the toxin molecule has become attached to the cell by its toxophore group, the toxophile group of the antitoxin molecule chemically binds the toxophore group of the toxin molecule, and thus prevents the union with the toxophile group of the cell. In this case, and that is the usual condition in the curative use of antitoxic sera, a much larger amount of antitoxin is needed than would have been required if the toxin were free in the circulation and no union with the living cell had taken place. Our present clinical and bacteriological knowledge, therefore, enables us to lay down certain limitations to the use of antitoxic sera in the treatment of disease produced by the toxic bacteria belonging to our first group. It is necessary:

1. That the bacteriological cause of the disease is positively identified and known.

2. That it be an organism which produces a free specific toxin, and virulent enough to be effective in the immunization of animals

3. That the experimental injection of the antitoxic serum in sufficient quantity is successful in saving animals from death, when injected with or immediately after a fatal dose of the toxin specific to the organism. Furthermore,

4. The bacterial cause and its toxin being both specific, the specificity of the action of the antitoxic serum follows as a natural sequence and must be recognized.

5. The combination between toxin and antitoxin being a chemical one there must be an absolute quantitative relation between the amount of toxin injected and the quantity of antitoxin required to neutralize it.

6. The antitoxin, when used for curative purposes, must be injected before the union of the toxin with animal cells has become sufficiently firm to cause pathological and destructive changes in the cells, tissues and organs. For the antitoxin only antagonizes and neutralizes free or partly free toxin. The time element is, therefore, of importance in antitoxic serum therapy. It must be remembered, however, that even where pathological changes have already occurred, the neutralization by antitoxin of subsequent toxin that may be developed prevents further pathological changes, and enables the system to cure those that have already occurred. The process is further aided in diphtheria by the use of local therapy to the site of the bacterial growth for the destruction of it and its pseudo membranous deposit.

It is on account of this last limitation that tetanus antitoxin serum therapy is so much less efficacious than the antitoxic serum therapy of diphtheria. In the latter disease the local throat lesion, with its clinical symptoms, appears somewhat before or early in the toxemia, so that the antitoxin is enabled to successfully antagonize the free toxin in the blood tissues. In tetanus, on the other hand, the infection occurs, but gives rise to no clinical symptoms until the toxin has entered into a close combination with the nerve cells and fibres of the brain, spinal cord and nerves for which this toxin has a selective affinity. Then only are clinical symptoms manifested, too late for the tetanus antitoxin to have any effect. Experimentally, it has been shown that a very short time (a few seconds) after tetanus toxin has been injected into the blood of animals it rapidly disappears from the circulation and becomes fixed in the central nervous system. As I have said before, this seems to be the keynote to the non-success of antitoxic serum therapy in the treatment of tetanus.

The first and second limitations which we have laid down require no amplification. It goes without saying that the identification of a bacterium is necessary before its toxin can be isolated or known, and such bacterium and its toxin must be identified as the specific bacteriological cause of a disease, before immunity can be established in an animal, and a specific antitoxic serum be produced. Infectious diseases whose bacteriological cause is not known cannot be treated by antitoxic sera. The use of diphtheria antitoxin, e.g., for the cure of infectious diseases of undetermined bacteriological pathogenesis is futile and illogical however much supported empirically by misleading statistics. It follows, too, that the effective preparation of antitoxic sera by immunization of animals with culture products obtained from non-toxin producing bacteria is impossible, as, for instance, the failure to produce a streptococcus antitoxic serum, although antistreptococcus serum is a logical and therapeutically somewhat effective product in certain diseases.

The logic of the third limitation follows from the nature of the chemical antagonism between toxin and antitoxin. Surely, if the life-saving effect does not occur under conditions present in the laboratory experiment, it cannot occur under the conditions present in disease. The fourth limitation, that the action of the antitoxic sera is absolutely specific, follows from the biological data which enter into its production. He is an enemy to the future progress of serum therapy who advocates the therapeutic utility of the antitoxic serum specific to one organism, for the cure of the toxic or microbic ravages of another.

There is no logic in such a recommendation. Rather is it the worst kind of empiricism. Preferable, by far, to adhere to the symptomatic treatment of disease than to rend asunder the complete logical chain upon which legitimate serum therapy depends. Such therapeutic experiments as the use of diphtheria antitoxin in the treatment of pneumonia, or diphtheria antitoxin in the treatment of epidemic cerebrospinal meningitis, have no bacteriological groundwork upon which they may rest, and are repugnant to the principles of scientific serum therapy. Both pneumonia and cerebrospinal meningitis vary from time to time in severity and in their death rate the results in a number of cases, even if large, treated on an illogical and inconclusive serum therapeutic basis, teach nothing as to the efficacy of such therapy. Such methods fall into disuse long before they have gained even a limited vogue. It is true that the injection, in limited quantity, of a heterologous serum, like horse serum, whether it be from an immunized or non-immunized animal, has a tendency, as Metschnikoff has shown, to stimulate phagocytosis, and may thus aid secondarily in the disintegration of any pathogenic organisms that happen to be floating in the blood. But this would be as readily accomplished by the injection of non-immunized horse serum. Even this is not probable, for reasons which we have no opportunity of discussing here.

The fifth limitation, as to the absolute quantitative relation between toxin and antitoxin, would give us exact indications for the dosage of antitoxic sera did we but know how much toxin has been produced and remained in the body of the patient. This we have, at present, no clinical means of estimating. The therapeutic indication is, therefore, to inject sufficient antitoxin to produce the desired result, provided no symptoms contraindicating further injections occur, and here the duration of time that the patient has been suffering from the disease becomes an important factor. For it is found in diphtheria that the longer the patient or animal has been suffering from the disease the larger the quantity of antitoxine required to produce a beneficial effect. It appears that an arithmetical progress in the time since the infection requires a geometrical progressive increase in dose of antitoxin necessary to antagonize the toxin that causes the disease. This is partly due to the increased amount of toxin in the body, but far more to the fact that toxin molecules that have entered into partial combination with the body cells require a large excess of antitoxin to drag them away from their union with the living cell.

Thus also clinical and bacteriological data derived from studies in immunity from infections due to organisms belonging to the second group, permit the formulating of certain essential prerequisites to the use of antimicrobic or bacteriolytic sera in the treatment of infectious diseases. These are:

1. The bacteriological course of the disease must be positively identified and known.

2. The experimental injection of the bacteriolytic serum in sufficient doses must be successful in saving animals from death when injected with or immediately after a lethal dose of a living corresponding bacterial culture.

3. The bacterial cause of the disease being specific, the specificity of the bacteriolytic serum follows as a natural sequence.

4. Since the antiserum has a destructive or bacteriolytic action upon the pathogenetic bacteria, this action being dependent upon the combined presence of two known substances, namely the alexin or complement (an unstable substance, present in the normal living body and in fresh serum) and the immune body (present in bacteriolytic sera), and since only a small amount of the alexin is present in the body, in quantity sufficient to produce only a very limited bacteriolysis, it follows that, unless the antibacterial serum be freshly drawn, thus securing the unchanged alexin present in the blood of the immune animal, the antimicrobic action of the bacteriolytic sera is limited by the insufficient amount of alexin present in the body of the patient. Wasserman, recognizing the impossibility of having the bacteriolytic sera freshly obtained for each case, advises for this purpose the injection of the fresh serum of the non-immunized horses or oxen in addition to the anti-serum itself. This recommendation, however, can hardly, for obvious reasons, be considered as having solved the problem. Under all circumstances it is absolutely necessary that the bacteriolytic serum be fresh.

5. The bacteriolytic sera have a quantitative relation to the amount of bacteria which they can destroy. At best the antisera protect only against a limited amount of bacterial infection. When this increases beyond a certain figure, no amount of antiserum will protect or cure the animal. Hence, very large doses are necessary, sometimes repeated. Thus the antistreptococcus serum is used in doses of 150 to 250 c.c., repeated if symptoms do not improve.

6. While enthusiasts might claim that the bacteriolytic action

of the antisera seen in animals, which are the subject of experimental infections, occurs also in patients suffering from infectious diseases, no curative effect can possible occur with regard to pathological changes which have already been produced by the bacterial infection. So that the later the antiserum is used, the less the chance of its having any curative effect.

Bacteriolytic sera have been prepared for the serum therapy of a number of the infectious diseases, but such sera have hitherto had little or no efficacy. Thus an antistreptococcus serum has been prepared for use in cases of septic infection by streptococcus pyogenes or erysipelatis. Pane has prepared an antipneumococcic serum, Calmette an antiplague serum, and antisera have been prepared for the treatment of typhoid fever, cholera, tuberculosis, anthrax, yellow fever, infections and suppurations due to pyogenes aureus and infections with the colon baccillus and the bacillus dysenteriæ. Attempts have been made to produce antisera in almost every infectious disease the bacterial cause of which is known. It is safe to generalize and say that none of these sera have been therapeutically effective, an occasional report of one or more apparently hopeless cases brilliantly cured to the contrary notwithstanding. These failures are probably due to one or more of the limitations inherent in all bacteriolytic sera, especially to the impossibility of providing sufficient alexin or complement, the difficulty of recognizing most of the infectious diseases until symptoms depending upon gross pathological changes have occurred, the serum therapy being thus applied too late, and finally to the fact that even the largest practicable doses of the bacteriolytic sera can destroy only a limited amount of bacteria, entirely insufficient to free the patient from the bacterial infection.

Such antimicrobic sera have, however, even been prepared for use in diseases the bacterial causes of which have not yet been identified or positively recognized. As, for instance, the antiserum prepared for the treatment of syphilis, which may be dismissed from serious contemplation. Time enough to speak of such a serum when the bacteriological cause of syphilis is known.

In scarlet fever, notwithstanding that the bacterial cause is not yet generally recognized, an antiserum has been prepared which may not thus summarily be dismissed from consideration, owing to the fact that eminent clinicians have ascribed to it remarkable efficacy in the treatment of this disease. Marmorek and Aronson both used an antistreptococcus serum in the treatment of scarlatina. The former used a streptococcus the virulence of which had been increased by repeated passage through animals. With this virulent culture of streptococcus horses were immunized, and the serum of such immune horses used for the treatment of scarlet fever, with the object of preventing the complications due to mixed infections with the streptococcus, and thus diminishing the death rate. Aronson's serum was prepared in a similar way, except that the original culture was from a streptococcus obtained from the bone marrow of a patient dead from scarlet fever. He also increased the virulence of the organism by repeated passage through animals. Tavel, and later Moser, prepared an antistreptococcus serum in which the streptococcus was taken from the blood of patients dying of virulent scarlatina. They did not attempt to increase the virulence of the organism by repeated passage through animals, claiming that such frequent passage through animals altered the biological character of the streptococcus, so that it was no longer identical with the species of streptococcus which complicated the scarlet fever. Neither Tavel nor Moser claims that the streptococcus is the bacteriological cause of scarlet fever, nevertheless, Moser ascribes to the antistreptococcus serum which he has thus prepared brilliant curative virtues in the treatment of scarlet fever.

Cases of scarlet fever treated in the St. Anna Kinderspital, in Vienna, were as follows:

Cases treated without serum in 1898........ 171, of which 22 died, 12.86%
"   "   "   "   " 1899........ 268,   "   44 "   16.41%
"   "   "   "   " 1900........ 265,   "   33 "   12.45%
"   " with serum (Moser) in 1901.. 389,   "   35 "   8.99%
"   "   "   "   " 1902.. 368,   "   25 "   6.70%

Ehrlich reports (*Wiener klinische Wochenschrift*, No. 23, 1903) 112 cases of varying severity treated by serum, with 17 deaths, or 15.17 per cent.

Pospischill (*Wiener klinische Wochenschrift*, No. 15, 1903) reports 26 severe cases treated, of which 12 died, almost 50 per cent. Moser himself reports 48 cases of varying severity treated by serum with 13 deaths, over 25 per cent. (*Wiener Med. Wochenschrift*, No. 44, 1903).

I may be permitted to compare these statistics with those of the Riverside Hospital, N. Y. In that institution there were treated, during the year 1904, 899 cases of scarlatina of every grade of severity, with 75 deaths; 17 of these deaths occurred within twenty-four hours of admission, the cases being admitted in a practically hopeless condition. They should properly be excluded, leaving a death rate of 6.45 per cent., or if included a death rate of 8.34 per cent.

From the statistics I have quoted it will be seen that this death rate, on classical lines of treatment and in a very large number of cases, is lower than the results from the Moser serum treatment in the St. Anna Kinderspital for 1901. And excluding the 17 practically moribund cases, the 6.45 per cent. death rate is better than the best reported results from the Moser treatment in St. Anna Kinderspital, those for 1902. It must not be forgotten that the Riverside service cannot select its cases but must take all that are offered, the hospital being in charge of the Health Department.

Nothwithstanding, however, that the statistics are not convincing nor impressive in favor of the Moser treatment, we would not be disposed to condemn this method of treating scarlet fever were there other good reasons in favor of its adoption. But there are unfortunately none such.

This serum violates the first logical essential for the production of an antiserum. The bacterial cause of scarlet fever is unknown, and while many of the complications are due to mixed infections with the pus organisms, surely the death rate in scarlet fever is not due wholly to the mixed infections. It is begging the question to inject a serum for the prevention of complications and leave the primary disease untreated. Indeed, Moser, in his latter reports, claims far more for his serum. He records a few temperature charts in which he shows that the fever curve, in these few cases, 24 hours after the injection underwent a critical drop, by which he implies, although he does not so state, that his serum antagonizes or neutralizes the toxic or bacterial cause of the fever in scarlet fever, in other words antagonizes the bacterial cause of the disease. In a few cases treated in the Reception Pavilion of the Willard Parker Hospital, in 1902, I did not observe any effect produced on the temperature curve by the injection of the serum. While it is the rule for the fever in scarlet fever to be maintained at the maximum temperature for the given case until the eruption has covered the body, and then gradually to resolve by lysis, it is not at all rare to observe in a case that begins with a high temperature, a critical drop before the third day when the eruption has scarcely covered the body. In these cases it will generally be found that the abnormally high temperature was due to the severity of the throat manifestations, and that the subsidence of these results in a critical drop of the temperature.

Furthermore, what has been said concerning the necessity of adding the unstable alexin, to enable the immune body to be effective in bacteriolytic serum therapy, must not be forgotten. If the labors of Buchner, Ehrlich, Morgenroth and Metschnikoff are of any value, the Moser and other similar sera must be absolutely worthless unless such antisera are accompanied by injections of fresh non-immunized horse serum to supply the alexin or complement. Again, while Moser uses large doses of his serum, 150 to 250 c.c., owing to the proven fact that the antisera only antagonize a limited amount of bacteria, yet in severe cases the bacterial mass must be so great that no amount of the bacteriocidal serum will antagonize it. It is true also that small quantities of a heterologous serum exert a phagocytic activity, yet large quantities of a heterologous serum, like horse serum, exert hemolytic properties. I believe that the body of even our youngest patient is able to dispose of 200 c.c. of heterologous serum, nevertheless, it does seem reasonable to believe that in such large doses of a foreign serum injected into very young patients, there is much that is objectionable. These and many other considerations prove the unscientific basis upon which the antistreptococcus serum therapy of scarlet fever rests.

These are some of the limitations of serum therapy at the present time. Many of them will be removed by future advances in bacteriological and biological knowledge. Let us not, as clinicians, hamper the master minds devoted to the solution of the intricate problems involved, and discredit the scientific structure which they are carefully erecting, fact on fact, by the empirical and premature use of such antisera in the treatment of disease for which there is not only no known scientific basis, but which on the contrary militate against the fundamental principles of immunity.

TWO CASES OF ACUTE YELLOW ATROPHY OF THE LIVER

By Albert Kohn, M.D.,
ADJUNCT ATTENDING PHYSICIAN.

The following two cases were observed on the service of Dr. Manges at Mt. Sinai Hospital during the year 1904.

Case I.—Fanny M., married, aged 28; born in Russia. Admitted March 30, 1904.

Family History.—Negative.

Previous History.—Has always been healthy. No history of rheumatism, tuberculosis, cardiac or kidney disease; no malaria. No previous jaundice. Had an attack of influenza six weeks ago which lasted three or four days, but with no complications. No history of previous gastric or hepatic disturbance. No sudden emotion or fright. Has two children; the last was born four and one-half months ago, nursed by the patient. Pregnancy and puerperium were normal. Menstruation has returned, the date of last period unknown.

Present History.—Three weeks ago the patient lost her appetite; had headache and muscular weakness, with vomiting. The vomiting was frequently repeated for about one week, when jaundice appeared. The icterus has progressively increased in intensity up to the present. There have been chilly sensations but no chills. No fever and no pain at any time. No delirium, twitchings, nor convulsions, but during the past three days the patient has been unconscious. The stools have been clay-colored. The urine not observed.

Physical Examination on Admission.—General condition fair. Body is well nourished. Patient is stuporous, almost comatose. She groans occasionally when disturbed. No twitchings.

Skin.—Whole body deeply jaundiced.

Throat.—Small white exudate on left tonsil.

Tongue.—Dry and moderately coated with a brown streak on either side.

Teeth.—In fair condition.

Gums.—On upper gum, anteriorly, is a rounded, small, hemorrhagic area, sharply circumscribed, about 3 mm. in diameter. On admission lower lip and the gum at lower right incisor were bleeding. There were no other hemorrhages in the mouth.

The *breath* had an odor of acetone.

Conjunctiva were markedly icteric and the vessels injected.

Pupils moderately dilated, equal, and reacted promptly to light, alternately contracting and dilating. Moderate mucous discharge from the eyes. No petechiæ.

Palpebral conjunctiva injected.

No facial paresis, no strabismus, no otorrhea, no mastoid tenderness.

Thyroid not enlarged.

There are palpable a few small, soft, postcervical glands; no auxillary glands; small inguinal glands.

Tips of fingers not clubbed. Superficial mammary veins dilated.

Breasts are enlarged, caked and milk can be expressed. Both forearms have a rash consisting of minute papules, somewhat faded.

Lungs.—*Anterior*, slight dullness at left apex. *Posterior*, negative. Dullness begins in tenth space.

Heart.—Right border at right border of sternum. Apex beat not visible nor palpable and best heard in fifth space, just inside the left border, which is 4½ inches to the left of the median line. Heart's action is regular, forcible, with sounds clear at the apex. There is an impurity of the first sound over the pulmonic area. The second aortic sound is clear. No thrill. Pulses equal, regular; somewhat accelerated (90), forcible, no increased tension, slight thickening, not tortuous.

Liver, Parasternal line.—Slight dullness in third space, well marked dullness in fourth and fifth spaces. Slight dullness in sixth space, tympanitic note below this. *Axilla*, well marked dullness in fifth, sixth and seventh spaces. In eighth and ninth a dull tympany. *Edge* of liver and gall-bladder not palpable.

Spleen.—Dullness in eighth and ninth space; tympanitic from there to free border. Not palpable.

Abdomen.—Somewhat rounded, moderately adipose, generally tympanitic; lax, not tender. Irregular fecal masses can be felt in the left iliac fossa. Kidneys not palpable. No change of note on changing posture.

Lower Extremities.—Knee-jerks exaggerated. Clonus of right ankle; none of left. Slight edema of left leg. No Kernig, no Babinski.

Vaginal Examination.—Uterus felt halfway to umbilicus. Cervix is soft, admits tip of finger, and is slightly lacerated. Appendages not felt.

Rectum full of soft fecal masses.

Pulse 90. Respiration 28. Temperature 99.2°F.

April 1: Stools clay-colored; urine deeply stained with bile. Urine report shows absence of leucin, tyrosin, acetone, diacetic acid, and indican.* Patient very stuporous; struggles somewhat when disturbed. Retches occasionally and regurgitates any fluid passed into the pharynx. Blood culture taken. Jaundice increased. Temper-

*Full urine report on collected urine by the pathological chemist, p. 92.

ature, 100.8°; pulse, 100; respirations, 20. A.M. Temperature, 102°; pulse, 140; respirations, 30. P. M.

Breathing is stertorous but regular. No new hemorrhages. Dullness which began posteriorly on right side in tenth space yesterday, is now first heard in eleventh space. With patient on left side, in right axilla, dullness begins at sixth rib extending to the tenth rib, a distance of about 12 cm. Anteriorly, in parasternal line, there is still dullness in third, fourth and fifth spaces, dull tympany in sixth space, a tympanitic note in seventh space. Liver not palpable.

Blood.—Hemoglobin, 93 per cent.; white blood count, 17,300; red blood count, 5,024,000.

April 2: General condition is somewhat worse. The jaundice is more intense. Patient is completely comatose. Breathing stertorous and rapid. Temperature, 104.4°; pulse, 134; respiration, 48. Patient is losing flesh. Ecchymotic spot on right arm, irregular in shape, purplish-green in color. Skin somewhat indurated on this arm. Sweetish odor to breath.

Lungs.—Few subcrepitant râles over right lung. Dullness in lower left axilla. Note low down posteriorly poor on both sides with harsh breathing.

Liver. Anteriorly.—Dullness in fourth and fifth space; flatness in sixth space; below this dull tympany. In right axilla with patient on left side dullness in fifth space, almost flatness in seventh space. In eighth space dull tympany which extends to free border.

Right kidney distinctly palpable. *Left kidney* lower pole felt on deep palpation.

Heart.—Unchanged.

Knee jerks present, not exaggerated. No edema. Involuntary urination and defecation.

Urine dark; has heavy odor; has bile, hyaline and granular casts. Sp. gr. 1036; albumin trace; urea, 2.4 per cent.

Vomitus looked bloody and showed red and white blood cells.

Milk is bile-stained.

There are two symmetrical, hemorrhagic streaks on buttocks, extending down the thighs.

About midnight the patient had a severe spasm of pectoralis major on right side and of the facial muscles. This lasted about fifteen minutes. The patient ceased breathing.

Leucin and tyrosin recovered.

URINE EXAMINATION, BY DR. S. BOOKMAN.

March 31: Quantity, 485 cc. Sp. gr., 1025.
April 1: Quantity, 585 cc. Sp. gr., 1021.
Both of the above were incomplete 24 hour specimens as involuntary emissions of urine occurred on both days.

Total N., 1.378 per cent. Ammonia, 0.09 per cent. Urea, 2.59 per cent. Total phosphoric acid, 0.29 per cent.

Tyrosin and leucin both present.

The liver tissue contained very little glycogen and showed no increase in phosphorus or sulphur contents.

PATHOLOGIST'S REPORT—EXAMINATION MADE BY DR. E. LIBMAN.

F. M., died April 3, 1904. Post-mortem examination eleven hours after death. Head not opened.

Acute degeneration of the liver.

Moderate rigor; body well nourished. Marked icterus. All organs are bile-stained. No petechiæ. Hemorrhagic gingivitis.

Esophagus shows post-mortem digestion.

Trachea and *bronchi* show marked blood imbibitions with marked hemorrhages. Contents, frothy dark blood.

Lungs.—Left is rather voluminous; brownish-red in color. It shows intense congestion with hemorrhagic areas. Upper lobe is more congested than lower. The bronchial nodes are enlarged and anthracotic. There is atelectasis of the lower lobe posteriorly. Right: same as left except that upper part of the lobe is hepatized, dark reddish-brown in color. In upper lobe there are several small bronchopneumonic areas. Bronchial nodes same as on left side.

Heart.—There is no increase of fluid in pericardium. Right auricle is dilated. Right ventricle is small, fatty overgrowth. Tricuspid is slightly thickened. Left auricle and ventricle are slightly dilated. There are signs of an old dilatation. Muscle is pale, yellow-brown, soft. Weight, 300 grams. Aortic flaps slightly thickened along semilunar lines. Coronaries negative.

Spleen.—Small, weighs 120 gms. Purplish-red on surface. On section pulp is soft, dark bluish-red in color. Connective tissue is prominent. Pulp is easily scraped off.

Adrenals cloudy.

Pancreas.—Firm, congested.

Kidneys.—Weight, 360 gms. together. Measure 20 x 7 cm. Left: capsule not adherent; on section shows congestion. Cut section looks granular, cloudy. Malpighian bodies are rather large. Pelvis negative. Right is larger and firmer than left and more congested. It shows a few petechiæ in pelvis. Otherwise same as left.

Liver.—Measures 20 x 14 x 9.5 cm. Weight, 840 gms. (1¾ lbs.). Organ is small, very soft. Surface is plum-red in color with ochre-yellow areas which are firmer and slightly elevated. The elevation is more marked in the areas on the under surface. On section the main part of the surface is taken up by irregular ochre-yellow areas between which are smaller dark brownish-red areas, which are somewhat depressed.

Gall-bladder contains yellowish-brown bile. There are small hemorrhages in the wall. Ducts and veins are negative.

Stomach.—Not dilated. Contains coffee-ground material and light yellowish fluid containing much thick mucus. The wall is digested but evidences of hemorrhage are distinct.

Intestines.—Small, collapsed. In upper two-thirds contents are tarry. There are hemorrhages in the wall. The vessels are injected. In the lower third the wall is practically negative. Contents are almost clay-colored.

Duodenum.—The mucosa contains many gaseous cysts (the bacillus aërogenes capsulatus was demonstrated).

Colon.—In the lower part, but not involving the rectum, are fibrinous deposits on the tops of the folds. Contents show much tenacious mucus. The mesenteric nodes are moderately enlarged and pale.

Bladder.—There are small hemorrhagic areas in the wall, especially at trigonum.

Uterus.—Slightly larger than normal. Shows evidences of previous pregnancies.

Ovaries.—Both are rather fibrous. Left contains small dermoid cysts. Right contains fibrous nodule (from corpus luteum probably). There are small hemorrhages into both ovaries.

MICROSCOPICAL REPORT, BY DR. MANDLEBAUM.

Adrenal.—Parenchymatous degeneration.

Liver.—Acute degeneration with necrosis. Fatty degeneration, bile pigment, proliferation of biliary ducts.

Spleen.—Perisplenitis. Acute interstitial inflammation.

Kidney.—Intense acute degeneration with necrosis of epithelium. Acute congestion.

Bladder.—Moderate necrosis of mucosa (P.M.).

Heart.—Parenchymatous degeneration. Cross striations almost absent.

Lung.—Right lower lobe: Intense, acute congestion. Lobular pneumonia.

Chemical examination of liver and intestinal contents by Dr. S. Bookman failed to reveal the presence of lead or arsenic.

CASE II.—G. D., male, aged 21 years, born United States, druggist. Admitted July 11, 1904.

Family and previous history unknown.

"Present illness began three weeks ago with jaundice, general malaise and loss of appetite. Jaundice has been increasing rapidly for the last three or four days. Has been more sleepy than usual for past week until last night; since then very restless. Early last evening had an attack of severe abdominal pain which lasted until 4 A.M., since then has been delirious. Has vomited three or four times during the last week, last time this morning. For the past week has also had complete loss of appetite with occasional headache. Bowels regular. Color of stools not noted. Urination frequent and urine high-colored. Fever last night; none before. Slight epistaxis three or four days ago. No other hemorrhages. No cough." History obtained from friend.

Physical Examination, July 12, 1904:

General condition: Fairly well nourished. Jaundice marked over entire body. Marked violent delirium. Small reddish spot on radial side of forearm which disappears on pressure. No rigidity of neck; no subcutaneous hemorrhages.

Glands.—Small ones palpable in axillæ and groins.

Ears and mastoids.—Negative.

Eyes.—Right pupil larger than left. Conjunctival icterus marked. No petechiæ. Pupils react to light.

Breath has an aromatic odor. Mucous membrane icteric. Teeth and gums in good condition. Throat negative.

Lungs.—Second rib on left side is prominent. Anterior and posterior negative.

Heart.—Systolic thrill at apex. Upper border third rib; right border at sternum. Left border at third space 11 cm. from median line. Apex beat in the fourth space just outside the nipple line 10 cm. from the median line. Action forcible. Systolic-diastolic murmur heard at apex. The diastolic follows a weak second sound. First sound markedly exaggerated at apex. Systolic murmur heard over base but no accentuation of second pulmonic. Systolic murmur heard over aortic area; second sound indistinct.

Liver.—Fifth space mammary line, dullness; sixth space flatness, (nearly so). No absolute flatness anywhere over the liver region. Seventh space slightly tympanitic. There is pure tympany two fingers above to the free border. In the axillary line dullness begins at the sixth rib, flatness at ninth space. Lower border obscured by tympany for a distance of two fingers.

Spleen.—Upper border cannot be determined. Lower border obscured by tympany and not palpable.

Abdomen slightly distended, generally tympanitic. Right side more rigid than the left. No masses palpable.

Extremities.—No edema.

Reflexes: Absent knee-jerks.

Rectal and genitals negative.

When patient is turned over on his abdomen liver dullness obtains to the free border.

July 13: General condition much worse. Stuporous; cannot be roused. Pressure over supra-orbital nerve elicits no pain.

Liver dullness begins in axillary line at sixth rib down to ninth rib. Marked tympany extends up above free border.

There is some bleeding from the mouth. No petechiæ. Pupils equal and react to light. Jaundice the same. Jaws are forcibly contracted. Lungs and heart unchanged.

July 14: Onset of delirium followed by coma after a three weeks' history of what seemed to be ordinary catarrhal jaundice. Liver became smaller from day to day while under observation. No leucin or tyrosin found in urine by microscopical test.

At 2.40 A.M. on July 14, the patient ceased to breathe.

The temperature on day of admission and for two days following was normal. On July 13 it rose rapidly to 103.2° and just before death, on July 14, was 104.4°.

Pulse during first two days between 68 and 82. On the third day between 82 and 120; just before death 142.

Respiration during first two days between 20 and 24; on the third day between 22 and 42; before death 48.

No autopsy was obtainable.

URINE EXAMINATION, BY DR. S. BOOKMAN.

Bile present in large amounts. Large amount pigmented epithelium. Many hyaline, hyalo-granular and coarsely granular casts. Calcium oxylate crystals and urates.

Color dark yellowish-brown with green fluorescence. Sp. gr. 1.0122. Total nitrogen, 0.588 per cent.; ammonia, 0.08 per cent.; total phosphoric acid, 0.25 per cent.; urea, 1.3 per cent.; total solids, 2.38 per cent.; inorganic solids, 0.803 per cent.

About 10 cc. of blood were obtained by venesection. This showed large amount of leucin present, but no tyrosin could be identified.

The above two cases of acute yellow atrophy of the liver are reported as supplementary to two cases described by Dr. Rudisch in the Mount Sinai Hospital Report of 1903, for, in spite of the fact that the number of cases in the medical literature is being continually increased, it is nevertheless true that acute yellow atrophy is a comparatively rare disease.

As regards the clinical history of these two cases one was at once struck by the classical course each ran. In each there was a period or first stage of gastro-intestinal symptoms with a gradually developing icterus, followed by a second stage of mental symptoms with rapidly increasing coma and death in a few days.

It is to be regretted that autopsy was refused in Case II.

The age of both patients was in accordance with the rule that about 50 per cent. of the reported cases occurred between the 20th and 30th years.

For a predisposing factor the second case has no history.

The first had her pregnancy as etiology, but in this differs from most of the cases occurring in pregnancy, the time usually being the fourth and the seventh months and in rare cases during the lying-in period; while this case occurred four and one-half months after the birth of the child.

In neither case could there be discovered any trace of poisoning, either organic or inorganic, nor were there any lesions suggested the possibility of a pre-existing syphilitic icterus.

In the physical examination both cases showed marked liver atrophy during the few days they were under observation. The decided tympany extending upward from the free border, especially when the patients were examined lying upon their left sides, was plainly due to the sagging back of the soft and flabby liver and bulging upward of the intestines.

The coma was never absolute until just before death. The patients showed a certain amount of resistance when aroused but immediately lapsed into their former state.

In neither case was there temperature until what might be considered an ante-mortem rise. The first case on admission had a temperature of 99.2° and on the second day a temperature of 100.8°, and on April 2, the day of death, a temperature of 104.4°. The temperature of Case II was normal for two days and only on the day preceding death rose to 103.2° In this lack of temperature again both cases adhere to the rule, the rise generally occurring in the catarrhal stage ushering in the disease and then falling to normal or subnormal.

The difficulty of all the studies on metabolism thus far encountered also applies here. The extremely short course of the cases after admission, together with the loses of urine from involuntary micturition, made simple percentage calculation the only one possible. The percentages of urea in both cases, especially in Case I, were above that ordinarily described, in some cases being present only in fractions of 1 per cent. The ammonia, on the other hand, has generally been described as existing in larger amounts than in either of these cases. Leucin and tyrosin were present in Case I, but cannot now be considered idiopathic of acute yellow atrophy either together or singly. In Case II leucin was recovered from the blood.

STATISTICAL REPORT—CHILDREN'S SERVICE.
1903.

ATTENDING PHYSICIAN.
HENRY KOPLIK, M.D.

ADJUNCT ATTENDING PHYSICIAN.
HENRY HEIMAN, M.D.

	Male.				Female.				
	Cured.	Improved.	Unimproved.	Died.	Cured.	Improved.	Unimproved.	Died.	Total.
Respiratory System.									
Bronchial Asthma	..	1	..	..	..	..	..	..	1
Bronchiectasis	..	..	..	..	..	1	..	..	1
Bronchitis	..	..	..	..	1	..	..	..	1
Empyema	9	6	..	3	5	1	..	1	25
" bronchopneumonia	..	..	..	2	1	..	..	1	4
" " varicella	..	..	..	..	..	1	..	..	1
" pertussis	..	..	..	1	..	..	..	..	1
" mumps	1	..	..	..	..	..	..	..	1
" retropharyngeal abscess	..	..	..	1	..	..	..	..	1
" erysipelas	..	..	..	..	..	1	..	..	1
" enteritis	..	..	..	..	..	1	..	..	1
" ileo-colitis	..	..	..	..	..	..	..	1	1
Lung, sarcoma of, and of vertebral column	..	..	..	1	..	..	..	..	1
Pleurisy, with effusion	3	..	..	..	3	..	..	..	6
Pneumonia, broncho	7	1	2	5	4	..	1	2	22
" " measles	..	..	..	1	..	..	..	..	1
" " rhachitis	..	..	..	1	..	..	..	..	1
" " double otitis media	..	..	..	..	..	..	..	1	1
" lobar	7	..	..	2	5	..	..	1	15
" " resolving	1	..	..	..	..	..	..	..	1
" " unresolved, gonorrheal proctitis	1	..	..	..	..	..	..	..	1
	29	8	3	16	22	2	1	7	88
Circulatory System.									
Endocarditis, chronic	..	6	..	1	..	9	1	1	18
" " acute rheumatism	..	..	..	..	..	1	..	..	1
" " pericarditis	..	1	..	..	..	1	..	2	4
" " chorea	..	..	..	..	..	1	1	..	2
" " chronic rheumatism	..	..	..	..	..	2	..	..	2
" " pericarditis, with effusion	..	..	..	..	..	1	..	..	1
" " nephritis: uremia	..	..	..	..	..	..	..	1	1
" " torticollis	..	1	..	..	..	..	..	..	1
	..	8	..	1	2	14	1	4	30

STATISTICAL REPORT—CHILDREN'S SERVICE, 1903.

	Male.				Female.				
	Cured.	Improved.	Unimproved.	Died.	Cured.	Improved.	Unimproved.	Died.	Total.
Diseases of the Blood.									
Leukemia, acute	..	..	..	1	..	..	..	..	1
Nervous System.									
Amaurotic family idiocy	..	..	..	..	..	..	1	2	3
Cerebral hemorrhage	1	..	..	..	..	..	..	..	1
Chorea	7	1	..	..	3	1	..	..	12
" insaniens	..	..	..	..	..	..	..	1	1
Exophthalmic goitre	..	..	..	..	..	1	..	..	1
Hydrocephalus and rickets	..	1	..	..	..	..	..	..	1
Idiocy, Mongolian	..	1	..	..	..	..	..	..	1
Meningocele	..	..	..	..	1	..	..	..	1
Muscular dystrophy	..	..	1	..	..	..	..	..	1
Neuritis, multiple	..	..	..	..	1	..	..	..	1
" optic	..	..	..	..	..	1	..	..	1
Neurosis, traumatic	..	..	..	..	..	1	..	..	1
Tic convulsif	..	1	..	..	..	..	..	..	1
	8	4	1	0	5	4	1	3	26
Gastro-enteric Tract.									
Colon, congenital dilatation of	..	1	..	..	..	..	..	..	1
Dysentery	..	..	..	1	1	..	1	..	3
Enteritis	2	..	..	..	2	..	..	..	4
" and marasmus	..	..	..	..	1	1	..	..	2
Entero-colitis	1	..	..	1	..	..	..	..	2
Intestinal intoxication	2	..	..	..	1	..	..	..	3
Gastro-enteritis	..	..	..	..	1	1	..	1	3
Intussusception	1	..	..	..	..	..	..	..	1
Stomach, perforated ulcer of, with general peritonitis	..	..	..	..	1	..	..	..	1
	6	1	0	4	6	1	1	1	20
Kidneys and Genito-Urinary System.									
Nephritis, chronic	1	1	..	..	..	5	..	2	9
" subacute	..	..	..	..	1	..	..	..	1
	1	1	0	0	1	5	0	2	10
Cutaneous Diseases.									
Desquamation after measles	..	..	..	..	..	..	1	..	1
" scarlatina form	..	..	1	..	..	..	..	..	1
Eczema	1	1	..	..	..	1	..	..	3
Lupus erythematosus	..	..	..	..	..	2	..	..	2
Urticaria	..	..	..	..	..	1	..	..	1
	1	1	1	0	0	4	1	0	8

	Male				Female				Total
Infectious Diseases.	Cured	Improved	Unimproved	Died	Cured	Improved	Unimproved	Died	
Diphtheria	1	..	..	..	1	..	..	..	2
" and rickets	..	..	..	..	1	..	..	..	1
Influenza	1	..	..	..	..	..	..	..	1
Lymphadenitis, tuberculous	..	..	..	..	..	1	..	..	1
Malaria	1	..	..	..	..	..	..	..	1
Meningitis, epidemic cerebro-spinal	3	..	..	2	1	..	..	4	10
" purulent, with marasmus	..	..	..	1	..	..	..	..	1
" tuberculous	..	..	..	7	..	..	1	7	15
Pertussis	..	..	1	..	..	..	..	..	1
Scarlet fever	1	..	..	..	..	..	..	..	1
Scarlet fever and chorea	..	..	1	..	..	..	..	..	1
Spondylitis, tuberculous	..	1	..	..	..	1	..	..	2
Tonsilitis, acute	1	..	..	..	2	..	..	..	3
Typhoid fever	13	..	..	..	14	..	..	..	27
" " ard relapse	..	..	..	..	3	..	..	..	3
" " " otitis media, purulenta	2	..	..	..	..	..	..	..	2
" " " general peritonitis	..	..	..	..	1	..	..	..	1
" " " pneumonia	..	..	..	..	..	..	..	1	1
" " " intestinal perforation	..	..	..	..	1	..	..	..	1
	23	1	2	11	23	1	2	12	75
Constitutional Diseases.									
Marasmus	3	..	..	1	..	..	..	1	5
Melena and icterus neonatorum	..	..	..	..	..	..	..	1	1
Morbus maculosus neonatorum	..	..	..	1	..	..	..	..	1
Rachitis	1	1	..	..	..	3	..	..	5
Rheumatic peliosis	1	..	..	..	..	..	..	..	1
Rheumatism, acute articular	2	..	..	..	..	..	..	..	2
Syphilis, congenital	..	..	..	..	1	..	..	..	1
" " with syphilitic hepatic cirrhosis	..	..	..	..	..	1	..	..	1
	7	1	0	2	1	4	0	2	17
Unclassified Diseases.									
Insolation	1	..	..	..	..	..	..	..	1
Liver, specific cirrhosis of	..	1	..	..	..	..	..	..	1
Mastoiditis, bilateral with tetany	1	..	..	..	..	..	..	..	1
Esophageal stenosis	..	..	..	..	..	1	..	..	1
Peritoneal adhesions	..	1	..	..	..	..	..	..	1
Peritonitis, traumatic	..	..	..	1	..	..	..	..	1
Purulent otitis media	..	..	..	..	..	1	..	..	1
Starvation	1	..	..	..	..	..	..	..	1
Tonsils, hypertrophy of	1	..	..	..	..	..	..	..	1
	4	2	0	1	0	2	0	0	9

Causes of Death.	Male.	Female.	Total
Amaurotic family idiocy	..	2	2
Chorea insaniens	..	1	1
Dysentery	1	..	..
Empyema	3	1	4
" bronchopneumonia	2	1	3
" pertussis	1	..	1
" retropharyngeal abscess	1	..	1
" ileo-colitis	..	1	1
Endocarditis, chronic	1	1	2
" " pericarditis	..	2	2
" " nephritis, uremia	..	1	1
Entero-colitis	1	..	1
Gastro-enteritis	1	1	2
Leukemia, acute	1	..	1
Lung, sarcoma of, and sarcoma of vertebral column	1	..	1
Marasmus	1	1	2
" meningitis	1	..	1
Meningitis, cerebrospinal	2	4	6
" tuberculous	7	7	14
Melena et icterus neonatorum	..	1	1
Morbus maculorus neonatorum	1	..	1
Nephritis, chronic	..	2	2
Pneumonia, broncho	5	2	7
" " rhachitis	1	..	1
" " double otitis media	..	1	1
" lobar	2	1	3
Peritonitis, traumatic	1	..	1
Pyopneumothorax	1	..	1
Typhoid, peritonitis	1	..	1
" pneumonia	..	1	1
	36	31	67

STATISTICAL REPORT—CHILDREN'S SERVICE.
1904.

ATTENDING PHYSICIAN,
HENRY KOPLIK, M.D.
ADJUNCT ATTENDING PHYSICIAN,
HENRY HEIMAN, M.D.

Specific Infectious Diseases.	Male Disch'd	Male Died	Female Disch'd	Female Died	Total
Diphtheria			1		1
Ephemeral fever	2		2		4
Influenza	1				1
Measles	1				1
Meningitis, epidemic cerebrospinal	9	9	8	11	37
" streptococcic		2			2
" tuberculous		9		4	13
Parotitis, infectious	1				1
Peritonitis, tuberculous	1	1	2		4
Syphilis, congenital				1	1
Tetanus	1				1
Tuberculosis, acute general miliary				1	1
Typhoid fever, uncomplicated	21		5		26
" complicated with empyema	1				1
" " " otitis media	1				1
" " " pleurisy with effusion			1		1
" " " scurvy	1				1
	40	21	19	17	97

Respiratory System.					
Bronchitis, acute	4		1		5
" chronic	1		1		2
Empyema	4		6		10
" with measles			1		1
Laryngismus stridulus		1			1
Pleurisy, with effusion	2				2
Pneumonia, acute broncho	9	5	4	2	20
" " " with double empyema			1		1
" " " " entero-colitis		1	1	2	4
" " " " otitis media	1		1		2
" " " " pericarditis				1	1
" " " " rickets	3	1			4
" " " " and diphtheria	1				1
" persistent broncho			1		1
" lobar	19	3	3	1	26
" " with empyema	3		1		4
" " " enteritis		1	1	1	3
" " " meningitis		1			1
" " " pleurisy	1				1
" " " pneumothorax			1		1
	48	13	22	8	91

Circulatory System.

	Male Disch'd	Male Died	Female Disch'd	Female Died	Total
Endocarditis, chronic	7	3	16	..	26
" " with acute exacerbation	2	2	2	..	6
" " " acute articular rheumatism	1	..	1	..	2
" " " cerebral embolism	..	1	..	..	1
" " " myocarditis	..	..	1	..	1
" " " nephritis and acute pericarditis	..	1	..	..	1
" " " acute pericarditis	1	..	..	..	1
" congenital	..	..	1	..	1
" " with bronchopneumonia	..	1	..	1	2
" septic	..	..	..	3	3
Pericarditis, with effusion	1	..	..	..	1
	12	8	21	4	45

Nervous System.

	Male Disch'd	Male Died	Female Disch'd	Female Died	Total
Amaurotic family idiocy	1	1	..	..	2
Cerebral palsy	1	..	..	..	1
" " congenital	1	..	..	..	1
Cerebral tumor	2	..	1	1	4
Chorea minor	6	..	4	..	10
" " with chronic endocarditis	..	..	2	..	2
Habit movements	..	..	1	..	1
Hydrocephalus, external	1	..	..	..	1
" internal	1	..	1	..	2
Idiocy, Mongolian	1	..	1	..	2
" " with broncho-pneumonia and congenital heart disease	..	1	..	..	1
Paralysis, post diphtheritic	..	1	..	..	1
Petit mal	1	..	..	..	1
Polio-encephalitis	1	..	..	..	1
	16	3	10	1	30

Diseases of the Blood.

	Male Disch'd	Male Died	Female Disch'd	Female Died	Total
Anemia	..	..	1	..	1
Leukemia	..	..	..	1	1
	..	..	1	1	2

Gastro-enteric Tract.

	Male Disch'd	Male Died	Female Disch'd	Female Died	Total
Autointoxication (intestinal)	..	..	2	..	2
Colitis, subacute	1	..	..	..	1
" chronic	1	..	..	..	1
Dyspepsia, acute intestinal	1	..	1	..	2
" chronic "	1	..	1	..	2
Enteritis, chronic catarrhal	1	..	1	..	2
Entero-colitis, acute	1	2	..	7	10
Gastro-enteritis	2	4	..	1	7
" " with erythema multiforme	..	..	1	..	1
Esophagus, stricture of	..	..	1	..	1
	8	6	8	9	31

Kidneys and Genito-Urinary System.

	Male Disch'd	Male Died	Female Disch'd	Female Died	Total
Kidney, sarcoma	..	..	1	..	1
Nephritis, acute, with purulent peritonitis	..	1	..	..	1
Nephritis, chronic, parenchymatous (post scarlatinal)	..	..	1	..	1
" " " with post diphtheritic myocarditis	1	..	..	..	1
" " " uremia and otitis media	1	..	..	..	1
Vulvovaginitis, gonorrheal	..	..	1	..	1
	2	1	3	..	6

Unclassified.

Marasmus	..	1	..	1	2

Causes of Death.

	Male	Female	Total
Cerebellar tumor	..	1	1
Entero-colitis	2	7	9
Endocarditis, chronic (acute exacerbation)	5	..	5
" " with cerebral embolism	1	..	1
" " " nephritis and acute pericarditis	1	..	1
" congenital, with bronchopneumonia	1	1	2
" septic	..	3	3
Gastro-enteritis	4	1	5
Idiocy, amaurotic family	1	..	1
Laryngismus, stridulus	1	..	1
Leukemia, acute lymphatic	..	1	1
Marasmus	1	1	2
Meningitis, epidemic cerebrospinal	9	11	20
" streptococcic	2	..	2
" tuberculous	9	4	13
Nephritis, acute, with purulent peritonitis	1	..	1
Paralysis, post diphtheritic	1	..	1
Peritonitis, tuberculous	1	..	1
Pneumonia, acute broncho	5	2	7
" " with double empyema	..	1	1
" " " entero-colitis	1	1	2
" " " pericarditis	..	1	1
" " " rickets	1	..	1
" lobar	3	1	4
" " with enteritis	1	1	2
" " . " meningitis	1	..	1
Syphilis, congenital, and malnutrition	..	1	1
Tuberculosis, acute general miliary	..	1	1
	52	39	91

POSTERIOR-BASIC MENINGITIS.

By Henry Koplik, M.D.,
ATTENDING PHYSICIAN.

This peculiar form of meningitis was first brought prominently to the notice of the profession by Gee and Barlow, who, in the *St. Bartholomew Reports* of 1878, described twenty-five cases of meningitis occurring in infants below two years of age. Some of these cases had existed from birth and others occurred sporadically at varying periods. The essential feature of all the cases described was, in the words of the authors, "the holding back of the head." In fact, they called this form of meningitis "cervical opisthotonos of infants," and laid special stress on the holding back of the head as the essential symptom of the disease. They also accentuated the fact that in tuberculous meningitis and other diseases the holding back of the head was an occasional occurrence, whereas in this form of meningitis it was a constant, unvarying symptom.

In some of their cases the onset had been gradual and in others sudden. In those cases in which the onset had been sudden the opisthotonos alone, or accompanied by fever, vomiting, rigidity of the limbs, and convulsions, seemed to be characteristic. The associated symptoms in their cases included rigidity of the limbs and convulsions throughout the course of the disease. The course of the disease in all these cases was chronic and only three of their twenty-five recovered. The duration of the disease, from its onset to the fatal termination, varied from twenty-seven days to nineteen months.

Post-mortem examination, in all cases in which it could be obtained, revealed the fact that no tubercle existed either in the brain or other organs of the body. There was lymph in varying quantities at the base of the brain, and the ventricles were dilated in most cases. In some cases there was otitis, but the other viscera showed no changes.

As to the etiology, these authors, at the time this paper was written, considered syphilis as a doubtful factor, and ventured the opinion that some of the acute cases with sudden onset resembled "epidemic cerebrospinal meningitis" of the sporadic variety.

In 1897 Carr described a number of cases of hydrocephalus with dilatation of the ventricles of the brain following meningitis, and ventured a theory, to which we will return, as to the cause of hydrocephalus in these cases. His cases resembled essentially those of Gee and Barlow.

In 1898, Still again called attention to this affection in an article in the *Journal of Pathology and Bacteriology* of that year. He mentioned the cases of Gee and Barlow, also stated that the disease occurs sporadically, and is uncommon in England and America, only forty-nine cases having presented themselves during the previous ten years in the Hospital for Sick Children in London. In this article he describes the findings in eight of the cases. He investigated post-mortem the exudate found in the ventricles and in the subarachnoid space, and isolated from these exudates a diplococcus which closely resembled the diplococcus intracellularis of Weichselbaum. He thought, however, that it grew more luxuriantly in broth and on agar-agar and glycerin-agar. He failed to find it in some of the chronic cases which had lasted several weeks, and he found it in the tendon sheaths in complicating arthritis in one case.

In describing the disease Still, in this article, considers it as not occurring in epidemics, but rather sporadically, and draws the distinction between epidemic cerebrospinal meningitis and these sporadic cases. In the cases he examined during life herpes and rash were absent. There were some minor differences also between these cases and the epidemic form of cerebrospinal meningitis. Still laid particular emphasis on the fact that cerebrospinal meningitis of the epidemic type was more rapidly fatal than the posterior-basic meningitis, but that they resembled each other in that they both seemed to affect, by predilection, the base of the brain. He concludes that posterior-basic meningitis is a disease of infancy of a non-tuberculous nature, due to a specific micro-organism, and that this micro-organism is almost identical with the diplococcus of Weichselbaum and Jäger. In other words, he did not think that this disease which we are describing could occur in epidemics. The periarthritis which complicated one of his cases was due to the essential cause—the diplococcus intracellularis.

In another article by Still in the *British Medical Journal*, 1898, he further describes the clinical features of these cases. Most of them occurred within the first two years, rarely after the second year of life, and he laid stress on the fact that many of these cases, in London, at least, have been reported as cases of tuberculous meningitis—an experience which the author has had in New York.

Still divides these cases distinctly into those which are fatal within six weeks, those which die after three or four months with hydrocephalus, and finally those which recover. In those cases which are fatal within six weeks post-mortem examination reveals lymph at the base of the brain and cord. In those which die after three or four months with hydrocephalus there is simply a thickening of the pia mater and arachnoid at the base of the brain, some adhesions between the cerebellum and medulla, and slight thickenings on the surface of the temporal or temporosphenoidal lobes. In the ordinary "suppurative vertical meningitis," as he calls it, there are complications elsewhere. In this form rarely so. In fifteen cases of suppurative meningitis there were as complications empyema, pleurisy, pneumonia, ulcerative endocarditis, membranous colitis, necrosis of the petrous portion of the temporal bone, and erysipelas. In two cases of fifteen of basic meningitis there was inflammation of the tendon sheaths, and in one there was an accidental tuberculous focus in some of the viscera. In some of the basic cases there was a mucopurulent secretion in the middle ear, but in none of them was there evidence of mastoid disease or of extension of the ear disease to the brain or meninges.

Still, in this article, laid stress on the bacteriological findings as described in his paper in the *Journal of Pathology and Bacteriology*, and again reiterates the fact that the tuberculous foci found by him in some cases of this disease had absolutely no connection with the primary affection.

In an article on posterior-basic meningitis in Allbutt's *System of Medicine*, Barlow and Lees defined more clearly the pathological changes found in these cases. The inflammation begins at the posterior part of the brain, in most cases, as the primary seat of inflammation, namely, the region where the brain and spinal cord meet and where the cerebellum overlaps the medulla. From this site the inflammation spreads down the cord to a varying degree, upward along the line of the ventricles, and forward along the base as far as the optic commissure and tips of the temporosphenoidal lobes; or the inflammation may begin in the transverse fissure and choroid plexuses. At an early stage of the disease the products of inflammation, though circumscribed, may be suppurative, but later on they may become absorbed and opacities of the meninges with adhesions result. These adhesions may unite the medulla and cerebellum, obliterate the foramen of Magendie and the fourth ventricle. This gives rise to an accumulation of fluid in the ventricles and consequent hydrocephalus. In some of these cases the ventricular fluid is clear and in others it contains flakes of fibrin and pus. In the latter the ependyma is thickened. In some cases the viscera were normal, in others the lungs were collapsed.

In the Cavendish lectures of Osler this author describes a case of posterior-basic meningitis occurring in an older child, considers the etiology and morbid anatomy, but ventures no definite opinion as to the identity or classification of these cases, at the same time noting the work of Still and Gee and Barlow.

The author of this paper has seen a number of cases of posterior-basic meningitis occurring sporadically throughout five years of continuous hospital service. He has never been able to establish, however, until recently, the fact, which was doubted by Still, that these cases may occur in epidemics of cerebrospinal meningitis. In the recent epidemic of 1904 the author saw thirty cases of cerebrospinal meningitis in his hospital service. Eight of these were typical cases of posterior-basic meningitis, admitted at various periods of the affection. Some of these cases were as young as four months of age; most of them were below two years of age.

Of the eight cases of posterior-basic meningitis admitted to my service during the recent epidemic of cerebrospinal meningitis the ages ranged from four months to five years. They were, respectively, two infants of four months, one of six months, one of nine months, one child of two years, one of three years, and one of five years. Most of these cases thus were below two years of age. The symptomatology of those above this age varied somewhat from these children and will be regarded in a separate rubric to which we will return later.

The previous history was negative in all of the cases. In other words, there was no history in any case of syphilis or tuberculosis, either in the child or in members of the family. In one case there was a history of ear trouble dating two months before admission and lasting for two weeks, but this had no connection with the illness. In another case the child had had measles three months before admission and scarlet fever a year before this. These diseases also had no connection with the illness for which the child was admitted.

As to the family history, it has been mentioned that there was no history of tuberculosis or syphilis or anything suggesting the disease in the child, father, mother, or other members of the family. In one case there was a history of miscarriage and of one child of the family having died of meningitis some years before the advent of the present case.

The duration of the disease before admission to the hospital varied in all the cases. One case was admitted the third day after the onset of the disease. This was the case of the child five years of age in which post-mortem examination revealed a form of posterior-basic meningitis, to which we will return. The other cases were admitted seven days, seventeen days, twenty-four days, four weeks, five weeks, and ten weeks after the onset of the initial symptoms.

The mode of onset, speaking now only of the cases below two years of age, which correspond accurately to those described by Gee, Barlow, and Still, in only one case was gradual; in all the others it was sudden. The child was taken with fever and vomiting, then it was noticed that there was rigidity of the neck, and in some cases convulsions occurred. These convulsions were repeated in one case daily for two weeks, the child being quiet in the interval of the convulsions. In other cases after the initial fever and vomiting the child became stupid; then the mother noticed that the fever continued or that the child became blind—in other words, did not notice or see things about it. Nourishment was taken by most cases at the time of the onset, unless rejected by vomiting. In the case in which the onset was gradual there is reason to suspect incorrect observation on the part of the mother, so that it may be said that in all cases the onset was sudden. In all cases the fever and vomiting were followed by rigidity of the neck, in some cases by convulsions, these symptoms being supplemented eventually by the so-called cervical opisthotonos.

When fully developed the picture of the disease as presented to us in the hospital was as follows: The children were emaciated; they lay quiet, seldom crying out; the head was retracted, there was marked or slight opisthotonos, the upper and lower extremities were adducted, the forearm being flexed on the arm, the thighs flexed on the abdomen, and the wrists and fingers flexed. In some cases the children presented the picture in the upper extremities seen in tetany, the so-called driving position of the hands. In other cases the lower extremities were extended and could not be bent, although the upper extremities would be strongly flexed. In the extended position of the lower extremities the thighs could not be flexed, nor could the lower extremity be flexed at the knee. The foot was strongly extended on the leg and the toes flexed into the plantar surface of the foot, resembling the tetany position. Sometimes the body would be curved to an extreme degree backward, the head assuming an angle of almost 90 degrees with the spinal cord. At times this opisthotonos and tetanus would relax and the spastic phenomenon would not be so apparent. As soon as disturbed, however, or if the back were rubbed, the patients assumed again a position of extreme opisthotonos. In other cases, in addition to the picture thus presented, there was a tendency to cross the legs; in others there were purposeless movements of the upper extremities in a sort of arc in front of the face. The fontanelles, if still open, were bulging and the sutures, in some cases in which hydrocephalus had supervened, were pressed apart by the accumulating fluid in the ventricles. In one case spasmodic contraction of the muscles of respiration occurred at intervals to such an extent as to cause a peculiar hissing sound in the larynx and also an extreme bulging anteriorly of the thorax. In some cases there was strabismus; in other cases this was absent. There was no pulsation to the bulging fontanelle above described. As a rule, the lungs, heart, liver, and spleen presented nothing positive. In all cases the emaciation was so extreme that the abdomen was retracted or rigid.

Some of the children presented, as an accidental find, marked rachitis and cranial tabes.

The temperature, in those cases which had lasted for some length of time, would not range above the normal until close to the final issue. In other words, they ran a temperature simulating what is seen in tuberculous meningitis. One case, in the hospital for five weeks, had a normal temperature for three weeks after admission and then presented wide excursions of temperature, as high as $106\frac{3}{4}°$, especially after lumbar puncture. These temperatures did not seem to be anything but cerebral temperatures, for lumbar puncture in the case just mentioned revealed nothing but sterile fluid. In another case, in which the post-mortem confirmed the diagnosis of posterior-basic meningitis, the range of temperature for fifteen days was normal with the exception of one day, when it rose to 102°. In one case, which does not belong to the rubric described by Gee and Barlow and Still, inasmuch as the child was three years of age, the patient died after twenty-four weeks of illness, and only during the first four weeks of the sojourn in the hospital was there any temperature. During these four weeks it ranged as high as $105\frac{3}{4}°$; during the remaining twenty weeks the temperature did not rise above the normal. In this case the child was admitted to the hospital on the seventh day of the disease, making a duration of twenty-five weeks.

Of the other symptoms of interest in these cases is, first, the condition of the fundus of the eye. In most of the cases below two years of age there was no change in the fundus; in other words, there was no optic neuritis, contrary to what is true of cases of tuberculous meningitis, in which, in the majority of cases, there are changes in the fundus. In all of the cases of the Still type there were other signs which are generally included in the symptomatology of meningitis, such as tâche cérébrale, with evanescent erythemas due to vasomotor paresis. Kernig's sign in these cases is of very little value for two reasons: first, that these infants or children lie in a spastic or flexed position, and second, that in children below two years of age the presence or absence of Kernig's sign is a very difficult matter to substantiate. As to the Babinski reflex, in most cases it was absent; in others it might have been established in the course of the disease.

The leukocyte count in most of these cases is of great interest. In one case the leukocytes ranged from 14,000 to 17,000 to the cubic millimetre. In another case the leukocytes ranged from 10,000 to 30,000, the latter being the count at the close of the disease. In another case the leukocyte count was 19,000, the child dying three days after admission. In the case of an infant twelve months of age, who was admitted on the twenty-fourth day of the disease, the leukocyte count on admission was 26,000. It can thus be seen from this simple enumeration of the leukocyte counts that they were, as a rule, low, similar to what is seen in tuberculous meningitis, and therefore of no diagnostic value.

Of especial interest are the results of lumbar puncture. Our experience has been that lumbar puncture in posterior-basic meningitis is not always successful in evacuating fluid. In some of our cases we have proved that the cause of the so-called dry tap on lumbar puncture is due to the closing up of the canal of Magendie by exudate, and also the matting together of the spinal canal in the vicinity of the cerebellum and pons to such an extent that the subarachnoid fluid cannot flow from the subarachnoid space and ventricles of the brain into the space of the cord and out, and thus through the cannula in the lumbar region. In cases in which hydrocephalus had supervened and in which the disease had lasted for weeks, lumbar puncture was of only negative value so far as diagnosis was concerned, inasmuch as repeated puncture in such cases revealed a sterile fluid. Although the fluid in some cases was not quite clear, no micro-organisms were found either by spread or culture. This must be explained by the fact that in these cases the micro-organisms have really died out, and the few that remained were found only post-mortem, as in one case, in the ventricles of the brain.

Of the six cases below two years of age, which correspond absolutely to those described by Still, one gave a negative result by lumbar puncture, that is, only a few drops of fluid being obtained during life. In this case post-mortem examination of the fluid of the ventricles revealed the meningococcus. In another case, four months of age, although typical of the disease which we are describing, the lumbar puncture gave but little fluid, two or three cubic centimetres at each puncture, sterile of micro-organisms. In this case unfortunately there was no post-mortem. In another case, which had lasted twenty-four days on admission, the puncture fluid revealed meningococci. In the fourth case, four months of age, admitted in the sixth week of the disease, the first puncture fluid was negative, the second revealed meningococci. In this case post-mortem examination confirmed the diagnosis. In the fifth case the puncture fluid revealed meningococci. In the sixth case, nine months of age, which sojourned in the hospital five months, a large number of punctures was made. The case was absolutely characteristic of the type described by Still, although no post-mortem was obtained. Hydrocephalus resulted and increased under observation. At one puncture no less than 250 c.c. of fluid were removed and yet the most patient search failed to reveal any micro-organisms. This being a chronic case, the cytology of the fluid was especially interesting. It resembled very closely what is seen in tuberculous meningitis. There was a mononuclear picture of leukocytes. I have explained this mononuclear picture elsewhere as being characteristic of so-called chronic cases of cerebrospinal meningitis.

In these cases, as in hydrocephalus, there is really a transudate rather than an exudate. The inflammation has run its course, but the hydrocephalus is the result of transudation of serum from the vessels rather than of exudation due to active inflammatory processes, and, according to Ribbert, a transudate would reveal a predominance of mononuclear lymphocytes.

In the second case, four months of age, there was a polynuclear picture, with sterile fluid. In the third case, four months of age, there was a marked polynuclear picture of the puncture fluid, and in this meningococci were found. In the fourth case, in which diagnosis was confirmed by post-mortem examination, there was a predominance of polynuclear elements in the puncture fluid, and in this case meningococci were found. In the fifth case, an infant nine months of age, the puncture fluid presented a polynuclear picture, and in this case also meningococci were found. It may be said, therefore, that the chronic cases yielded negative results so far as micro-organisms in the puncture fluid are concerned, and that the mononuclear picture resembled what is seen in tuberculous meningitis.

Post-mortem examinations were obtained in three of the six cases occurring in children below two years of age. In one, an infant six months of age, post-mortem examination showed that the superior surface of the brain was pale, that the convolutions were flattened, and that at the base there was a small amount of organizing, purulent exudate. The floor of the fourth ventricle was bulging and ready to burst. The foramen of Magendie was almost $\frac{2}{3}$ cm. in diameter. The fluid aspirated from the ventricle showed meningococci. The cord presented hemorrhages in the cervical, mid-dorsal, and lumbar regions.

The thymus was large, the lungs showed simple congestion, the heart muscle was pale, the spleen was moderately large, the Malpighian bodies quite large, and the liver was congested and somewhat fatty; the gall-bladder and duct were negative, the kidneys negative, the adrenals and pancreas negative; the stomach showed a few hemorrhagic areas in the fundus; the intestines showed follicular enteritis, swelling of the mucosa, vessels markedly injected, and the mesenteric nodes moderately enlarged.

In another case, an infant nine months of age, admitted on the seventeenth day of the disease, there was some purulent exudate over the vertex, but it was most marked at the base, completely surrounding the cord. There was considerable increase of the subarachnoid fluid, there was hydrocephalus, and marked dilatation of the ventricles.

In the third case, two years of age, admitted in the sixth week of the disease, post-mortem made at the end of the sixth week, examination of the brain revealed the dura adherent to the calvarium and the pia adherent to the dura mater over the motor areas on both sides. The brain was edematous, with marked injection of the blood-vessels. There was an organized exudate of a yellowish-gray color on the surface of the brain. At the base, over the chiasm and anterior surface of the medulla and pons, and to a slight extent over the cerebellum anteriorly, there was a thick, grayish-yellow exudate. No tubercle. The ventricles were moderately dilated and contained some turbid fluid. The choroid plexus was congested, and a few petechiæ were scattered over the surface of the brain.

Case I.—Male infant, aged four months; admitted May 31, 1904, in the twenty-fourth day of the disease.
Family History.—Negative.
Previous History.—Negative. Labor normal.
Present History.—Child became ill twenty-four days before admission, with fever, crying out, painful rigidity of the neck, erythema over the general surface; eyes turned upward; no convulsions; occasional vomiting; fontanelles bulging; bowels and urination normal. There has been increasing loss of weight and slight cough. On admission, general condition fair, child well nourished. Head retracted to an extreme degree, no opisthotonos, feet drawn up on the abdomen, arms extended. Child cries when disturbed, otherwise quiet. Seems to notice objects. Sutures of the head still open, anterior fontanelle open and bulging; pupils react to light, no strabismus, no facial paralysis, no paralysis of the extremities. There is a Babinski reaction on both sides, often automatic; knee-jerks increased, no clonus; there is tâche cérébrale; distinct trismus of the lower jaw, preventing a view of the throat. Skin, heart, lungs, liver, and spleen negative; abdomen rigid, without any palpable abnormality. There is shallow breathing, irregular in rhythm; pulse is of fair quality, but irregular.

Under observation there was occasional vomiting, this increasing until the child vomited after every feeding, always of projectile character. The rigidity and retraction of the head did not diminish. The fundus of the eye, examined by Dr. Gruening, gave a negative result.

On June 4 child's condition became worse to a marked degree; the pulse became very weak and rapid; the respirations, though rapid, continued irregular. The child took no nourishment, became slightly cyanotic, and lay with upper extremities in a condition of overextension, the fists clenched in the tetany position.

Lumbar puncture was made in this case on three different occasions, the first two punctures being negative, the third yielding 5 c.c. of a turbid fluid showing a marked preponderance of polynuclear leukocytes and numerous extracellular and intracellular Gram-negative diplococci, both by culture and stain. (Examination by Dr. E. P. Bernstein.)

The temperature in this case was normal until six hours before the exitus, which took place June 4, five days after admission. At this time, just before death, the temperature rose to $105\frac{1}{2}°$. The range of pulse was very irregular—from 100 to 180 per minute. The respirations were irregular, ranging from 30 to 50 per minute. The leukocytosis in this case was 26,000 to the cubic millimetre. No post-mortem.

CASE II.—Male infant, aged four months; admitted to the service June 25, 1904, in the fifth week of the disease.

Family History.—Negative.

Previous History.—Negative, both as to infectious diseases and ear complications.

Present History.—Infant became suddenly ill five weeks before admission, with fever, convulsions, and rigidity of the neck. Two weeks before admission the child went into a condition in which it lay quiet, with occasional contractions of the muscles of the arms and legs. At this time the mother noticed that the child no longer saw objects. Emaciation became marked, bowels constipated.

On admission, physical examination revealed an infant the general condition of which was poor. It lay very quiet, seldom cried. The head was retracted and there was some opisthotonos. The upper and lower extremities were adducted toward the trunk; the forearm, wrists, and fingers were flexed, the hands in the tetany driving position. The spastic condition of the lower extremities was so great that they could not be flexed beyond a slight angle, in which they were constantly held. There were periods of relaxation, however, in which the lower extremities could be flexed. The spastic condition of the upper extremities was very marked. There were purposeless movements of the upper extremities, and a tendency to cross the legs. Reflexes at the knee were present, the great toe held in the Babinski position most of the time, but no true Bakinski could be obtained; there was no clonus. The pupils reacted to light, of equal size; no strabismus. No facial paralysis. Anterior fontanelle prominent, posterior fontanelle closed; head not enlarged. No Macewen; ears and mastoid negative; marked signs of rachitis on the chest. Heart, lungs, liver, and spleen presented nothing of interest.

June 26.—Examination revealed an infant with body in a condition of spastic rigidity, with arching of the back, retraction of the head, with intervals in which the rigidity and opisthotonos are not so pronounced; fontanelles bulging; craniotabes marked. A Babinski was obtained at this time; the hands still continued in the tetany position;

arms rigid and extended; knees sometimes relaxed, at other times rigid. The occasional spasm which caused marked rigidity and arching backward of the head and body also affected the muscles of respiration, so that there was, when these spasms occurred, a crowing sound heard, formed in the larynx on inspiration. Trismus was present at times. A lumbar puncture was made on June 27, and 1.3 c.c. of a yellow, cloudy fluid obtained. The report on this fluid showed a cytological picture of a polynuclear type, but no meningococci. Spreads and culture negative. (Examination by Dr. Bernstein.)

The child died nine days after admission. During the whole stay in the hospital the temperature was normal with the exception of the second day, when it mounted to 101°. The pulse was very irregular, ranging from 104 to 150 during the stay in the hospital. The respirations ranged from 18 to 30.

CASE III.—Female infant, aged six months; admitted in the fourth week of the disease.

Family History.—Negative. Mother has three other children.

Previous History.—Negative, with the exception of a diarrhea, at the age of two months, which lasted two weeks.

Present History.—Infant has been sick four weeks. Illness began suddenly with fever and convulsions. Convulsions lasted two weeks and were repeated daily. Infant vomited once or twice. In the interval of the convulsions child lay perfectly quiet and did not cry. For the past two weeks there have been no convulsions. Mother thinks infant is blind and that the head is increasing in size. Slight cough for the last few days. Infant takes nourishment well. Bowels and urination normal. Child has lost in weight.

Physical examination shows condition good, well nourished, infant restless, head and extremities in constant motion. Skin presents nothing peculiar; small glands are felt in the neck and groin, none elsewhere. There is rigidity of the neck; no Kernig, no Babinski; kneejerk present; no clonus; strabismus, pupils react to light, are equal, moderately dilated; no facial paralysis; tâche cérébrale; tongue slightly coated. Heart, liver, and spleen normal. Abdominal wall rigid; abdominal contents present nothing peculiar. Child vomits its nourishment. Respiration irregular; at times child does not appear to breathe. Fontanelles bulging, head retracted. Child continued in this condition without very much change until just before death, which occurred quite suddenly.

While in the hospital on the first day the temperature reached 101°, on the second day 102⅖°, and on the third day of the sojourn in the hospital it dropped to normal and remained there until the exitus. The pulse was quite irregular, ranging from 100 to 130, respirations from 30 to 34.

Both eyes, examined by Dr. Gruening, showed optic atrophy.

Culture of the cerebrospinal fluid during life gave a negative result.

but that removed after death showed meningococci and a polynuclear leukocytic picture. (Examination by Dr. Bernstein.)

Post-mortem.—(By Drs. E. Libman and Dr. Bernstein.) Thymus enlarged; lungs somewhat congested; heart muscle pale, foramen ovale open; spleen moderately enlarged, Malpighian bodies enlarged; kidneys negative; adrenals and pancreas negative; stomach, a few hemorrhagic areas in the fundus; intestines showed follicular enteritis, mucosa congested, and nodes enlarged. Brain surface pale, convolutions flattened; ventricles distended with fluid, at the base a small amount of purulent exudate; floor of the fourth ventricle ready to burst, foramen of Magendie 2.3 cm. Cord showed hemorrhages in the cervical and dorsal regions underneath the pia.

CASE IV.—Female infant, aged nine months; admitted May 12, 1904, in the seventeenth day of the disease.

Family History.—Negative.

Previous History.—Negative, with the exception that there was a discharge from the right ear two months ago which lasted four weeks.

Present History.—Infant was taken suddenly ill seventeen days ago, with fever, 104° according to the statement of the physician in charge. There was no cough and no convulsions. Rigidity and retraction of the head present for the last fifteen days. There was occasional vomiting; intestinal movements normal at first, but lately have become green, containing mucus.

Physical examination shows well-nourished infant; head retracted; neck rigid; pupils contracted, react to light. No Kernig, no Babinski; knee-jerks markedly increased; no clonus. Tâche cérébrale; hyperesthesia; no meningeal cry; no rash on extremities, body, or mucous membranes. Fontanelles depressed. Respirations very irregular. Lungs, heart, and liver normal; spleen palpable below the borders of the ribs; abdomen relaxed.

Child continued very much in the same condition during its stay in the hospital, with the exception that on May 23 physical examination revealed the head more and more retracted, so that it formed almost a right angle with the spine. Respirations shallow and very irregular, fontanelle not bulging; there is slight convergent strabismus; no facial paralysis. Child cries out without any cause, takes its food very poorly. There is marked tâche cérébrale, increased knee-jerks; opisthotonos is marked, though there are periods of relaxation during which the opisthotonos disappears. The retraction of the head, however, remains constant.

Examination of the blood showed leukocytosis ranging from 15,000 to 30,000 to the cubic millimetre.

Lumbar puncture revealed cerebrospinal fluid decidedly cloudy, showing a preponderance of polynuclear leukocytes, Gram-negative staining diplococci intracellular and extracellular both by spread and culture. (Examination by Dr. Bernstein.)

The temperature during the stay in the hospital was normal with the exception of the seventh day, when it rose, without apparent cause, to 101°, then dropped to normal, finally falling to subnormal just before death. The pulse was quite irregular, ranging from 80 to 160 per minute. The respirations were 20 to 38 per minute.

The urine showed amorphous urates and a few leukocytes.

Post-mortem examination (by Dr. Bernstein) made of the brain only, showed a purulent exudate over the vertex and a marked exudate at the base, completely surrounding the cord. The ventricles were dilated and contained an increased amount of fluid. Brain not opened.

CASE V.—Female infant, aged nine months; admitted March 29, 1904, in the tenth week of the disease.

Family History.—Negative.

Previous History.—Difficult and prolonged labor. Child was born perfectly normal.

Present History.—Infant was taken suddenly ill ten weeks before admission, with fever, stupor, and retraction of the head. The child continued from this time on with occasional fever and in a stuporous condition. Three weeks before admission it developed general convulsions, these convulsions being frequently repeated. The head became a great deal larger, there was a slight cough, and marked emaciation.

On admission the general condition of the child was very poor, emaciated, head retracted to extreme degree, marked opisthotonos. Forearm flexed on the arm, hands held in the driving position; lower extremities extended and the feet in the equinovarus position. Eyes prominent, head considerably enlarged, marked prominence of forehead and occiput; anterior and posterior fontanelles open, with bulging of the anterior fontanelle; separation of the bones of the cranium at the sutures. Macewen percussion note obtained on both sides of the skull. Incisors of the lower jaw present; slight trismus of lower jaw. Tâche cérébrale. Examination of the fundus of the eye negative.

This child was punctured eight times, from 40 to 250 c.c. of fluid being withdrawn at each puncture. The puncture fluid was carefully centrifuged and repeatedly examined, with a view to finding meningococci, but none were found, nor were tubercle bacilli found. Cultures were made, with negative results, as were also injections into animals. (Examinations by Dr. Kramer.)

This infant was in the hospital six months, during most of which time the temperature was normal. There were periods, however, of a week in which the child ran a very irregular temperature, especially the first week of its sojourn in the hospital, when it ranged from subnormal to 104.6°. These temperatures were higher after lumbar punctures. After the second week the temperature remained normal.

The blood count, taken during the course of the disease, showed leukocytosis ranging, in the first week, from 9,000 to 17,000, after which it remained low, not exceeding 10,000.

The pulse was very irregular, ranging from 100 to 160 per minute on different days. Respirations also were irregular both in rhythm and depth, ranging from 15 to 30 per minute.

Although the infant continued in the hospital for six months the head steadily enlarged in spite of the withdrawal of fluid. The emaciation came to a standstill at a certain point, and then the infant increased very slightly in weight, remaining thus until its withdrawal from the hospital.

Unfortunately there was no post-mortem, but the whole picture of the disease clinically was that of hydrocephalus following cerebrospinal meningitis, with extreme retraction of the head and opisthotonos which were constant, accompanied by tetany in the extremities and trismus of the jaw.

CASE VI.—Female child, aged two years; admitted April 25, 1904, in the fifth week of the disease.

Family History.—Negative.

Previous History.—Normal labor, breast-fed child. One year before admission had an abscess in the neck extending over three weeks; otherwise has been a bright, healthy child.

Present History.—Five weeks before admission child was taken suddenly ill, with fever, general convulsions. Since the onset there have been, at times, remissions of the fever, though it has continued more or less up to the present time. The child has gradually become stupid, though the father thinks it is not blind. It vomits occasionally, and for the past three days there have been constant movements of the upper and lower extremities. The child has emaciated markedly. Bowels and urination normal. The father has noticed that the child's head has perceptibly enlarged during the illness.

Physical examination of the child shows that it lies with the head retracted, eyes wide open, head turned to the left. The body is arched and the neck rigid. There are occasional purposeless movements of the forearm and arms and sometimes of the lower extremities. At times there seem to be coarse tremors of the upper extremities. The child starts at the least sound. The respirations are irregular and shallow. At times the extremities are held in a spastic condition, the feet being in a condition of extension, the arms flexed at the elbow, the fingers and toes flexed. In other words, the hands are clenched and the lower extremities are in a spastic condition similar to that seen in tetany. The pupils are equal, though widely dilated, but react to light. There is slight nystagmus. At times the arching of the back relaxes, but as soon as the muscles of the back are irritated the arching becomes extreme. Macewen's sign is marked, especially on the right side. The eyes show no optic neuritis or change in the fundus. Lung, heart, and liver negative; spleen congested, palpable below the free border; abdomen rigid, scaphoid in shape. On account of the trismus of the lower jaw the mouth cannot be opened or the throat examined.

Lumbar puncture reveals fluid in which there is an abundance of polynuclear elements, to the extent of 73 per cent., and 27 per cent. mononuclear. There are extracellular and intracellular diplococci not staining with Gram.

The child died suddenly without any change in the symptoms four days after admission.

The blood count the day after admission showed a leukocytosis of 19,200 to the cubic millimetre.

The temperature was normal during the child's stay in the hospital, with the exception of one day, when it rose to $101\frac{1}{2}°$ without any apparent cause. The pulse ranged from 100 to 140, and the respirations from 26 to 48.

Post-mortem examination, by Dr. E. Libman, showed that the dura mater was adherent to the calvarium and the pia mater to the dura mater over the motor areas on both sides. The brain was markedly edematous, with pronounced injection of the vessels. There was a moderate amount of organized exudate of a yellowish-gray color on the surface of the brain. There was an increase of the subarachnoid fluid at the base of the brain; over the chiasm, anterior surface of the medulla, pons, and, to a slighter extent, over the cerebellum anteriorly, there was a thick, grayish-yellow exudate. The ventricles were moderately dilated, containing a turbid fluid. The choroid plexus was injected and there were a few petechiæ scattered over the surface of the brain.

Meningococci were found in the exudate at the base of the brain.

The above six cases are a series occurring in children two years of age and below, corresponding quite closely to what has been described recently by Still. All the clinical features of these cases were similar, and all presented the marked head retraction described by Gee, Barlow, Lees, and Still as characteristic of these cases. They all occurred in the course of an *epidemic of cerebrospinal meningitis* of a very extensive nature, prevalent among both children and adults, and were admitted, with twenty-four other cases of cerebrospinal meningitis, to my hospital service. These cases were admitted at more or less advanced periods of their affection, as may be seen by reference to the histories, and none of them recovered. One case was discharged with increasing symptoms of hydrocephalus, as may be seen from the notes. It was, however, in a very poor physical condition at the time of its discharge.

The leukocyte count, as may be seen, was not very high in any case, and the lumbar punctures were unsuccessful in those cases in which the canal of Magendie was proved post-mortem to have been either narrowed or completely obliterated.

The question has arisen as to the exact causes of the peculiar features of these cases—that is, first, the retraction of the head, and, second, the hydrocephalus. Carr, in the *Medical and Chirurgical Transactions* of 1897, has attempted to explain the hydrocephalus as due, first, to obliteration of the foramen of Magendie, thus allowing an accumulation of fluid in the ventricles for which there is no escape; and second, to pressure of the exudate at the base, and in some cases thrombosis of the veins of Galen, resulting in a transudation or dropsy, so to speak, of the ventricles.

As to the retraction of the head, it has been explained by Still and his predecessors as due to an irritation of the cervical nerves as they emerge from the intervertebral notches, thus causing a contraction of the smaller deep muscles of the neck.

Whatever the cause of the head retraction and the hydrocephalus in these cases, these two features are peculiar to them, and do not necessarily occur in forms of basic meningitis at a later period of life; nor does the fact that this form of meningitis is peculiar to infants necessarily exclude its occurrence at a later period.

I have been fortunate to observe a case of basic meningitis occurring in a boy five years of age, in which post-mortem examination revealed a typical meningitis of the Still type, due to streptococcus infection. In this case there was no retraction of the head; in fact, as will be seen from a study of the history of the case, the signs of meningitis were almost equivocal. Only slight rigidity of the neck, increasing stupidity, a Kernig sign, and tâche cérébrale led to the suspicion that meningitis might be present. In other words, basic meningitis may occur at a later period in life without the characteristic symptoms seen in infants below two years of age.

CASE.—*Basic meningitis due to streptococcus infection, occurring in a boy aged five years.*

Family History.—Negative.

Previous History.—Normal birth; no traumatisms. Measles at age of one year; slight attack of pneumonia at two years of age. When four years old (one year before admission) he fell; was not unconscious, but was confined to bed for three weeks with high fever, loss of appetite; vomited once, immediately after the fall; no other symptoms. Boy recovered completely.

Present History—The boy came under observation September 2, 1904. At that time he complained of headache and had a slight cough.

Examination revealed that the boy had febrile movement from 103° to 105½°; pulse from 120 to 128; respirations 20 to 24. Examination of the lung gave equivocal signs. There was slight dullness over the right lung and diminished breathing behind.

Fever continued in the remittent curve from 101° to 104½°, and reaching 105½°. Respirations 20 to 24. Leukocyte count of 8,000. Aside from headache there were no signs of meningitis before admission.

On admission of the boy to the hospital physical examination showed that he was slightly stupid, complained of sore throat, which was negative on inspection; temperature had the same curve as noted above. There was dullness of the right lower lobe, behind and in the axilla; slightly diminished breathing. Heart was negative.

So slight were the signs of meningitis that the boy was rather suspected to have had typhoid, but the Widal test was made with negative results. The leukocyte count, however, mounted to 25,400. On the fourteenth day of the disease the boy became semi-stupid, developing rigidity of the neck and a Kernig sign. Lumbar puncture was made and a turbid fluid obtained, showing a preponderance of polynuclear leukocytes; abundant streptococci, both on spread and culture. (Examination by Dr. Bernstein.) The boy became more stupid, developed strabismus of the left eye, and there was considerable hyperesthesia and irritability.

Examination of the fundus showed optic neuritis of the left eye. Strabismus was supplemented with flatness on one side of the face. Patient developed conjunctivitis; the pupils were uneven and did not react to light. The lung developed a few subcrepitant râles over the upper part of the right lung in front and behind, with small areas of dullness. Spleen not palpable. Heart and liver negative. There was a leukocyte count before death of 18,000 to the cubic millimetre. The temperature of this case during the stay in the hospital was exceedingly irregular. It was of the remittent type, at times reaching 104₄° and falling as low as 99°. On some days the temperature did not fall to normal; on other days it fell to normal, but immediately rose again to the figures mentioned. The pulse was extremely irregular, varying from 96 to 140 at various stages of the disease. The respirations were 24 to 32.

Post-mortem (by Dr. Buerger) revealed a pure type of basic meningitis, the exudate at the base extending as far forward as the tips of the temporo-sphenoidal lobes. There was absolutely no exudate on the superior and lateral surfaces of the brain, although there was marked congestion of these areas. The purulent exudate did not extend down into the spinal cord. The ventricles were dilated and contained a turbid fluid. Lungs showed hemorrhagic areas of broncho-pneumonia scattered through both lungs.

Here was a case, it will be seen, of classical basic meningitis due to streptococcus infection, possibly from the lungs. A careful examination of the ears post-mortem throughout the bony construction showed absolutely nothing abnormal, nor could the avenue of infection be traced in this case. During life the symptoms of meningitis in this case were so non-characteristic as to lead two physicians whose powers of observation are undoubted to think of typhoid fever, or of some obscure disease other than meningitis. It was only in the later stages of the meningitis, when the stupor became evident and the rigidity of the neck marked, accompanied by Kernig's symptom, tâche cérébrale, and paresis of the facial nerves and ocular muscles, that meningitis was thought of. Lumbar puncture confirmed the suspicion. At no time in the course of the disease was there retraction of the head.

There are thus, according to the author's interpretation, two forms of basic meningitis. The first, which is primary, corresponds to the type described by Still, in which there is a primary inflammation of the meninges, as described in his paper, caused by the diplococcus intracellularis of Weichselbaum; and the second, occurring in older children, in which the symptoms in no way resemble those of the cases described by Still and the set described in this paper.

The cases occurring in older children may be complicated with pneumonia, as in the case last quoted, or may be secondary to a pneumonia. The characteristic symptomatology is evidently lacking, but there may occur certain symptoms which will point to a basic involvement, as in our case, such as facial paresis and paralysis of the muscles of the eye.

It is interesting, however, to note that cases of basic meningitis of the type described by Gee, Barlow, Lees, and Still may occur in epidemics of cerebrospinal meningitis, and be due to the same essential cause as the disease which occurs in older children. In fact, it seems that in the majority of cases of children attacked by cerebrospinal meningitis below two years of age the symptomatology is so closely allied—in reality identical—with that described by Gee, Barlow, and Still that the conclusion is inevitable that cerebrospinal meningitis, both epidemic and sporadic, in young children takes the form described by these authors in a certain set of cases.

BILATERAL EMPYEMA IN CHILDREN—A REPORT OF TWO CASES.

By Henry Heiman, M.D.,

ADJUNCT ATTENDING PHYSICIAN TO THE CHILDREN'S WARD.

In the clinical features and course of empyema in children there are to be noted certain important differences from the disease in adults.

I. In children, and especially in infants, empyema is sometimes very insidious. In a child, for example, convalescent from lobar pneumonia, recovery may appear to be complete, the temperature may be normal, the physical signs may have disappeared almost entirely. The child may apparently be well for several days or more, but then the physician is called and is surprised to find considerable pus in the affected chest. It is wise, therefore, in those cases in which empyema is liable to occur as a sequela, to observe the children more carefully and for a longer time than would be necessary in adults.

II. Occasionally spontaneous absorption of small quantities of pus occurs in children, whereas recovery in adults without operative interference occurs almost never.

III. Operative interferences in children is easier, and recovery after operation is more rapid. Because of the thin chest wall persistent sinuses occur less frequently, and because of the softness, elasticity, and rapid growth of the ribs, the wounds heal more rapidly. Even in bilateral empyema in children, with prompt and proper surgical treatment the prognosis in fairly good.

Because of the comparative rarity of double empyema and the meagreness of the literature on this subject, the report of these two cases, treated in the children's service of Dr. Koplik, may prove of interest. According to Holt, bilateral empyema occurs in about 3 per cent. of all cases of empyema in children. Of Koplik's 120 cases, only two were bilateral.

Case I.—J. S., male, age two years, born in Russia, admitted to the hospital July 8, 1904, with the diagnosis of double pneumonia and enteritis. One week later, when the temperature was normal and the general condition excellent, the patient was discharged because of a suspicious desquamation of the skin. Three days after discharge the patient was readmitted with the diagnosis of empyema. After leaving the hospital there had been continued cough and profuse perspiration, but no fever or vomiting. Pus had been aspirated from the left chest on the day previous to readmission. Examination of the patient (July 18, 1904) showed:

The leukocyte count was 26,400. The general condition was much poorer than on discharge. There were cough, dyspnea and cyanosis.

Examination of the *lungs* showed dullness and diminished breathing over entire left chest anteriorly. Posteriorly there were numerous râles over both chests; over the whole of the left chest, marked dullness and diminished breathing; and similar signs over the right chest from the scapular spine to the base of the lung.

Heart.—The upper and left borders were obscured by pulmonary dullness. The right border was one finger to the right of the right sternal border. The heart's action was rapid, but regular. No murmurs. The pulse was of poor quality.

Liver.—The free edge was palpable three fingers below the free costal border.

The spleen, abdomen, genitals, extremities, and rectal examination were negative. The urine was negative throughout the illness, except for a trace of albumin during the first few days.

Soon after readmission exploratory puncture of the pleural cavities showed the presence of pus in both chests, spreads and cultures of which showed pneumococcus. On the following day, employing the surgical procedure usual in these cases, I resected a portion of the eighth rib on the left side, evacuating considerable greenish pus and draining the pleural cavity with two rubber tubes. The patient reacted fairly well after the operation. During the next three days there were high temperatures, rapid heart action and a leukocytosis; vigorous stimulation was resorted to. Then the general condition began to improve and the temperature dropped to normal. Drainage from the wound, which was dressed daily, was free; the discharge continuously diminished; and the lung expanded well.

Nine days after the resection on the left side an intercostal incision was performed on the right side, pus having been aspirated from the right chest twice in the meantime.

Recovery was now rapid and uninterrupted. The patient gained in weight, the hemoglobin increased from 50 per cent. after the first operation to 70 per cent. just before discharge, and the wounds healed rapidly.

Six weeks after the first operation the wounds were entirely healed and the patient was discharged cured.

CASE II.—S. T. L., female, age one year, admitted to the hospital July 8, 1902, with the diagnosis of empyema on the right side. The child had been ill eleven days with fever and slight cough.

Physical examination showed the child to be in poor general condition. There were dyspnea and cyanosis of the ears, lips and finger tips.

Lungs.—At the base of the *right lung* posteriorly were flatness, absent breathing, and diminished voice and fremitus; higher up, as well as in the right axilla, were marked dullness, compression breathing and numerous râles.

The breathing was rapid and diminished.

Liver.—The free edge of the organ was palpable 3½ fingers below the free costal border in the mammary line.

Spleen.—Palpable two fingers below the free costal border.

Both *kidneys* could be distinctly palpated. Otherwise examination of the abdomen was negative.

On the day of admission the patient looked very sick, the fever was moderately high, the stools were green, examination of the urine showed nothing noteworthy. The leukocyte count was 47,000. On exploratory puncture of the right chest thick greenish pus was withdrawn, the bacteriological report of which was pneumococcus.

Because of the poor general condition of the child and the small amount of pus in the right chest, immediate operation was not deemed advisable. The patient was carefully observed, put on stimulation, and a week after admission as much pus as could be obtained (only 1 c.c.) was aspirated from the right chest. There continued high fever, the leukocytosis and little change in the physical signs. When, however, twelve days after admission, the general condition had improved somewhat and the signs in the right chest had increased, under local anesthesia an intercostal incision was made below the right scapular angle, a small quantity of pus was evacuated, and a drainage tube inserted. The child went into collapse after the operation, but after heroic stimulation the patient gradually rallied. Drainage from the wound was free and the general condition improved for four days. Then new signs were found in the left chest, on aspiration of which pus was withdrawn. On the same day, fifteen days after admission, an intercostal incision was performed on the left side. The child stood this operation well and for the next ten days seemed to be getting on fairly well. Then there developed an ileo-colitis; there were frequent diarrheal movements with mucus and blood. The vitality of the patient had already been taxed to the utmost, and this intercurrent affection probably contributed largely to the ultimately fatal termination.

In the first case the diagnosis of double empyema having been made at the outset, the indications for treatment were plain. The left side was relieved at once by operation; while the child was recovering from this operation, as much pus as could be obtained was aspirated from the right chest. Then, when the child had recovered sufficiently, the right side was operated upon. Most authorities agree that the sooner the left side is operated upon, the better is the prognosis. By relieving the left chest the pressure on the heart is minimized, and there is less liability to a complicating pericarditis, cases of which have been recorded. Occasionally an unfortunate outcome of opening both pleural cavities at the same time has been the collapse of both lungs. On that account it is advisable to operate only on one side at first and then, before operating upon the other side, to wait seven to ten days so that firm adhesions may form.

The rarity of bilateral empyema and meagre mention of the subject in the literature seemed to us sufficient warrant for the publication of these cases.

REPORT OF THE DEPARTMENT OF GENERAL SURGERY.

INTRODUCTORY REMARKS.

By Arpad G. Gerster, M.D.

Since May, 1904, the two divisions of the surgical service have been installed in their magnificent new home. It seems appropriate to describe the conditions under which their work is done at the new hospital.

The space occupied by the surgical service consists of one children's ward, two half wards, and two full wards, to each of which are attached a number of subsidiary smaller rooms containing one bed each. These small rooms are used for the isolation of noisy or dying patients. Attached to each ward is an examining room, fully equipped as a small operating room, and provided with excellent north light. In these examining rooms all that work is done that might disturb the repose or the routine of the wards. Anesthesia for purposes of examination, or for the incision of an abscess, the change of large dressings or the change of dressings on nervous and noisy patients, and many other manipulations involving a certain degree of disturbance or soiling, are now done to great advantage in these examining rooms. Thus, by the aid of our detached rooms and by that of our examining rooms, we manage to have cheerful, quiet and cleanly wards. One year's experience has abundantly demonstrated the fact that the elimination from the ward proper of the work now done in these subsidiary spaces represents an innovation of enormous value to the surgeon and especially to the patient.

Another important improvement is to be noted in our operating plant, occupying the entire fifth floor of the administration building. Our large and truly magnificent operating theatre is flanked on each side by two smaller operating rooms, all of them provided with splendid diffused light, vertical and horizontal, entering from the north by day, and very adequate electric lighting during the night. The operating theatre and two of the smaller operating rooms are used exclusively in non-septic cases, while all the infectious work is done in the other two operating rooms, each of which has its independent supply of instruments and sterilizers. Opposite the row of operating rooms are situated two anesthetizing and two recovery rooms, the large sterilizing room, where all the dressing materials, gowns, towels, ligatures and sponges are sterilized daily, for all the services of the hospital. Then there is a completely equipped Roentgen apparatus and developing room, a dressing room with bath room attached for the use of the visiting surgeons, a dressing room for the house staff, and another dressing room for the nurses employed at operations, each of these various dressing rooms being amply provided with washstands.

In immediate connection with the amphitheatre is, on one side a room containing two sets of sterilizers for producing hot and cold water for solutions and irrigation, then a sterilizer for larger vessels, such as basins, dishpans, pus-basins, pitchers, etc., and a blanket warmer. All these apparatus are worked by steam, furnished from central boilers. The other side of the operating theatre has an extension containing the large instrumentarium.

Telephones connect all the wards with the operating plant; maintain, in fact, connection with every part of the institution, so that, for instance, the pathologist can be summoned, and does appear without delay to make frozen sections of a doubtful tumor, and to pass his opinion, while the pertinent operation is in progress.

Another beneficent innovation, and a great boon to our sick and convalescent, is the heated solarium and "garden," situated on the roof of every building containing patients.

Last, but not least, is the "reception department," also an innovation, which might be aptly called a filter through which every patient must pass before being installed in any one of the hospital wards. This department consists of three small wards, each containing beds, one for men, one for women and another one for children. There are two ample bathrooms and a small, but perfectly equipped operating room. This department has a separate entrance from without, where ambulance cases are received, and is strictly isolated from all the other parts of the hospital. Here each patient is divested of his clothes, which are immediately sent to be disinfected, after which they are stored in a system of individual lockers, in an adjoining space. Here each patient is subjected to a thorough examination, after which he receives such a bath and cleansing as his condition admits. Surgical, notably accident cases, undergo here a preliminary cleansing and disinfection before they are sent up to the operating plant. Minor accident cases also are here taken care of by the medical men in charge at hours when the dispensary is not working. After his bath, the patient is clothed in clean linen and placed in bed to rest a while, after which he is transferred to the ward to which he had been assigned. Thus, it is seen, that the clothes and the filth adhering to them and to the person of a patient never reach the wards of the hospital, but are retained in this, what we may call a filter.

Another extremely important advantage accrues to the inmates of the hospital from the reception department. It is the possibility of observing for a sufficient while febrile cutaneous eruptions, especially in children, to determine their contagious or harmless nature. The latter, after the matter is settled, are transferred to their respective ward, contagious cases are sent off to the hospitals destined for their reception. Thorough disinfection follows the appearance of every case of contagion, and in these small spaces is an easy matter.

Contagious cases originating in the hospital are transferred to and treated in our isolating pavilion.

On entering the new hospital Dr. Lilienthal and Dr. Gerster agreed to divide the service in the following manner:

Dr. Lilienthal's, that is the second surgical division, to consist of

Female ward T..................................with	25	beds
" " " 6 subsidiary rooms............ "	7	"
Male ward R.................................... "	14	"
" " " 5 subsidiary rooms............ "	5	"
One-half children's ward...................... "	8	"
Total	59	"

Dr. Gerster's, that is the first surgical division, to consist of

Male ward Q..................................with	25	beds
" " " 4 subsidiary rooms............ "	4	"
Female ward M.................................. "	11	"
One-half children's ward...................... "	8	"
Total	48	"

Thus it is seen that during the year ending May 1, 1905, Dr. Gerster's service had eleven beds less than Dr. Lilienthal's. Furthermore, that while one division has more men, the other has more women. These inequalities are to be straightened out by the agreement that each May 1st the surgeons will exchange wards. Thus, beginning from May 1, 1905, Dr. Gerster will take possession for one year of those wards that were in charge of Dr. Lilienthal since May 1, 1904.

STATISTICAL REPORT OF THE FIRST SURGICAL DIVISION, 1903.

Arpad G. Gerster, M.D.,
ATTENDING SURGEON.

A. A. Berg, M.D., and A. V. Moschcowitz, M.D.,
ADJUNCT SURGEONS.

Diseases of the Head and Face.—23 CASES, 2 DEATHS.	Total	Cured	Improved	Unimproved	Died
Cerebral tumor (Gumma?)	1	1	..	..	..
Jacksonian epilepsy	1	..	1	..	..
Compound depressed fracture of skull	1	1	..	..	..
Simple " " " middle meningeal hemorrhage, coma	1	..	..	..	1
Compound comminuted fracture of skull, traumatic meningitis, abscess of frontal lobe	1	..	..	..	1
Fracture of base of skull	2	1	..	1	..
Trigeminal neuralgia (2d Division)	1	..	1	..	..
Retarded mental development	1	..	..	1	..
Carcinoma of mastoid region	1	..	..	1	..
Double hare lip	1	1	..	..	..
Gingivitis	1	..	..	1	..
Glossitis	1	..	1	..	..
Burns on face and hands	3	3	..	..	..
" " " chest and upper extremity	1	1	..	..	..
Epithelioma of face	1	..	1	..	..
Necrosis of inferior maxilla	1	..	..	1	..
Melano sarcoma of inferior maxilla	1	1	..	..	..
Osteomyelitis of lower jaw (syphilitic)	1	1	..	..	..
Recurrent giant cell sarcoma of lower jaw	1	1	..	..	..
Sarcoma of lower jaw	1	1	..	..	..

Diseases of the Neck.—24 CASES, 5 DEATHS.

	Total	Cured	Improved	Unimproved	Died
Phlegmonous inflammation of submaxillary gland	2	2			
Abscess of neck	1	1			
Tubercular glands of neck	4	3	1		
Carbuncle of neck	1	1			
Cyst of neck (lymphangioma)	1	1			
Dermoid cyst of neck	2	2			
Persistent thyroglossal duct	1	1			
Carcinomatous cervical adenitis	1				1
Cystic goitre	5	5			
Adenoids	1	1			
Carbolic burn of throat (asthenia)	1				1
Epithelioma of tonsil and fauces	1				1
Sarcoma of tonsil	1	1			
Carcinoma of larynx, sepsis	1				1
Edema of larynx	1				1

Diseases of Upper Extremity.—16 CASES, 1 DEATH.

	Total	Cured	Improved	Unimproved	Died
Simple fracture of clavicle	1	1			
Fibroma of shoulder	1	1			
Dislocation of shoulder	1	1			
Fracture of humerus	1		1		
Giant cell sarcoma of humerus	1	1			
Gonorrheal arthritis of elbow	1			1	
Tubercular " " " (general tuberculosis)	1				1
Compound fracture of radius and ulna	1	1			
Recurrent myxofibroma of forearm	1	1			
" sarcoma " "	1	1			
Tubercular synovitis of wrist	2	2			
Phlegmon of hand	2	2			
Carbolic gangrene of finger	1	1			
Enchondroma of finger	1	1			

Diseases of the Thorax.—30 CASES, 6 DEATHS.

	Total	Cured	Improved	Unimproved	Died
Empyema	3	3			
Pyopneumothorax	1				1
Persistent thoracic fistula	4	4			
Pleurisy with effusion	1	1			
Melano sarcoma of back	1	1			
Fracture of twelfth dorsal vertebra	1	1			
Tubercular spondilitis with mediastinal abscess	1			1	
" " " " and extradural abscess	1				1
Tumor of spinal cord	1				1
Mammary abscess	2	2			
Chronic mastitis	1		1		
Fibroma of breast	2	2			
Carcinoma of breast	5	4		1	
Recurrent carcinoma of breast	1	1			

Diseases of the Thorax—Continued.

	Total	Cured	Improved	Unimproved	Died
Angio-sarcoma of breast	1	..	1	..	..
Carcinoma of Esophagus	4	3	..	..	1

Diseases of the Abdominal Wall.—3 CASES, 0 DEATHS.

	Total	Cured	Improved	Unimproved	Died
Actinomycosis of abdominal wall	1	..	..	1	..
Sarcoma of rectus sheath	1	..	..	1	..
Irritating silk-worm gut suture	1	1	..	..	..

Diseases of the Stomach.—14 CASES, 1 DEATH.

	Total	Cured	Improved	Unimproved	Died
Toxic gastro-enteritis	1	1	..	..	..
Ulcer of stomach, spastic stenosis of pylorus	3	3	..	..	..
Perforated ulcer of stomach, diffuse peritonitis	1	..	..	..	1
Benign stenosis of pylorus	2	2	..	..	..
Peripyloritis	1	1	..	..	..
Carcinoma of pylorus	3	..	3	..	..
" " body of stomach	2	..	..	2	..
" " cardia	1	..	1	..	..

Diseases of the Liver.—8 CASES, 5 DEATHS.

	Total	Cured	Improved	Unimproved	Died
Amebic colitis with amebic abscess of liver	3	..	..	..	3
Abscess of liver	2	1	1	..	..
Cirrhosis of liver, pancreatitis and nephritis	1	..	..	..	1
Carcinoma of liver	2	..	..	1	1

Diseases of the Gall Bladder.—27 CASES, 4 DEATHS.

	Total	Cured	Improved	Unimproved	Died
Cholecystitis	2	..	1	..	1
" and pneumonia	1	..	..	..	1
Cholelithiasis and chronic cholecystitis	6	6	..	..	..
" cholecystitis, stones in common duct	4	3	1	..	..
" " hydrops of gall bladder, and pericholecystic abscess	2	2	..	..	..
" with empyema of gall bladder	3	3	..	..	..
" and acute gangrenous cholecystitis	3	3	..	..	..
" with gangrenous perforative cholecystitis and diffuse peritonitis	2	..	..	..	2
" pericholecystitis, cholangitis	1	1	..	..	..
" cholecystitis, stone in common duct, cholecysto-duodenal fistula	1	1	..	..	..
Pericholecystitis	1	1	..	..	..
Carcinoma of gall bladder	1	..	..	1	..

Diseases of Pancreas.—4 CASES, 3 DEATHS.

	Total	Cured	Improved	Unimproved	Died
Peripancreatic hemorrhage	1	1	*1		
" " subphrenic abscess	1				1
" fat necrosis with sero-purulent peritonitis	1				1
Sarcoma of tail of pancreas, peripancreatic abscess	1				1

Diseases of the Spleen.—1 CASE, 0 DEATHS.

	Total	Cured	Improved	Unimproved	Died
Primary splenomegaly	1			1	

Diseases of the Intestines.—19 CASES, 5 DEATHS.

	Total	Cured	Improved	Unimproved	Died
Chronic peritonitis with adhesions	1	1			
" intestinal obstruction due to adhesions	1				1
Intestinal obstruction, cause unknown	1				1
" " due to lympho-sarcoma of mesentery	1		1		
Volvulus of sigmoid flexure	2	2			
Carcinoma of sigmoid flexure	2	1		1	
Tuberculosis of the cecal junction	1		1		
Actinomycosis of cecum and abdominal wall	1	1			
Gangrenous amebic colitis	1				1
Colitis	2	1		1	
Perforation and gangrene of intestine due to band, peritonitis	1				1
Cecal fistula following appendicitis	1	1			
Gangrene, perforation of sigmoid flexure, with peritonitis from mesenteric thrombosis	1				1
Enteroptosis	1			1	
Chronic constipation	2	1	1		

Diseases of the Vermiform.—109 CASES, 11 DEATHS.

	Total	Cured	Improved	Unimproved	Died
Acute catarrhal appendicitis	11	10		†1	
" appendicitis with abscess	7	6			1
" gangrenous or perforative appendicitis	54	51			3
" " " " with sero-purulent peritonitis	1				1
Acute gangrenous or perforative appendicitis with diffuse purulent peritonitis	2	2			
Acute gangrenous appendicitis with mesenteric thrombosis	1				1
" " " pylephlebitis, liver abscess	1				1
" " " with thrombosis of mesentereolum	1	1			
Appendicitis, acute gangrenous, with abscess and diffuse peritonitis	11	7			4
Appendicitis, empyema of appendix	8	8			
" chronic	6	2		*4	
" " with endometritis and curettage	1	1			

*Recurrence of this case reported under head "cured."
†This case not operated.

Diseases of the Vermiform—*Continued.*

	Total.	Cured.	Improved.	Unimproved.	Died.
Appendicitis, chronic, with ovarian cyst	2	2			
" " " fibroid uterus	1	1			
" " " twisted fallopean tube and hematoma of ovary	1	1			
" carcinoma of appendix, pregnancy and sepsis	1	1			

Diseases of Peritoneum.—2 CASES, 0 DEATHS.

	Total.	Cured.	Improved.	Unimproved.	Died.
Abdominal tumor	1			*1	
Tuberculous peritonitis	1			*1	

Hernia.—78 CASES, 4 DEATHS.

	Total.	Cured.	Improved.	Unimproved.	Died.
Hernia, inguinal (double hernia counted as 2)	48	46		*2	
" " bladder	2	2			
" " undescended testis	2	2			
" " (double) and epigastric	1				1
" " " " umbilical	1	1			
" " strangulated	5	3			2
" " " and purulent peritonitis	1				1
" femoral	6	4		*2	
" " strangulated	4	4			
" umbilical, "	2	2			
" ventral	6	6			

Diseases of Perineum and Male Genitals.—117 CASES, 2 DEATHS.

	Total.	Cured.	Improved.	Unimproved.	Died.
Vesical calculus	4	3		*1	
Chronic cystitis	1			*1	
Tubercular cystitis and diabetes	1		*1		
" " ren mobilis	1	1			
" "	1			*1	
Cystitis and pyelonephritis	1				1
Hypertrophy of prostate	4	3			*1
" " " and vesical calculus	1			*1	
Acute gonorrheal prostatitis	1	*1			
Peri-urethral abscess	3	1	1	*1	
Perineo-urethral fistula, abscess of scrotum	1		1		
Prostatic abscess, epididymitis	1	1			
Stricture of urethra	3	3			
" " " cystitis, prostatic calculi, pyelonephritis, and abscess of penis	1		1		
False passage of urethra	1	*1			
Stricture of urethra, extravasation of urine	1	1			
Hydrocele	1	1			
Double hydrocele	2	2			
Varicocele	5	5			

*Unoperated.

Diseases of Perineum and Male Genitals—Continued.

	Total.	Cured.	Improved.	Unimproved.	Died.
Spermatocele	1	1			
Epididymo-orchitis	1		*1		
Tubercular epididymitis	2	1	1		
Endothelioma of testis and cord	1	1			
Perineal recto-vesical fistula	1			*1	
Carcinoma of rectum and chronic intestinal obstruction	1		1		
Recurrent carcinoma of rectum	1			*1	
Carcinoma of rectum	3	1		*2	
Adenoma "	1	1			
Papilloma "	1	1			
Epithelioma of perineo-femoral fold	1	1			
Ulcerated scar after excision of rectum	1	1			
Syphilis of rectum	1			*1	
Prolapsus recti	3	3			
Rectal incontinence	1	1			
Fistula in ano	16	16			
Hemorrhoids	36	36			
" papilloma of vocal chord	1			*1	
" with diabetes	1			1	
Ischio-rectal abscess	8	8			
Rectal polyp	1	1			
Chronic endometritis	1	1			

Diseases of Kidneys and Ureter.—20 CASES, 3 DEATHS.

	Total.	Cured.	Improved.	Unimproved.	Died.
Chronic nephritis	1		*1		
Ren mobilis	1	1			
Nephralgia	1			*1	
Nephrolithiasis	2		*2		
Pyelitis, tubercular	1			*1	
Calculus pyelonephritis	1	1			
Acute "	1		*1		
Left hydronephrosis and calculus, atrophied right kidney	1				1
Acute ascending pyonephritis, gonorrheal	1	1			
Pyonephrosis	2	1		*1	
" and calculus	1	1			
Double tubercular pyonephrosis	1				1
Genito-urinary tuberculosis	1			*1	
Tumor of kidney	1			*1	
Perinephritic abscess, empyema, subphrenic abscess and purulent peritonitis	1				1
Perinephritic abscess, pyonephrosis, suppurative infarction of kidney	1	1			
Ureteral calculus	1	1			
" " vesical calculi	1	1			

*Unoperated.

Diseases of the Lower Extremity and Pelvis.
53 CASES, 4 DEATHS.

	Total	Cured	Improved	Unimproved	Died
Toe.—Arteriosclerotic gangrene	2	1	1		
Diabetic gangrene	2			*1	*1
Perforating ulcer	1	*1			
" " diabetic	1	1			
Tuberculosis	1	1			
Hallux valgus, bilateral	1	1			
Foot.—Arteriosclerotic gangrene	2	2			
Diabetic gangrene	1			*1	
Traumatic gangrene	1		1		
Diabetic cellulitis	1				1
Wound of foot	1	1			
Traumatic necrosis of os calcis and astragalus	1	1			
Paralytic club-foot	1	1			
Ankle Joint.—Tuberculosis	2	1	1		
Leg.—Diabetic gangrene	1				*1
Ulcer	1		*1		
Varicose ulcer	1	1			
Wound of leg	2	2			
Phlegmon of leg	1		1		
Tibia.—Osteomyelitis	1	1			
Sarcoma	1	1			
Knee Joint.—Suppuration of	2	2			
Chronic synovitis	1	1			
Patella.—Fracture	1	1			
Thigh.—Abscess	1	1			
Contusion	1	*1			
Recurrent sarcoma	1	1			
Tuberculosis	1			*1	
Sciatica	1			*1	
Femur.—Sarcoma	1	1			
Fracture	2	2			
Fracture and dislocation	1		*1		
Deformed callus	1		*1		
Syphilis	1	1			
Acute osteomyelitis	1				1
Buttock.—Abscess	1	1			
Lipoma	1	1			
Lumbar abscess	1		1		
Gluteal Artery.—Aneurism	1	1			
Humerus.—Acute osteomyelitis	1	1			
Tuberculosis	1	1			
Pubis.—Tuberculosis	1		1		
Inguinal Glands.—Tuberculosis	1	1			
Bubo	1	1			
Sacrum.—Infected dermoid cyst	1	1			
Infantile contractions of lower extremities	1			*1	

*Unoperated.

Diseases of Female Genitalia.—24 CASES, 0 DEATHS.

	Total.	Cured.	Improved.	Unimproved.	Died.
Bartholin's Glands.—Abscess	1	1			
Vagina.—Cyst of	1	1			
Retained secundines	1	1			
Relaxed vaginal outlet	1	1			
" " " with lacerated cervix	1	1			
Uterus.—Endometritis	2	2			
Prolapse and retroversion	1	1			
Carcinoma	1	1			
Fibroids	3	2		*1	
Fallopian Tubes and Ovaries.—Tubo-ovarian abscess	1		1		
Salpingo-öophoritis	1		*1		
Chronic "	1	1			
Double pyosalpinx	1	1			
Ovarian cyst	4	4			
Twisted ovarian cyst	1	1			
Cystic ovary	1	1			
Ectopic gestation	1	1			
Pelvic abscess	1	1			

Miscellaneous Diseases.—9 CASES, 0 DEATHS.

	Total.	Cured.	Improved.	Unimproved.	Died.
Acute articular rheumatism	1			*1	
Progressive anemia	1			*1	
Chronic myocarditis	1			*1	
Neurasthenia	1			*1	
Enteroptosis	1			*1	
Syphilis	1		*1		
Acute miliary tuberculosis	1			*1	
Metastatic multiple glandular sarcoma	1			*1	
Multiple myelomata	1			*1	

Operations on Head and Neck.—29 OPERATIONS, 5 DEATHS.

	Total.	Cured.	Improved.	Unimproved.	Died.
Elevation of depressed fracture of skull	1	1			
Craniectomy for compound depressed fracture of skull with cerebral abscess and meningitis	1				1
Double hare lip, plastic	1	1			
Removal of melano-sarcoma of alveolar margin of inferior maxilla	1	1			
Sequestrectomy for syphilitic osteomyelitis of inferior maxilla	1	1			
Resection of horizontal ramus of lower jaw for recurrent giant cell sarcoma	1	1			
Excision of giant cell sarcoma of inferior maxilla	1	1			
Incision and drainage of phlegmonous submaxillary adenitis	2	2			
" " " " abscess of neck	1	1			

*Not operated.

Operations on Head and Neck—*Continued.*

	Total.	Cured.	Improved.	Unimproved.	Died.
Excision of tubercular glands of neck	3	3			
Incision of carbuncle of neck	1	1			
Excision of lymphangioma of neck	1	1			
" " dermoid cyst of neck	2	2			
Extirpation of persistent thyro-glossal duct	1	1			
" " carcinomatous cervical glands	1				1
" " cysts of thyroid	4	4			
Partial thyroidectomy for cystic and parenchymatous goitre	1	1			
Removal of adenoids	1	1			
Langenbeck's operation for epithelioma of tonsil and fauces	1				1
" " " sarcoma of tonsil	1	1			
Laryngectomy for carcinoma of larynx	1				1
Tracheotomy for edema of larynx	1				1

Operations on Upper Extremity.—13 OPERATIONS, 1 DEATH.

	Total	Cured	Improved	Unimproved	Died
Excision of fibroma of shoulder	1	1			
Amputation through shoulder joint for giant-celled sarcoma of humerus	1	1			
Incision and drainage of tubercular abscess of elbow joint	1				1
Suture of compound fracture of radius and ulna	1	1			
Excision of recurrent myxofibroma of forearm	1	1			
" " " sarcoma " "	1	1			
" " tuberculous ganglion of wrist	2	2			
Incision and drainage of phlegmon of hand	1	1			
Amputation of finger	3	3			

Operations on Thorax.—23 OPERATIONS, 3 DEATHS.

	Total	Cured	Improved	Unimproved	Died
Excision of rib and drainage for empyema	4	4			
Thoracoplasty for chronic empyema	3	3			
Excision of rib and drainage for pyopneumothorax	1				1
" " sarcoma of back	1	1			
Incision and drainage of tuberculous mediostinal abscess	1			1	
Laminectomy for extradural tuberculous abscess from spondylitis	1				1
Laminectomy for tumor of cord	1				1
Incision and drainage of mammary abscess	2	2			
Excision of fibroma mammæ	2	2			
Amputation of breast for malignant neoplasm	5	4	1		
Excision of recurrent cancerous nodule	1	1			
Tracheotomy for malignant stenosis	1		1		

Operations on Abdominal Wall.—1 OPERATION, 0 DEATHS.

	Total	Cured	Improved	Unimproved	Died
Removal of buried silk-worm gut suture from abdominal wall	1	1			

Operations on the Stomach.—14 OPERATIONS, 2 DEATHS.

	Total	Cured	Improved	Unimproved	Died
Gastrostomy for carcinoma of esophagus	3		2		1
Posterior gastro-enterostomy for ulcer of stomach	2	2			
Suture of perforated ulcer of stomach, diffuse peritonitis	1				1
Posterior gastro-enterostomy for benign pyloric stenosis	2	2			
Gastrolysis for peripyloritic adhesions	1	1			
" " hour-glass stomach	1	1			
Posterior gastro-enterostomy for pyloric cancer	3		3		
" " " and gastrostomy for malignant, pyloric, and cardiac stenosis	1		1		

Operations on Liver.—7 OPERATIONS, 5 DEATHS.

	Total	Cured	Improved	Unimproved	Died
Incision and drainage of amebic liver abscess	3				3
" " " " liver abscess	1	1			
Omentopexy and cholecystostomy for cirrhosis of liver	1				1
Laparotomy for carcinoma of liver	2			1	1

Operations on Gall Bladder and Ducts.

23 OPERATIONS, 3 DEATHS.

	Total	Cured	Improved	Unimproved	Died
Cholecystectomy for acute gangrenous cholecystitis and cholelithiasis	3	2			1
Cholecystectomy for acute gangrenous perforative cholecystitis with peritonitis	2	1			1
Cholecystostomy and drainage for empyema of gall bladder	1	1			
Cholecystectomy and drainage for acute ulcerative cholecystitis, empyema, and cholelithiasis	1	1			
Cholecystectomy and drainage for acute ulcerative cholecystitis and cholelithiasis	2	2			
Cholecystectomy and drainage for chronic cholecystitis and cholelithiasis	5	5			
Cholecystectomy for pericholecystitis	1	1			
" and drainage for chronic cholecystitis and cholelithiasis	1	1			
Cholecystostomy and choledochotomy for cholecystitis and common-duct stones	2	2			
Cholecystostomy and drainage for hydrops gall bladder and cholelithiasis	1	1			
Secondary closure of biliary fistula	1	1			
Cholecystectomy and choledochotomy for cholelithiasis and common-duct obstruction by stone; suture of duodenum for cholecystitic duodenal fistula	1	1			
Retroduodenal choledochotomy and drainage for multiple calculi in common and hepatic ducts	1	1			
Cholecystostomy and drainage for pyophlebitis due to gangrenous appendicitis	1				1

Operations on Pancreas.—2 OPERATIONS, 1 DEATH.

	Total	Cured	Improved	Unimproved	Died
Laparotomy and drainage of peripancreatic hematoma	1	1	..	..	..
Incision and drainage of peripancreatic abscess	1	..	..	..	1

Operations on Spleen.—1 OPERATION, 0 DEATHS.

	Total	Cured	Improved	Unimproved	Died
Exploratory laparotomy for primary splenomegaly	1	..	..	1	..

Operations on Intestines.—10 OPERATIONS, 3 DEATHS.

	Total	Cured	Improved	Unimproved	Died
Incision and drainage for retro-cecal abscess due to tuberculous ileo-cecal junction	1	..	1	..	..
Multiple operations, incision and drainage, for actinomycosis of cecum and abdominal wall	1	1	..	..	..
Incision and drainage for acute gangrenous perforative amebic colitis	1	..	..	..	1
Exploratory laparotomy for carcinoma sigmoid flexure	1	..	..	1	..
Ileocolostomy for fecal fistula following appendectomy	1	1	..	..	..
Resection sigmoid flexure for carcinoma	1	1	..	..	..
Celiotomy and drainage for diffuse peritonitis, due to perforation sigmoid flexure	1	..	..	..	1
Laparotomy and reduction of volvulus of sigmoid flexure	2	2	..	..	..
Entero-enterostomy for intestinal obstruction, due to adhesion	1	..	..	..	1

Operations on Appendix.—122 OPERATIONS, 9 DEATHS.

	Total	Cured	Improved	Unimproved	Died
Appendicectomy for acute catarrhal appendicitis	7	7	..	..	..
" " chronic " "	3	3	..	..	..
Incision and drainage for appendicular abscess	5	5	..	..	..
Appendicectomy and drainage for acute catarrhal appendicitis and abscess	2	2	..	..	..
Appendicectomy and drainage for acute gangrenous or perforative appendicitis with abscess	47	45	..	..	2
Appendicectomy for acute gangrenous appendicitis	2	2	..	..	..
" and drainage for acute gangrenous appendicitis and thrombosis mesenteriolum and portal vein	3	1	..	..	2
Appendicectomy and drainage for acute gangrenous and perforative appendicitis, with serous peritonitis	3	3	..	..	..
Appendicectomy and drainage for acute gangrenous appendicitis with sero-purulent peritonitis	1	..	..	..	1
Appendicectomy and drainage for acute gangrenous or perforative appendicitis with diffuse peritonitis	1	1	..	..	..
Rectal counter incision for appendicular pelvic abscess	1	1	..	..	..
Vaginal counter incision for appendicular pelvic abscess	1	1	..	..	..
Appendicectomy and drainage for acute gangrenous appendicitis with abscess and diffuse peritonitis	11	7	..	..	4
Appendicectomy and drainage for empyema of appendix	8	8	..	..	..

Operations on Appendix—*Continued.*

	Total	Cured	Improved	Unimproved	Died
Appendicectomy for chronic appendicitis.	22	22			
" " " " and oöphorectomy for ovarian cyst	2	2			
" " " " " myomectomy	1	1			
" " " " " salpingo-oöphorectomy	1	1			
" " cancer of appendix and accouchement force for pregnancy	1	1			

Operations for Hernia.—80 OPERATIONS, 4 DEATHS.

	Total	Cured	Improved	Unimproved	Died
Hernia, Bassini, for inguinal	53	51		2	
" " " strangulated inguinal	4				2
" " " inguinal and castration for undescended testicle	2	2			
" " " " " transplantation for undescended testicle	1	1			
" double inguinal and plastic for epigastric	1				1
" laparotomy for strangulated inguinal and purulent peritonitis	1				1
" herniotomy for strangulated inguinal	1	1			
" Bassini for femoral	4	2		2	
" laparotomy for strangulated femoral	1	1			
" Bassini for strangulated femoral	3	3			
" for strangulated umbilical	2	2			
" " umbilical	1	1			
" " ventral	6	6			

Operations upon Kidney and Ureter.—12 OPERATIONS, 3 DEATHS.

	Total	Cured	Improved	Unimproved	Died
Nephropexy	1	1			
Nephrectomy for calculus pyelonephritis	1	1			
" " atrophied kidney	1				†1
" " pyonephrosis, gonorrheal	1	1			
" " calculus pyonephrosis	1	1			
Nephrotomy " " hydronephrosis	1				†1
" " ureteral calculus	1	1			
Double nephrotomy for tubercular pyonephrosis	1				1
Exploratory nephrotomy, nephropexy for ren mobilis	1	1			
Nephrotomy and litholopaxy for ureteral calculus and vesical calculi	1	1			
Incision and drainage for pyonephrosis	1	1			
" " " " perinephric abscess, empyema, subphrenic abscess, and purulent peritonitis	1				1
Incision and drainage and nephrectomy for perinephric abscess and pyonephrosis	1	1			

†Two operations on one patient.

Operations on Perineum and Male Genitals.

101 OPERATIONS, 1 DEATH.

	Total	Cured	Improved	Unimproved	Died
Suprapubic cystotomy for vesical calculus	1	1			
Litholopaxy for vesical calculus	1	1			
Perineal cystotomy for vesical calculus	1	1			
" prostatectomy for hypertrophy of prostate	2	2			
Suprapubic " " " " "	1	1			
Incision and drainage for abscess of prostate	1	1			
" " " " peri-urethral abscess	2	1	1		
" " " " " " and tubercular epididymitis	2	1	1		
" " " " fistula in ano	15	15			
" " " " ischio-rectal abscess	8	8			
Urethroplasty for perineo-urethral fistula	1		1		
External urethrotomy for stricture of urethra	2	2			
" " " " " " and extravasation of urine	1	1			
" " " " cystitis and pyelonephritis	1				1
Resection of urethra for traumatic stricture of urethra	1	1			
External urethrotomy, prostatectomy, for stricture of urethra and prostatic calculi	1		1		
Injection of and irrigation with carbolic acid for hydrocele	1	1			
Winkelman for hydrocele	2	2			
Volkman's " "	1	1			
Excision of sac for spermatocele	1	1			
" " veins for varicocele	5	5			
" " epithelioma of perineo femoral fold	1	1			
" " carcinoma of rectum, vaginal route	2	2			
Orchidectomy for endothelioma of testis and cord	1	1			
Colostomy for inoperable carcinoma of rectum and chronic intestinal obstruction	1		1		
Cauterization for papilloma of rectum	1	1			
Cauterization for ulcerated scar after excision of rectum	1	1			
Linear cauterization for prolapsus recti	2	2			
Sigmoidopexy " " " "	1	1			
Clamp and cautery for hemorrhoids	35	35			
Ligature for hemorrhoids	2	2			
" " renal polyp	1	1			
Elastic ligature for fistula in ano	1	1			
Perineorrhaphy for rectal incontinence	1	1			
Curettage for endometritis	1	1			

Operations on Lower Extremity and Pelvis.

39 OPERATIONS, 3 DEATHS.

	Total	Cured	Improved	Unimproved	Died
Amputation of toe for gangrene. 1. Arteriosclerotic	1	1			
" " " " " 2. Diabetic	1		1		

Operations on Lower Extremity and Pelvis—Continued.

	Total	Cured	Improved	Unimproved	Died
Perforating ulcer, diabetic	1	1			
Osteotomy and drainage for tuberculosis of toe	1	1			
Resection for hallux valgus	1	1			
Amputation through knee joint for arteriosclerotic gangrene	1	1			
" of thigh for arteriosclerotic gangrene	1	1			
" through thigh for sarcoma of tibia	1	1			
Incision and drainage for diabetic cellulitis of foot	1				1
Plastic for wound of foot	1	1			
Removal of tarsus for traumatic gangrene of foot	1		1		
Resection of os calsis and astragalus for necrosis	1	1			
Tendon transplantation for paralytic club foot	1	1			
Drainage of ankle joint for tuberculosis	1	1			
Incision " " " " "	1		1		
Skin-graft for wound of leg	2	2			
Excision of ulcer of leg and ligation of varicose veins	1	1			
Sequestrectomy for osteomyelitis of tibia	1	1			
Mayo operation for suppuration of knee joint	2	2			
Incision and drainage for chronic synovitis of knee joint	1	1			
Incision and drainage for phlegmon of leg	1		1		
Fixation for fracture of patella	1	1			
Incision and drainage for abscess of thigh	1	1			
Exarticulation at hip for sarcoma of thigh	1	1			
Reduction of fracture of femur	2	2			
Osteotomy for syphilis of femur	1	1			
" " acute osteomyelitis of femur	1				1
Excision of lipoma of buttock	1	1			
Ligation of internal iliac artery for aneurysm of gluteal artery	1	1			
Osteotomy for acute osteomyelitis of ilium	1	1			
Osteotomy for acute tuberculous osteomyelitis of ilium	1	1			
Incision and drainage for tuberculosis of pubis	1		1		
" " " " abscess of buttock	1	1			
" of infected dermoid cyst of sacrum	1	1			
" and drainage for tuberculosis of inguinal glands	1	1			
" " " " inguinal bubo	1	1			
" " " of lumbar abscess	1		1		

Operations for Diseases of Female Genitalia.

21 OPERATIONS, 0 DEATHS.

	Total	Cured	Improved	Unimproved	Died
Incision and drainage of abscess of Bartholin's glands	1	1			
Excision of cyst of vagina	1	1			
Curettage for retained secundines	1	1			
Plastic for relaxed vaginal outlet, trachelorraphy	1	1			
" " " " "	1	1			
" Alexander, trachelorraphy for prolapse retroversion	1	1			
Curettage for endometritis	2	2			
Hysterectomy for carcinoma of uterus	1	1			

Operations for Diseases of Female Genitalia—*Continued.*	Total.	Cured.	Improved.	Unimproved.	Died.
Hysterectomy for fibroids	1	1			
" " cyst of ovary	1	1			
Myomectomy for fibroids	1	1			
Salpingo-oöphorectomy for tubo-ovarian abscess	1		1		
Pyosalpingo-oöphorectomy for double pyosalpinx	1	1			
Oöphorectomy for chronic oöphoritis	1	1			
Salpingo-oöphorectomy for ovarian cyst	2	2			
Plastic operation for cystic ovary	1	1			
Oöphorectomy for ovarian cyst	1	1			
Salpingo-oöphorectomy for ectopic gestation	1	1			
Incision and drainage of pelvic abscess	1	1			

STATISTICAL REPORT OF THE FIRST SURGICAL DIVISION 1904.

Arpad G. Gerster, M.D.,
ATTENDING SURGEON.

A. A. Berg, M.D., and A. V. Moschcowitz, M.D.,
ADJUNCT SURGEONS.

Diseases of Head and Neck.—TOTAL, 56; DEATHS, 8.	Total.	Cured.	Improved.	Unimproved.	Died.
Scalp.—Carcinoma of	1	1			
Skull.—Fracture of base	2		1		*1
Depressed fracture	1	1			
" " with laceration of brain	1				1
Compound and depressed fracture	1	1			
Brain.—Concussion	1	1			
Tumor	1				1
Tumor of cerebellum	2		2		
Epilepsy	1		1		
Nerves.—Trigeminal neuralgia	2	2			
Face.—Burns with sepsis	1				*1
Lip.—Hare	1	1			
Epithelioma	1	1			
Upper Jaw.—Epulis	1			*1	
Lower Jaw.—Osteomyelitis	4	3	1		
Sarcoma	1			*1	
Tongue.—Carcinoma	2				2
Tonsils.—Adenoids	1	1			
Syphilis	1				1
Carcinoma	1			*1	
Peritonsilar abscess	1	1			
Tonsil, Pharynx and Larynx.—Carcinoma	1			*1	
Submaxillary Glands.—Abscess	1	1			
Endothelioma	1	1			

*Not operated.

Diseases of Head and Neck—*Continued.*

	Total.	Cured.	Improved.	Unimproved.	Died.
Neck.—Abscess	3	2			1
Infralingual and suprahyoid abscess	1	1			
Acute adenitis	2	2			
Tuberculous adenitis	12	8	1	*3	
Cervico-pharyngeal fistula	1	1			
Lymphangiectasia cysticum	1	1			
Thyro-glossal cyst	2	2			
Thyroid Gland.—Cyst	3	3			

Operations on Head and Neck.—49 OPERATIONS, 6 DEATHS.

	Total	Cured	Improved	Unimproved	Died
Extirpation of dermoid thyro-glossal cyst	1	1			
" " thyroid cyst	2	2			
Hemithyroidectomy	1	1			
Extirpation of cystic lymphangioma of neck	1	1			
" " cervico-pharyngeal fistula	1	1			
" " tuberculous glands of neck	8	7	1		
" " carcinoma of submaxillary gland	1	1			
" " adenoids	1	1			
" " carcinomatous glands of neck	1	1			
" " carcinoma of lip	1	1			
" " " " scalp	1	1			
" " lipoma of neck	1	1			
Elevation of depressed fracture of skull	3	2			1
Trephining for cerebellar tumor	3	2			1
" " epilepsy	1	1			
Cheiloplasty for hare lip	1	1			
Resection of inferior dental nerve for neuralgia	1	1			
Lossen Braun operation for trigeminal neuralgia	1	1			
Excision of tongue for carcinoma	2				2
Tracheotomy for syphilitic laryngeal stenosis	1				1
Plastic on ear for congenital deformity	1	1			
Extirpation of cervical lymph nodes, Hodgkins	1	1			
Incision of peritonsilar abscess	1	1			
" and drainage of submaxillary abscess	1	1			
" " " " abscess of neck	7	6			1
Osteotomy and drainage for osteomyelitis of lower jaw	4	4			
Plastic for fistula of cheek	1	1			

Diseases of Thorax.—TOTAL, 35; DEATHS, 3.

	Total	Cured	Improved	Unimproved	Died
Abscess of breast	3	2	1		
Chronic mastitis	1	1			
Fibro-adenoma of breast	2	2			
Carcinoma " "	11	9	1	*1	

*Not operated.

Diseases of the Thorax—*Continued*.

	Total.	Cured.	Improved.	Unimproved.	Died.
Sarcoma of breast	1	1			
Tuberculosis of chest wall	2	2			
" " ribs	2	2			
Fractured ribs	1		1		
Empyema of pleura	2	1			1
Interlobar empyema	1		1		
Thoracic sinus following empyema	1			*1	
Pyopneumothorax	2	1	1		
Tuberculous pleurisy	1			*1	
Carcinoma of esophagus	3		2		1
" " " with perforation into trachea	1				1
Stricture of esophagus, luetic	1		1		

Operations on Thorax.—32 OPERATIONS, 1 DEATH.

	Total.	Cured.	Improved.	Unimproved.	Died.
Incision and drainage of abscess of breast	3	2	1		
Amputation of breast for chronic mastitis	1	1			
" " " " fibro-adenoma	2	2			
Radical operation for carcinoma of breast	10	9	1		
" " " sarcoma " "	1	1			
Secondary " " recurrent carcinoma of breast	3	3			
" " " " sarcoma " "	1	1			
Resection of ribs and thoracic fascia for tuberculosis	2	2			
" " " for empyema	4	1	1		‡2
" " " " pyopneumothorax	2	2			
" " " " tuberculosis	2	2			
Incision and drainage for subphrenic abscess	1				†1

Diseases of Stomach.—TOTAL, 27; DEATHS, 8.

	Total.	Cured.	Improved.	Unimproved.	Died.
Ulcers of stomach	4	4			
Perforated gastric ulcer with serofibrinous peritonitis	1	1			
" " " " localized abscess	1	1			
Gastric ulcer with spastic ileus	1				1
" " and chronic appendicitis	1	1			
Peripyloritis, probably due to gastric ulcer	1	1			
Benign stenosis of pylorus	2	2			
" " " " and cholecystitis	1				1
" " " " " umbilical hernia	1				1
Lympho-sarcoma of stomach	1				1
Carcinoma of cardiac end of stomach	3		1		2
" " stomach	10	1	5	2	2

*Not operated.
‡One death recorded under appendicitis.
†Death recorded under appendicitis.

Operations on Stomach.—33 OPERATIONS, 9 DEATHS.

	Total	Cured	Improved	Unimproved	Died
Posterior retro-colic gastro-enterostomy, Murphy button	12	7	2		3
" ante-colic " " " "	4		3		1
Pylorectomy for benign stenosis of pylorus	1	1			
Gastrectomy, partial, for carcinoma of stomach	1	1			
Gastrostomy, Kader	8		4		4
Pyloroplasty, Finney	3	2			1
Gastrorrhaphy for perforated ulcer	1	1			
Laparotomy for inoperable carcinoma of stomach	2			2	
Incision and drainage for perigastric abscess	1	1			

Diseases of Intestine.—TOTAL, 13; DEATHS, 6.

	Total	Cured	Improved	Unimproved	Died
Large.—Volvulus of cecum and peritonitis	1				*1
Carcinoma of sigmoid	2				2
Papillary colitis	1		1		
Small.—Intussusception	3	2			1
Perforated typhoid ulcer	2	1			1
Acute lymphadenitis of mesenteric glands	1	1			
Sarcoma of	1				*1
Suspected intestinal obstruction	1	1			
Tumor of intestine	1			*1	

Operations on Intestine.—19 OPERATIONS, 5 DEATHS.

	Total	Cured	Improved	Unimproved	Died
Large.—Colostomy	3	1			§2
Ileo-sigmoidostomy for closure of artificial anus	1	1			
Sigmoidopexy for prolapse of rectum	1	1			
Resection of sigmoid for carcinoma	1				1
Laparotomy for inoperable carcinoma of sigmoid	1				1
Resection of ascending and transverse colon for gangrenous intussusception	1				1
Closure of fecal fistula	1	1			
Resection of transverse colon for injury of transverse meso-colon in gastrectomy operation	1	†1			
Small.—Laparotomy and reduction of intussusception	2	2			
Laparotomy and suture of perforated typhoid ulcer	2	1			1
Resection of intestine for fecal fistula, Murphy button	1	1			
Enteroenterostomy for viscious circle after gastroenterostomy	1	1			
Enterotomy for removal of Murphy button	1				‡1
Laparotomy for suspected intestinal obstruction	1	1			
" " lymphadenitis of mesenteric glands	1	1			

*Not operated.
§One death recorded under resection of sigmoid. One operation for carcinoma of rectum.
†Recorded under gastrectomy (partial).
‡Death recorded under anterior ante-colic gastroenterostomy.

Diseases of Appendix Vermiformis.—TOTAL, 106; DEATHS, 6.

	Total.	Cured.	Improved.	Unimproved.	Died.
Acute catarrhal appendicitis	4	4			
" appendicitis with abscess	7	7			
" catarrhal appendicitis with thrombosis of omentum	1	1			
" gangrenous and perforative appendicitis	33	32			1
" " appendicitis with thrombosis of mesentery	1	1			
" " perforative appendicitis and pyelophlebitis	1				1
" " " " with multiple abscess, subphrenic abscess and pleural empyema	1				1
Acute gangrenous perforative appendicitis with multiple abscesses	1	1			
Acute gangrenous appendicitis with diffuse purulent peritonitis	11	9			2
" " " " " sero-purulent peritonitis	4	4			
Empyema of appendix	2	2			
" and diverticulum of appendix	1	1			
Subacute catarrhal appendicitis	5	3		*2	
Chronic appendicitis	34	32		*1	1

Operations for Appendicitis.—121 OPERATIONS, 6 DEATHS.

	Total.	Cured.	Improved.	Unimproved.	Died.
Appendicectomy for acute catarrhal appendicitis	3	3			
" " chronic appendicitis	54	52			†2
" " subacute catarrhal appendicitis	2	2			
" " acute empyema of appendix	2	2			
" " gangrenous appendicitis	4	4			
" and drainage for acute appendicitis and abscess	5	5			
" " " " " gangrenous or perforative appendicitis	31	29			2
" " " " chronic appendicitis	1	1			
" " " " acute gangrenous or perforative appendicitis with diffuse purulent peritonitis	11	9			2
" " " " acute gangrenous or perforative appendicitis with diffuse sero-purulent peritonitis	3	3			
" " " " acute gangrenous appendicitis and pyelophlebitis	1				1
" " " " empyema and diverticulum of appendix	1	1			

Diseases of Liver.—TOTAL. 3; DIED, 1.

	Total.	Cured.	Improved.	Unimproved.	Died.
Liver abscess, multiple abscesses	1				1
" " amebic	2	1	1		

*Refused operation.
†One death recorded under resection of colon. One death from peritonitis following inadequate ligature of appendix.

Diseases of Pancreas.—TOTAL, 2; DEATHS, 1.

	Total	Cured	Improved	Unimproved	Died
Chronic pancreatitis and cholangitis	1	1			
Carcinoma of head of pancreas and obstruction of common duct	1				1

Operations on Liver.—3 OPERATIONS, 1 DEATH.

	Total	Cured	Improved	Unimproved	Died
Transpleural hepatotomy and drainage for liver abscess	1				1
" " " " " amebic liver abscess	2	1	1		

Operations on Pancreas.—1 OPERATION, 1 DEATH.

	Total	Cured	Improved	Unimproved	Died
Laparotomy for carcinoma of pancreas	1				1

Diseases of Gall Bladder and Bile Ducts.

TOTAL, 25; DEATHS, 5.

	Total	Cured	Improved	Unimproved	Died
Cholecystitis	7	2		*5	
" cholelithiasis, calculi in gall bladder, empyema of appendix	1	1			
" calculi in gall bladder and cystic duct	2	2			
" carcinoma of gall bladder, calculi in gall bladder and cystic duct	1				1
Empyema of gall bladder, cholelithiasis, calculi in gall bladder and cystic duct	2	2			
Cholecystitis, cholelithiasis, calculi in gall bladder, cystic and common duct	2	1			1
Cholecystitis, cholelithiasis, calculi in gall bladder, cystic duct, common and hepatic ducts	1	1			
Cholecystitis, cholelithiasis and calculi in common duct	1			†1	
Acute gangrenous cholecystitis, bact. ærogenes capsulatus	1				1
" " " cholelithiasis, calculi in gall bladder and cystic duct	3	2			1
Persistent biliary fistula following cholecystostomy	1	1			
Cholecystitis and chronic pancreatitis	1	1			
Acute septic cholangitis	1	1			
Cholecystitis, cholangitis, pyelophlebitis	1				1

Operations on Gall Bladder.—19 OPERATIONS, 4 DEATHS.

	Total	Cured	Improved	Unimproved	Died
Cholecystectomy	12	7		1	‡5
Cholecystostomy	4	4			
Cholecystectomy and Choledochotomy	2	2			
Secondary cholecystectomy	1	1			

*Not operated.   †Not operated on account of cardiac.
‡One death recorded under Finney pyloroplasty.

Diseases of Female Genitals.—TOTAL, 28; DEATHS, 1.

	Total.	Cured.	Improved.	Unimproved.	Died.
Fibroid uterus	4	4			
Prolapse of uterus	1			*1	
Retroflexion of uterus	2	2			
Carcinoma of bladder and fibroid uterus	1		1		
Ovarian cyst	3	3			
Twisted ovarian dermoid cyst and chronic appendicitis	1	1			
Carcinoma of ovary	2		2		
Sarco-carcinoma of ovary	1		1		
Tubal pregnancy	1	1			
Bilateral pyosalpinx	2	2			
Pyosalpinx and appendicitis	4	4			
" " ventral hernia	1	1			
Hydatidiform degeneration of chorion	1	1			
Lacerated cervix	1	1			
Rectocele and cystocele	1	1			
Traumatic laceration of rectovaginal septum	1	1			
Carcinoma vulvæ	1				†1

Operations on Female Genitals.—30 OPERATIONS, 1 DEATH.

	Total	Cured	Improved	Unimproved	Died
Salpingo-oöphorectomy for pyosalpinx	4	4			
" " " ruptured ectopic gestation	1	1			
" " " sarco-carcinoma of ovary	1		1		
" " " twisted dermoid cyst	1	1			
" " " ovarian cyst	3	3			
Double salpingo-oöphorectomy for metastatic carcinoma of ovaries	2	2			
" " " " diseased appendages	2	2			
Hystero-salpingo-oöphorectomy for fibroid uterus and diseased appendages	4	4			
Hysterectomy for fibroid uterus with suprapubic cystotomy for carcinoma of bladder	1	1			
Hystero-salpingo-oöphorectomy for double diseased appendages	1	1			
Trachelorrhaphy	1	1			
Anterior and posterior colporrhaphy	1	1			
Perineorrhaphy	1	1			
Ventral fixation for retroflexion	1	1			
Alexander for retroflexion	1	1			
Curettage of uterus	3	3			
Myomectomy	1	1			
Excision of labia minora for carcinoma	1				1

Diseases of Abdominal Wall.—TOTAL, 7; DEATHS, 1.

	Total	Cured	Improved	Unimproved	Died
Intramural abscess	2	2			
Fat necrosis	1	1			
Myxofibroma	1	1			

*Not operated. †Myocarditis diabetes.

Diseases of Abdominal Walls—*Continued.*

	Total.	Cured.	Improved.	Unimproved.	Died.
Abscess surrounding urachus	1	1			
Recurrent carcinoma	1			*1	
Retroperitoneal sarcoma	1				1

Operations on Abdominal Wall.—5 OPERATIONS, 1 DEATH.

Incision and drainage of intramural abscess	3	3			
Extirpation of myxofibroma of abdominal wall	1	1			
Exploratory incision for retroperitoneal sarcoma	1				1

Hernia.—TOTAL, 68; DEATH, 4.

Inguinal	30	30			
" and varicocele	1	1			
" " hydrocele of canal of Nuck	1	1			
" " undescended testicle	3	3			
" superficial, Kuester	1	1			
" double	9	9			
" " and chronic appendicitis	1	1			
" and femoral hernia with varicocele	1	1			
" strangulated	10	9			1
Femoral	2	2			
" strangulated	3	2			1
Ventral hernia	3	2		*1	
" traumatic	1	1			
" strangulated	1				1
Umbilical, strangulated	1				1

Operations for Hernia.—80 OPERATIONS, 4 DEATHS.

Inguinal Hernia.—Radical operation, Bassini, for inguinal hernia†	54	54			
Radical operation, Halstead, for inguinal hernia	4	4			
Herniotomy and radical cure, Bassini, for strangulated inguinal hernia	9	8			1
Herniotomy for strangulated inguinal hernia	1	1			
Femoral Hernia.—Radical operation, Bassini, for femoral hernia	1	1			
Radical operation, Lenhard, for femoral hernia	1	1			
Herniotomy and radical operation, Bassini, for strangulated femoral hernia	1	1			
Herniotomy and radical operation, Lenhard, for strangulated femoral hernia	1	1			
Herniotomy for strangulated femoral hernia	1				1
Umbilical Hernia.—Radical operation for umbilical hernia	1	1			
Herniotomy for strangulated umbilical hernia	1				1

*Not operated.
†10 operations bilateral.

Operations for Hernia—*Continued.*

	Total.	Cured.	Improved.	Unimproved.	Died.
Ventral Hernia.—Radical operation for ventral hernia	3	3			
Herniotomy for strangulated ventral hernia	1				1
Extirpation of hydrocele of canal of Nuck	1	1			

Diseases of Kidney and Ureter.—TOTAL, 27; DEATHS, 4.

	Total.	Cured.	Improved.	Unimproved.	Died.
Hydronephrosis	1	1			
Intermittent hydronephrosis due to kinking of ureter and nephroptosis	1	1			
Hydronephrosis due to congenitally narrow ureter	1	1			
Pyonephrosis	3	2		*1	
Double pyonephrosis	1			*1	
Pyelonephritis	1	1			
Pyonephrosis, perinephritic and subphrenic abscess	1	1			
Calculous pyonephrosis	3	1	1		1
Renal colic	1	1			
" calculus	2			*1	1
Tuberculous kidney	1		*1		
Movable kidney	2	1		*1	
" parovarian cyst	1	1			
Cystic adenoma of kidney	1				1
Chronic nephritis, decapsulation	1				1
Perinephritic abscess	2	2			
Stricture of ureter	1	1			
Purulent ureteritis due to stricture	1		1		
Calculus in ureter	1	1			
Calculous anuria, calculi in both ureters	1	1			

Operations on Kidney and Ureter.—28 OPERATIONS, 4 DEATHS.

	Total.	Cured.	Improved.	Unimproved.	Died.
Nephrectomy	10	8			2
Nephropexy	3	3			
Nephrotomy, double	1	1			
" for renal calculus	1	1			
Incision and drainage of perinephric abscess	5	5			
Nephrolithotomy	1				1
Ureterectomy	2	2			
" sacral route	1	1			
Ureterotomy for calculus	2	2			
Uretero-lisathorsis	1	1			
Decortication of kidney	1				1

Diseases of Perineum and Male Genitals.
TOTAL, 105; DEATHS, 1.

	Total.	Cured.	Improved.	Unimproved.	Died.
Carcinoma of bladder	2		1	1	
Vesical calculus	1	1			

*Not operated.

Diseases of Perineum and Male Genitals—*Continued*.

	Total	Cured	Improved	Unimproved	Died
Hypertrophied prostate	4	3	*1		
Prostatic abscess	1	1			
Stricture urethra	1	1			
Urethral fistula	1	1			
" sepsis	1	1			
Tuberculous testicle	1	1			
" " bilateral	1	1			
Gumma of testicle	1	1			
Sarcoma "	1	1			
Gonorrheal epididymo-orchitis	1		*1		
Hydrocele	2	2			
Carcinoma of rectum	4	2		*1	1
Incontinence of rectum after extirpation	1	1			
Prolapse of rectum	2	1		*1	
Ulcer " "	2	1		*1	
Hemorrhoids	45	43		*2	
" and fistula in ano	5	5			
" " ischio-rectal abscess	2	2			
Fistula in ano	15	13		*2	
Ischio-rectal abscess	8	8			
Fissure of anus	1	1			
Eczema of perineum	2	1		*1	

Operations on Male Genitals and Perineum.

117 OPERATIONS, 0 DEATHS.

	Total	Cured	Improved	Unimproved	Died
Orchidectomy for tuberculous testicle	1	1			
" " gumma	1	1			
" " sarcoma	1	1			
" " undescended testicle	1	1			
Orchidopexy " " "	3	3			
Suprapubic cystotomy, exploratory	3	2		1	
" " for carcinoma of bladder	1		1		
" " and division of prostatic obstruction with cautery	1	1			
Winkelman operation for hydrocele	3	3			
Volkman " " "	1	1			
Incision and drainage of ischio-rectal abscess	10	10			
Cauterization of fissure in ano	2	2			
Excision of fistula in ano	4	4			
Incision and curettage of fistula in ano	15	15			
Cauterization of ulcer of rectum	3	3			
Ligature operation for hemorrhoids	2	2			
Clamp and cautery for hemorrhoids	54	54			
Excision of rectum for carcinoma	1	1			
Gersuny operation for incontinence after resection of rectum	1	1			

*Not operated.

Operations on Male Genitals and Perineum—*Continued.*

	Total.	Cured.	Improved.	Unimproved.	Died.
External and internal urethrotomy	2	2			
Plastic for defect of perineal urethra	1	1			
Perineal prostatectomy	2	2			
Litholopaxy	1	1			
Incision and drainage of pelvic abscess	1	1			
" " " " prostatic abscess	1	1			
" " " " tuberculous epididymitis	1	1			

Diseases of Upper Extremity.—TOTAL, 28; DEATHS, 1.

	Total.	Cured.	Improved.	Unimproved.	Died.
Shoulder Joint.—Dislocation of	1	*1			
Tuberculosis of	1	1			
Clavicle.—Fracture of	1	*1			
Scapula.—Sarcoma	1	1			
Axilla.—Recurrent carcinoma of	1	1			
Lymphadenitis, suppurative	2	2			
"	1	1			
Traumatic division of bronchial plexus	1		1		
Humerus.—Tumor of head	1			*1	
Fracture of	1	*1			
Osteomyelitis of, acute	1		1		
" " chronic	2	1			1
Humerus, Radius and Ulna.—Fracture of	1	*1			
Forearm.—Recurrent myxofibroma of	1	1			
Traumatic aneurysm of radial artery	1	1			
Ulcer	1	1			
Radius.—Fracture of, Colles	1	*1			
Osteomyelitis, acute	3	2	1		
Hand.—Tuberculosis of extensor tendons	1	1			
Phlegmon	1	1			
Fingers.—Cicatricial web	1	1			
Diabetic gangrene of	1	1			
Wound of flexors	1	1			
Phlegmon	1	1			

Operations on Upper Extremity.—25 OPERATIONS, 1 DEATH.

	Total.	Cured.	Improved.	Unimproved.	Died.
Osteotomy and drainage for osteomyelitis of humerus	4	3			1
" " " " " " radius	3	2	1		
Amputation of finger for diabetic gangrene	1	1			
Resection of shoulder joint for tuberculosis	1	1			
Reduction of dislocation of shoulder joint	1	1			
Extirpation of scapula for sarcoma	1	1			
" " tuberculous axillary glands	2	2			
Secondary operation for carcinomatous axillary glands	1	1			
Incision and drainage of axillary abscess	2	2			
Extirpation of recurrent myxofibroma of forearm	1	1			

*Not operated.

Operations on Upper Extremity—*Continued.*

	Total	Cured	Improved	Unimproved	Died
Extirpation of traumatic aneurysm of ulna artery	1	1			
Excision of ulcer of forearm	1	1			
Extirpation of extensor tendon sheaths for tuberculosis	1	1			
Incision and drainage of phlegmon of hand	2	2			
Plastic operation for cicatricial web fingers	1	1			
Tenoplastic for divided flexor tendons	1	1			
Nerve anastimosis for traumatic division of brachial plexus	1		1		

Diseases of Lower Extremity.—TOTAL, 81; DEATHS, 7.

	Total	Cured	Improved	Unimproved	Died
Contractures after anterior poliomyelitis	1	1			
Groin.—Inguinal adenitis	1	1			
Femoral adenitis	1	1			
Inguinal and femoral adenitis	1	1			
Hip Joint.—Tuberculosis of	1			*1	
Thigh.—Infected hematoma	1	1			
Metastatic sarcoma	1			*1	
Femur.—Acute osteomyelitis	2				2
Fracture.—Of neck	4	*1	*2		*1
Mal-united of middle third	1			1	
Of middle third	1	*1			
Of lower third	1	*1			
Posterior dislocation of	1	*1			
Patella.—Ununited fracture of	1	1			
Knee Joint.—Prepatella bursitis	1	1			
Acute suppuration of	3	3			
Tuberculosis of	2	2			
Lipochondroma	1	1			
Floating cartilage	1	*1			
Traumatic arthritis	1		*1		
Contracture	1		*1		
Bow legs	1			*1	
Ankylosis	1	1			
Tibia.—Osteomyelitis, acute	5	3	1		1
Chronic	4	4			
Fibula.—Osteomyelitis, acute	1	1			
Subacute	1	1			
Tibia and Fibula.—Gumma	2	1		*1	
Fracture, Potts	1	*1			
Leg.—Phlegmon	1	1			
Ulcer	4	*2	*1	*1	
" syphilitic	1		*1		
" sepsis	1				*1
Gumma	1	1			
Gangrene, diabetic	1				1
Hematoma	1	*1			

*Not operated.

Diseases of Lower Extremity—*Continued*.	Total	Cured	Improved	Unimproved	Died
Ankle Joint.—Suppurative arthritis	1	1			
Tuberculosis	1	1			
Sprain of	1	*1			
Foot.—Phlegmon	2	2			
Perforated ulcer	1	1			
Gangrene, arteriosclerotic	2			*2	
Wounds, contused and lacerated	4	3			1
Leg and Foot.—Gangrene, embolic	1	1			
Erythromelalgia	1			*1	
Veins.—Varicose	3	2		*1	
Thrombophlebitis	3	3			
Arteries.—Popliteal aneurysm	1	1			
Toe.—Phlegmon	2	2			
Gangrene, arteriosclerotic	2		*1	*1	
Gangrene, diabetic	1			*1	
Lacerated wound	1			*1	

Operations on Lower Extremity.—58 OPERATIONS, 5 DEATHS.

	Total	Cured	Improved	Unimproved	Died
Osteotomy and drainage for osteomyelitis of femur	2				2
" " " Neuber, for osteomyelitis of tibia	5	4	1		
" " " for osteomyelitis of tibia	7	6			1
" " " Bier, for osteomyelitis of tibia	1	1			
Mayo operation for pyarthrosis of knee joint	2	2			
Refracture of femur for mal-union	1	1			
Suture of patella for ununited fracture	1	1			
Resection of knee joint	2	2			
Amputation of thigh	2	2			
Resection of knee joint for contracture	1	1			
Osteoplastic operation for viscious union of tibia and fibula following pathological fracture	1	1			
Amputation of leg	2	2			
Osteoplastic amputation of foot for trauma	1	1			
Amputation of toes for trauma	1				1
" " big toe	2	2			
Arthrodasis of knee joint for deformity	1	1			
" " ankle " "	1	1			
Extirpation of inguinal glands	2	2			
" " femoral "	1	1			
" " prepatellar bursa	1	1			
" " lipochondroma of knee joint	1	1			
" " gumma of leg	1	1			
Exarticulation at knee joint for diabetic gangrene	1				1
Incision and drainage of abscess of thigh	1	1			
" " " " " foot	1	1			
" " " " phlegmon of leg	4	4			
" " " " " foot	2	2			

*Not operated.

Operations on Lower Extremity—*Continued*.

	Total	Cured	Improved	Unimproved	Died
Incision and drainage for perforating ulcer of foot	1	1			
Curetting of ulcer of leg	1	1			
Plastic operation on foot for traumatic defect	1	1			
Skin graft	1	1			
Excision of varicose veins	4	4			
Ligature of femoral artery for popliteal aneurysm	1	1			

Diseases of Pelvis and Spine.—TOTAL, 7; DEATHS, 0.

	Total	Cured	Improved	Unimproved	Died
Contusion of spine	1	*1			
Tuberculosis of spine	1			*1	
" " sacrum	1		*1		
Spina bifida, sacral meningocele	1	1			
Osteomyelitis of pelvis	1	1			
Tuberculosis " "	1			1	
Sarcoma " "	1			*1	

Operations on Pelvis and Spine.—3 OPERATIONS, 0 DEATHS.

	Total	Cured	Improved	Unimproved	Died
Extirpation of meningocele and plastic for spina bifida	1	1			
Incision and drainage of pelvic abscess	1	1			
" " " for tuberculosis of pelvis, repeated operations	1			1	

Unclassified Diseases.—TOTAL, 21; DEATHS, 1.

	Total	Cured	Improved	Unimproved	Died
Extensive burns of trunk and extremities	1	*1			
Acute enteritis	2	*2			
" gastritis	1	*1			
Nephritis	1		*1		
Colitis	1			1	
Constipation	2	*2			
Hodgkin's disease	2	1		*1	
Furunculosis	1			*1	
Multiple abscesses of skin	2	1			1
Coprostasis	1	*1			
Erysipelas	1			*1	
Influenza	1	*1			
Neurasthenia	1		*1		
Pneumonia	1			*1	
Climacteric symptoms	1			*1	
Chronic plumbism	1	*1			
Probable tuberculosis of ileum	1			*1	

Operations on Unclassified Diseases.—2 OPERATIONS, 1 DEATH.

	Total	Cured	Improved	Unimproved	Died
Incision and drainage of multiple abscesses	2	1			1

*Not operated.

ACCIDENT SERVICE.

600 Cases,* December 1, 1903–December 1, 1904.

Head and Neck.—210 cases.

Wounds.—Scalp wounds	86
Lacerated wound of face	43
Incised wound	9
Lacerated wound of tongue	2
" " " ear	1
Blank cartridge wound of face	5
Contusions.—Of eye	7
Of nose	1
Foreign Body.—In eyes	22
In eyes and burn of cornea	2
" nose	5
" throat	3
" ear	2
Fractures.—Inferior maxilla	1
Nasal bone	3
Malar "	1
Superior maxilla	1
Compound fracture of nasal bones	1
Abscess of face	1
Alveola abscess	2
Burns of neck	3
Frostbite, ears	1
Hematoma of scalp	1
Epistaxis	2
Toothache	1
Acute otitis media	1
Conjunctivitis	1
Tongue tie	1
Dog bite of face	1

Upper Extremity.—294 cases.

Wounds.—Lacerated wound of wrist	6
Lacerated wound of hand	27
Phlegmon of finger	32
Incised wound of finger	13
Lacerated " " "	64
Cellulitis of arm	11
Contusion of hand	30
Blank cartridge wound of hand	11
Lacerated wound of axilla	1
Contusion of shoulder	3
" " wrist	7

*This includes both Surgical Divisions.

Upper Extremity—*Continued.*

Burns.—Burn of hand	17
Burn of arm and shoulders	1
Dislocation.—Finger	1
Shoulder	3
Elbow joint	3
Fracture.—Fracture of shaft of radius	3
Colles fracture	13
Clavicle	6
Olecranon	2
Finger, compound	2
Radius and ulna	4
Internal condyle of humerus	2
Neck of humerus	1
Metacarpal bone	2
Foreign Body.—In finger	5
In hand	13
Dog bite of hand	13
Sprained elbow	2
Separation of epiphysis of lower end of radius	1
Mosquito bite	2
Abscess in axilla	1

Lower Extremity.—70 CASES.

Fracture.—Malleolus of tibia	1
Internal condyle of femur	1
Patella	2
Middle third of tibia	3
Tibia and fibula	1
Third metatarsal	1
Foot	1
Sprain.—Ankle	5
Knee joint	5
Wound.—Lacerated wound, toe	3
Crushed foot	5
Infected wound of foot	15
Ulcer of foot	2
Lacerated wound on lower leg	6
Foreign Body.—In knee joint	1
Burn of foot	6
Traumatic effusion into knee joint	1
Contusion of leg	9
Ingrowing toe nail	1
Hydrops of knee	1

Chest.—6 CASES.

Fracture of ribs	2
Pleurisy	1
Lacerated wound of chest wall	1
Burn of chest	1
Contusion of chest	1

Miscellaneous.—20 cases.

Erythema bullosa	1
Rheumatism	1
Rat bites	2
Retention of urine	8
Carbolic acid burn	1
Abdominal cramps	1
Ring worm	1
Acute gastritis	1
Ischio-rectal abscess	1
Lacerated wound of base of penis	1
Arsenic poisoning	1
Coal-gas poisoning	1

First Surgical Division.

December 1, 1903–December 1, 1904.

Anesthesias.—594.

Gas and ether	476
Chloroform	60
N_2O	20
Gas and ether to chloroform	8
Chloroform to gas and ether	4
Local to ether	2
Local, eucaine, Schleich	24

REPORT ON THE DISEASES OF THE KIDNEY AND URETER FOR 1903-1904.

TREATED IN THE FIRST SURGICAL DIVISION.

By Arpad G. Gerster, M.D.,
ATTENDING SURGEON.

```
Patients ................................................. 43
   "   operated on  .................................... 28
   "   not   "   "  .................................... 15
```

	Total.	Cured.	Improved.	Unimproved.	Died.
Ren mobilis	3	2	..	1	..
Chronic nephritis	2	..	1	..	1
Nephralgia	2	1	..	1	..
Hydronephrosis*	3	3	..	..	..
Nephrolithiasis	4	..	2	1	1
Ureteral lithiasis†	3	3	..	..	..
Calculus hydronephrosis and atrophy of other kidney	1	..	..	..	1
" pyelonephritis	1	1	..	..	..
" pyonephrosis	3	3	..	..	..
Pyonephrosis	7	5	..	2	..
Pyelonephritis	2	..	1	..	1
Tuberculosis of kidney	5	..	1	3	1
Tumor of kidney (unoperated)	1	..	..	1	..
Congenital cystic adenoma	1	..	..	..	1
Metastatic suppurative infarction of kidney	1	1	..	..	..
Stricture of ureter	1	1	..	..	..
Chronic suppurative ureteritis and stricture	1	1	..	..	..
Perinephritic abscess	2	2	..	..	..

*One patient subsequently contracted tuberculous pyonephrosis.
†One case calculi in both ureters

OPERATIONS ON THE KIDNEY AND URETER FOR 1903-1904.

35 operations on 28 patients; 6 deaths.

	Total.	Cured.	Improved.	Unimproved.	Died.
Nephropexy	2	2			
Nephrotomy, single, for anuria combined with nephrectomy of opposite atrophic kidney	1				1
Nephrotomy, double, for anuria	2	1			1
" " for calculus*	4	3			1
" " pyonephrosis	1	1			
Nephrectomy for hydronephrosis	2	2			
" " suppurating kidney	10	9			1
" " congenital cystic adenoma	1				1
" " metastatic infarction	1	1			
Suprapubic cystotomy and dilatation of ureter for stricture	1	1			
Ureterolysorthosis	1	1			
Ureterolithotomy, double	1	1			
Ureterectomy	1	1			
Parasacral exploration of ureteral stump	1	1			
Decapsulation of kidney	1				1
Incision and drainage of perinephritic abscess	2	2			

GENERAL REMARKS.

Before entering upon the recital of the histories of our cases, we may render an account of the routine measures adopted for arriving at diagnosis, and for the shaping of a safe indication.

During the time embraced by this report every patient admitted for a disorder of the urinary apparatus is methodically subjected to cystoscopy and catheterism of the ureters. The urines, separately collected from each ureter, are submitted to chemical and miscroscopical analysis, and their freezing point is determined. In addition the freezing point of the blood is ascertained.

Expanded experience has tended to heighten our appreciation of the great value of cystoscopy and of the analysis of the separated urines. But cryoscopy has been found valuable only as an additional aid in the estimation of the resistance of the patient to operative measures, when supported by other important clinical facts.

A more detailed report on cryoscopy will subsequently be published.

*In one case litholapaxy was done subsequently for vesical calculus, with success.

1902-1903, vol. iii., page 369. *Movable kidney; nephropexy; cure.*—Hannah F., æt. 23, symptoms of six months' standing. Nephropexy with chromic gut sutures. July 27, 1902. Discharged cured August 26.

1903-1904, vol. iii., page 385. *Movable kidney; nephropexy; cure.*—Minnie R., æt. 24, symptoms of 14 months' standing. Operation January 22, 1903. Discharged cured February 20.

1902-1903, vol. iv., page 377. *Left hydronephrosis; calculus; atrophy of right kidney; uremia; left nephrotomy; right nephrectomy; death.*—Fanny I., æt. 26, admitted September 5, 1903. Forty-eight hours before was suddenly taken with agonizing pain in left lumbar region. Passed no urine within the last twenty-four hours, nor did the catheter draw any urine. On admission internal organs were found normal. Rigidity of left half of abdominal wall. A smooth, rounded, tender mass was felt in left hypochondriac and lumbar region. Bladder empty. General condition bad, anxious face. Pulse, 110, good; temperature, 99°. Immediate nephrotomy of left side. Renal pelvis dilated and contained stones. Parenchyma thinned, containing a number of cysts. Stones removed. Drainage. Reacted well, but within the subsequent days the general condition and pulse deteriorated, while the secretion of urine, comprising thirteen ounces on September 6, amounted on September 7 to seven ounces, while on September 9 there was complete anuria. At the same time symptoms of increasing uremia manifesting themselves, so that on September 9 the right kidney was exposed. After considerable search a small, round, soft mass, about 2 inches long and 1 inch wide, and connected with the ureter, was identified as the remnant of the right kidney. This was extirpated. Uremia was relieved, sufficient quantities of urine escaping through the external wound, and were withdrawn by catheter. But, unfortunately both wounds became infected, extensive necrosis of the tissues followed, sepsis causing the death of the patient on September 22.

1903-1904, vol. iii., page 393. *Bilateral ureteral calculi; bilateral hydronephrosis; suppression of urine; double nephrotomy; suprapubic cystotomy; bilateral ureteric lithotomy; cure.*—Morris L., æt. 48, bookmaker, admitted November 25, 1903. During five years past had attacks of kidney colic on right side. Noticed small stones in his urine. Nine days before admission had a severe, sudden pain in left lumbar region. Since three days before admission passed no urine whatever. On admission examination showed a well nourished body, urinous odor of breath, internal organs normal; pulse, 100, of good quality; temperature, 99°. Catheterism produced no urine. Immediate double nephrotomy. On the left side a dilated pelvis, and no stones were found. About 7 inches from the pelvis an obstruction was met in the ureter. On the right side hydronephrosis was well marked. The ureter was obstructed six inches below the pelvis of the kidney. Drainage of both kidneys. The following morning the dressings contained abundant urine and from then on the renal function was unimpaired, all the urine escaping through the wounds. The patient did very well. December 30, 1903, cystoscopy revealed normal bladder, normal right ureteral orifice, and from the mouth of the left ureter a small whitish mass of the size of a pea was seen to protrude. January 4, 1904: Suprapubic cystotomy being done, no stone was found where the cystoscope had indicated its presence. An incision similar to the one employed for exposure of the common iliac artery exposed the right ureter, and the calculus was found within it at the brim of the pelvis. The ureter being incised, a calculus ¾ of an inch long was extracted. Catgut suture of the ureter, drainage and closure of the external wound followed. The operation was borne very well. January 5: Twice voided two ounces of urine each time. January 18: By a similar procedure, a stone about one-half inch long was removed from the left ureter. Within a few days he voided spontaneously increasing quantities of urine. January 27: He passed 21 ounces by urethra. As the lumbar wounds closed, he passed all the urine by the normal channel. Discharged cured February 8, 1904.

1902-1903, vol. iv., page 392. *Double tuberculous pyonephrosis; uremia; double nephrotomy; death.*—Mollie W., æt. 21, admitted June 25, 1903, had been entirely well up to her second confinement six weeks before. She then began to be troubled with frequent urination, vulvar pain, chills and fever, vomited occasionally, and had lost much strength and flesh. During the past week drowsiness and hiccoughs set in. On admission the general condition was poor, respiration stertorous, pupils widely dilated, internal organs normal, abdominal walls very rigid, marked pain and tenderness in left hypochondriac and lumbar region, where a tumor was to be felt. Some tenderness in right lumbar region. Vaginally, ureters could be felt to be much thickened. Catheter withdrew no urine from bladder. Pulse, 120; temperature, 100°. The diagnosis of bilateral pyelonephritis and uremia was made. Six hours after admission both kidneys were incised and drained. They were much enlarged, the pelvis dilated, containing small quantities of purulent urine. The cortices studded with numerous abscesses. June 26: General condition unimproved. Two ounces of turbid, bloody urine withdrawn by catheter. After this no more urine descended to the bladder, though the lumbar dressing appeared to be moist. June 27: Coma, followed by convulsions. June 28: Death.

Autopsy.—Both kidneys the seat of marked cheesy tuberculosis, likewise both ureters.

1902-1903, vol. iv., page 397. *Nephrolithiasis; nephrolithotomy; cure.*—Daniel D., æt. 47, admitted July 15, 1903. Had had attack of renal colic on the left side the past fifteen years, the last one twelve days before admission. No constitutional symptoms were present. *On admission:* General condition good; internal organs normal, pulse and temperature normal; urine normal, except that it contained a few pus cells. Urea, 1½ per cent. July 17: Nephrolithotomy and suture of kidney. Two small stones were extracted from the ureter, where, two inches below the renal pelvis, they were found impacted. August 11: Discharged cured.

1902-1903, vol. iv., page 398. *Multiple ureteral calculi; vesical calculus; nephrolithotomy; litholapaxy; cure.*—Morris T., æt. 31, admitted July 15, 1903. For the past three and a half years had attacks of renal colic on left side. Passed three calculi, since when the colics had ceased. Three days before admission began to feel colicky pain in right side, which was present on admission. General condition good, internal organs normal, abdominal walls rigid, marked tenderness in right iliac and lumbar regions. Cystoscopy revealed a stone in the bladder. Both ureteral orifices normal, and catheters could be passed up to the renal pelvis. The catheter withdrawn from the right side, brought away phosphatic debris lodged in its eye. Combined urine alkaline, 1020; trace of albumin, numerous pus and red blood cells; 1.3 per cent. of urea. Urine from right kidney acid, contained pus and a few red blood cells, and 1.3 per cent. of urea. July 20: Nephrolithotomy. The renal pelvis and upper segment of ureter were impacted with a large number of small phosphatic calculi. In the extraction of the ureteral calculi the pelvis was slightly rent, and the rent immediately sutured. Drainage. August 15: Litholapaxy under cocaine. September 2: Discharged cured.

1903-1904, vol. iii., page 383. *Nephrolithiasis; (coronary endarteritis); nephrolithotomy; death.*—Alfred A., æt. 61, admitted October 9, 1904. For one year had suffered from renal colic of right side. Had had three attacks of hematuria. On admission: A short, stout body, fairly well nourished; pulse and temperature normal; internal organs, including the physical appearances of the heart, normal; urine abundant, and practically normal. Considering these findings a favorable prognosis was made. October 10: Nephrolithotomy. A small triangular-shaped stone was removed from the pelvis. For five days after the operation the patient was doing apparently well, passing large quantities of bloody urine containing hyaline and granular casts; his temperature not rising above 100.6°, and the highest pulse being 94. October 15: Abdomen became much distended, though not painful. Gases were easily expelled in large quantities. Hiccoughing set in. Bowels were easily moved by laxatives and enemata. The pulse became progressively more rapid and feeble, and the patient somnolent. The wound was healthy. October 17: Distention very marked, extremities cold and cyanosed; pulse thready, 120-130; somnolency more pronounced. Died under symptoms of heart failure. Autopsy.

1903-1904, vol. iii., page 369. *Hydronephrosis; nephrectomy; cure.*—Betsie K., æt. 19, admitted November 2, 1903. Present illness, similar to another attack six months ago, was of two weeks' duration. Had pain in right side and back, chilly feelings and nausea. On admission: General condition good, internal organs normal. In right flank large, movable, smooth, tender mass. Urine contained a faint trace of albumin, was otherwise normal. Temperature and pulse normal. November 6, 1903: Exploration revealed an enormously distended kidney and pelvis, there being hardly any trace of parenchyma. Removal of the organ. Uninterrupted recovery. December 12: Discharged cured.

1903-1904, vol. iii., page 371. *Hydronephrosis with congenitally narrow ureter; nephrectomy; cure.*—Sarah S., æt. 25, admitted March 30, 1904. Illness of two to three years' duration, with weekly attacks of headache, nausea and constipation. On admission: General condition good, internal organs normal, right kidney palpable. Temperature, 103°; pulse, 120. Urine normal. April 2: Exploration revealed enlarged kidney, much distended pelvis, the ureter exceedingly small. Cortex very thin, here and there cystic. As the smallness of the ureter precluded any plastic measure for attaining natural drainage, the kidney was removed. Uninterrupted recovery. April 26: Discharged cured.

1902-1903, vol. iii., page 374. *Calculus pyelonephritis; nephrectomy; cure.*—Jennie S., æt. 18, admitted December 20, 1902. For five years periodical pain in right loin. Urine cloudy, becoming clearer at rare intervals. During last two weeks fever, chills, frequent micturition, constant pain in right loin, with night sweats and loss of strength and weight. On admission: General condition fair. Temperature 101.6°; pulse, 84. Internal organs normal. In right loin a large rounded tumor, which was tender to pressure. Cystoscopy showed a large amount of pus issuing from right ureter. Urine: Acid, 1018, albumin, much pus. December 22, 1902: Nephrectomy. The kidney was much enlarged, pelvis distended by fluid, containing a large, rough, black calculus, and foul pus. Cortex one-half inch thick, whitish in appearance. No tubercle bacilli. Uninterrupted convalescence. January 17, 1903: Discharged cured.

1902-1903, vol. iv., page 378. *Acute ascending (gonorrheal?) pyo-*

nephrosis; nephrectomy; cure.—Albert B., æt. 23, admitted April 27, 1903. Had gonorrhea one and a half years ago. Four months before had an attack of grippe. Sudden onset of pain in right loin. Ever since gonorrhea had very frequent urination, night sweats, and had lost twenty-nine pounds. On admission: general condition good, internal organs normal, in right loin a non-movable, tender, rounded mass of uneven surface could be felt. Urine: Acid, 1028, albumin, pus abundant. Cystoscopy: Bladder normal, both ureteral orifices congested, clear urine descending from left ureter, masses of pus from the right one. Catheter passed easily into left ureter, but was arrested in right ureter one-half inch from bladder. Deep urethral stricture of large calibre. Left kidney discharged acid, albuminous urine, with one and a half per cent. of urea, pus cells and a few red blood cells. Right kidney yielded only pus. May 1, 1903: Nephrectomy. Kidney very large, lobulated, everywhere adherent. Its structure entirely disintegrated by numerous abscesses. Pelvis much dilated by pus. Ureter thickened, edematous, its lumen narrowed, its mucous lining hyperplastic and ulcerated. Uninterrupted recovery. May 31: Discharged cured.

1902-1903, Vol. iii., page 390. *Calculus pyonephrosis; nephrectomy; cure.*—Yetta C., æt. 35, admitted March 20, 1903. Illness of three months' duration. Acute onset with pain in right loin, radiating down along ureter. Urine turbid. Vomited frequently, had fever and chills and frequent urination. On admission: General condition fair, internal organs normal. The whole right side of abdomen rigid and tender; in the loin down to the crest of ilium a firm, nodular, tender mass, movable with respiration. Urine: Intermittently cloudy, containing traces of albumin, acid, 1031, and pus when cloudy. Diagnosis: Calculus pyonephrosis. March 23, 1903: Nephrectomy. Kidney large, cortex thick, pale and edematous, with small punctate, yellow foci; spreads from these foci showed pus, no bacteria. Pelvis and calices much dilated, containing gray fibrinous clots and a rough, brown stone. Uninterrupted recovery. May 4, 1903: Discharged cured.

1903-1904, Vol. iii., pages 370 and 373. *Intermittent hydronephrosis, due to kinking of ureter from periureteric adhesions; ureteral lysorthosis; cure. Tuberculosis of kidney; nephrectomy; cure.*—Sophie S., æt. 21, admitted December 30, 1903: had been operated upon two years ago for floating kidney. Since then had been entirely well until six months ago, when she commenced to have attacks of pain in the right loin, during which her urine was very scanty. As the attacks passed off the urine increased. Micturition frequent, urine clear, no cough. On admission: General condition fair, internal organs normal. During an attack of pain the right kidney became large. Cystoscopy showed a normal bladder, internal organs normal. Urine: From right kidney clear, acid, trace of albumin, a few pus cells, no tubercle bacilli, nine-tenths per cent. urea; from left kidney clear, acid, trace of albumin, few red blood and pus cells, urea seven-tenths per cent. January 1, 1904: Ureteral lysorthosis. Ureter dilated in its upper segment, tortuous and fixed by dense adhesions. Renal pelvis somewhat dilated; cortex appeared normal. Liberated ureter from adhesions, and sewed up outer wound. Tumor subsequently disappeared. February 9: Discharged cured. Readmitted, February 23, 1904: Since her discharge had suffered from constant lumbar pain, chills and fever, vomiting and very frequent urination. Right kidney again much enlarged, and very tender. Temperature, 104.2°; pulse, 140. Leucocyte count, 28,000. February 25: Aspiration of tumor yielded pus. Incision of perinephric abscess, drainage. Gradual improvement. March 5: Tubercle bacilli in urine. March 14: Nephrectomy: in upper pole of kidney abscess cavity, one inch in diameter. Uninterrupted recovery. April 19: Discharged cured.

1903-1904, Vol. iii., page 374. *Pyonephrosis; sympathetic inflammation of the opposite kidney; nephrectomy; cure.*—Esther S., æt. 25, admitted June 1, 1904. Illness of one year's duration. Suffered with continuous pain in left loin, cloudy urine and painful micturition. On admission: General condition poor, fairly well nourished; internal organs normal, left kidney enlarged and palpable; white bloodcell count, 25,800. Temperature 101.4°; pulse, 104. Combined urine: Acid, 1020, numerous pus cells. Cystoscopy: Right ureteral orifice dilated, left ureteral mouth plugged with pus, an ulcer on the vesical mucosa above and behind it. Urine, from right kidney: A few red bloodcells and hyaline casts. Its freezing point, 2.06; that of the blood, 0.61; urea of combined urine, 2.2 per cent. In spite of the low freezing index of the blood, it was decided to give the patient a chance for recovery by operation, because the other ascertained factors indicated a functional adequacy of the right kidney. June 4: Nephrectomy. Kidney was double the normal size, attached everywhere by adhesions, in the separation of which the kidney being ruptured, a large quantity of foul pus escaped. Recovery uninterrupted. July 14: Discharged cured.

1903-1904, Vol. iii., pages 376 and 392A. *Pyonephrosis; perinephric abscess; empyema of ureter; incision and drainage of perinephric abscess; nephrectomy; ureterectomy; fecal fistula; cure.*—Morris M., æt. 38, admitted July 29, 1903. Present illness began two months ago with severe sticking pains in right loin, chills, fever, sweating and constipation. On admission: Internal organs normal; no tumor could be felt in right loin, but he complained there of marked tenderness and pain. Urine: Acid, cloudy, with much pus; no tubercle bacilli.

Leucocyte count, 7,000. Temperature, 103.1°; pulse, 130. July 31: Incision and drainage of perinephric abscess. Suppuration of the abscess cavity diminished, but discharge became distinctly urinous, and pyuria continued unabated. September 10: Nephrectomy. Kidney lobulated, enlarged, pale; pelvis and calices much distended by pus; cortex extremely thin. The wound healed normally, but pyuria still continued. October 16: Cystoscopy revealed thick pus descending from right ureter. Left ureter appeared normal; considerable cystitis. October 19: Ureterectomy for empyema of ureter, which was found to be a thick-walled, elongated sac of the dimensions of a small intestine, filled with thick pus. Its extirpation offered great difficulty on account of intimate adhesions to the peritoneum and to the posterior wall of the ascending colon, demanding the constant use of the knife. The after treatment was complicated by considerable sloughing, as a consequence of which, on October 29, a colic fistula established itself. January 11, 1904, this fistula was closed by a plastic operation. General condition improved visibly after this, though intense cystitis persisted, and remained rebellious to every known form of treatment. February 9: Discharged improved (with cloudy urine). April 26: Readmitted on account of the cystitis. Cystoscopy demonstrated only a very intense cystitis. Under the assumption that a stump of the right ureter, left behind, might be the cause of the continued trouble, on May 2 the posterior surface of the bladder was exposed by the parasacral route. Careful exploration revealed that our assumption was unfounded. June 6: Discharged with unabated cystitis.

1903-1904, Vol. iii., page 377. *Pyonephrosis; nephrectomy: cure.*—Julia T., æt. 22, admitted February 6, 1904. Present illness of one month's duration, characterized by dull pain in right hypochondrium and loin, by frequent voiding of cloudy urine, night sweats, fever and loss of flesh. Before onset, had had paronychia of the thumb, which was looked upon as the primary focus of the infection. On admission: General condition fair, internal organs normal. In right loin an ovoid, smooth, hard and tender mass. Urine: Acid, 1020, trace of albumin, 2.5 per cent. urea, a few hyaline casts, some pus. Cystoscopy: Normal bladder, ureteral orifices normal, catheterism of both ureters easy. No urine obtained from right side; that from left kidney was acid, clear, had a trace of albumin and some hyalogranular casts. Its cryoscopic index was 1.7. February 8, 1904: Nephrectomy. The kidney was bathed in a perinephric abscess, its parenchyma totally disorganized by many abscesses, so that the organ had to be removed piecemeal. March 12: Discharged cured.

1903-1904, Vol. iii., page 378. *Calculus pyonephrosis; insufficiency of opposite kidney; nephrotomy; improvement of insufficiency; nephrectomy; cure. Readmission, four months later, in uremic coma;*

death.—Abraham L., æt. 61, admitted October 15, 1903. Present illness of three months' standing. Great frequency of and pain in urination, urine very cloudy. On admission: general condition poor, general arteriosclerosis, emphysema of lungs, liver large, heart slightly dilated. In left loin a large, tender, rough mass. Cystoscopy: Severe cystitis, preventing view of ureteral orifices. Urine: Acid, cloudy, 1018, much albumin, much pus. Urea, 1.9 per cent. Total of urea for twenty-four hours, 138 grains. October 26, 1903: Nephrotomy, removal of a large number of renal calculi and evacuation of much foul pus. On account of insufficient kidney action, nephrectomy was refrained from. Immediate improvement followed, the quantity of excreted urea rising, by November 18, to 483 grains, the quantity of daily urine having also doubled. The temperature, which had become normal after October 26, began to be febrile beginning from November 29, in consequence of which nephrectomy was done on December 4. This was followed by cessation of the fever. The parendyma of the kidney was atrophic, its pelvis and calices still containing a number of stones. He made an uninterrupted recovery, and was discharged with the wound healed on January 18, 1904, when his urine still contained traces of albumin and some hyaline casts, excreted urea being 411 grains. Four months later he was readmitted moribund, suffering from uremic coma, to which he succumbed two hours after admission.

1903-1904, Vol. iii., page 379. *Calculus pyonephrosis; nephrectomy; cure.*—Meyer K., æt. 21. Six months before admission, a vesical calculus had been removed in his case by suprapubic section at this hospital. Two weeks after his discharge, began to experience pain in left lumbar region. On admission, January 22, 1904: Internal organs normal. Cystoscopy: Pus descending from left ureter. Urine: Acid, cloudy, albumin, pus. Temperature and pulse normal. January 25: Nephrectomy. Kidney large, soft, large abscess in lower pole, pelvis filled with calculi. Discharged cured, February 17.

1903-1904, Vol. iii., page 380. *Nephrectomy; death.*—Male, M., æt. 46, admitted June 27, 1904. Five years before perinephric abscess had been incised. Renewed formation of abscesses in the region of the scar, which were either incised or evacuated spontaneously. Was wearing a drainage tube at the time of his admission. Urine: Acid, 1010, albumin, much pus. No cystoscopy was done. July 1: Nephrectomy. Kidney degenerated, cortex containing several foci of pus. The other kidney failed, the total quantity of urine passed after operation not exceeding 12 ounces. Died July 4 of uremia. No autopsy.

1902-1903, Vol. iv., page 396. *Metastatic pyonephrosis; perinephric* abscess; *nephrectomy; cure.*—Walter B., æt. 24, admitted July 15, 1903. Six weeks before onset of renal trouble had had a small infected wound of a toe. Two weeks later began to feel pain in left iliac region, radiating toward the groin, with chills and fever. Urination not disturbed. July 3: His family attendant had incised an abscess pointing in the rectum. Had lost much flesh and strength. On admission: Poorly nourished, internal organs normal. In left loin a large, tender mass. Temperature, 103.2°; pulse, 96. Combined urine: Acid, 1018, trace of albumin, much pus, few red bloodcells; 2.5 per cent. urea. Cystoscopy: Normal bladder, except for some injection around left side of trigonum. Both ureteral orifices normal. Right catheter easily introduced; left catheter impeded one-half inch from orifice. Urine: Right kidney—acid, faint trace of albumin, 2.0 per cent. of urea. July 18: Incision and drainage of perinephric abscess. Transient abatement of fever. July 27: Severe chill, temperature 104.6°. Frequent repetition of chills with high fever, determined nephrectomy; done August 1. Kidney enlarged, containing two large purulent infarcts, one in the lower section, the other in the middle of the organ. Immediate recession of fever. Uninterrupted recovery. September 21: Discharged cured.

1903-1904, Vol. iv., page 388. *Congenital cystic adenoma of kidney: nephrectomy; died.*—Helen R., six months old, admitted July 4, 1904. The baby was well until six weeks before, when the mother noticed that the abdomen was becoming larger and tender. Urination normal. On admission the infant was well nourished. Its internal organs were normal. The abdomen was much enlarged, owing to the presence therein of a large, smooth, firm, elastic tumor, which occupied the right loin, extending from the free border of the ribs above to the pelvis below, and reaching over to the left umbilical and hypogastric regions. Urine normal. July 4, 1904: Nephrectomy. The tumor was easily removed by a combined lumbar and abdominal incision, after its size had been reduced by the evacuation of its fluid contents. The operation lasted about 20 minutes, but in spite of all precautions to prevent shock the child died therefrom two hours after the operation.

1903-1904, Vol. iii., page 392. *Stricture of lower segment of right ureter; suprapubic cystotomy and ureteral dilatation; methodical maintenance of cystoscopic dilatation; cure.*—Israel L., æt. 35. admitted July 13, 1904. Since two days, sharp, constant, right lumbar pain; nausea. On admission: General condition good, internal organs normal, moderate arteriosclerosis; abdominal wall rigid on right side, where there was marked tenderness, as also in right loin. Moderate fever, normal pulse. Leucocyte count, 14,000. Combined urine: Acid. 1012, trace of albumin, few red bloodcells. Cystoscopy: A few hemorrhagic areas of mucosa near right ureteral orifice. Catheter passed readily into left ureter; urine drawn therefrom was normal, its cryoscopic index 1.49. In right ureter catheter arrested one inch above orifice. July 18: Suprapubic cystotomy, followed by gradual rapid dilatation of strictured ureter up to full size. The ureteral catheter was left *in situ* for eighteen hours, its distal end being brought out of the bladder by way of the urethra. The suprapubic wound was closed by a vesical and a superficial suture. It healed by first intention. Four weeks after operation methodical dilatation, by the aid of the cystoscope, was begun. Discharged cured, September 15.

1903-1904, Vol. iii., page 389. *Chronic nephritis; chronic endocarditis; decapsulation; death.*—Sarah F., æt. 29, admitted October 27, 1903. Renal malady of ten years' duration. On admission: general condition poor, pronounced anemia, ascites, anasarca, hydrothorax; heart enlarged, mitral insufficiency; albuminuric retinitis. Internal treatment having failed, decapsulation was done December 11, 1903, under ether. Just when the kidney had been exposed patient expired.

1903-1904, Vol. iii., page 390. *Perinephric abscess; incision and drainage; cure.*—Matthew L., æt. 21, admitted August 31, 1904. Seven weeks before had small superficial abscess on left forearm. One week later began to have pain in left loin, with chills and fever. Urination normal. On admission: Internal organs normal. In left loin marked pain and tenderness, but no tumor could be made out. Temperature, 103.6°; pulse, 112. Leucocyte count, 25,600. Separated urines normal. Cryoscopic index: Right side, 2.83; left side, 3.83. September 3: Incision and drainage of perinephric abscess after successful aspiration. October 10: Discharged cured.

1903-1904, Vol. iii., page 391. *Perinephric abscess; negative puncture; exploratory laparotomy; lumbar incision and drainage and cure.*—Edward F., æt. 18, admitted July 13, 1904. Four weeks ago sudden onset of abdominal pain below and to the right side of umbilicus, radiating to the back and groin; slight fever. On admission: General condition fair; internal organs normal, except the heart, where systolic murmur was present at apex. Abdominal parietes rigid, but no pressure pain could be elicited anywhere. Temperature, 103°; pulse, 100. Widal reaction negative; leucocyte count, 16,000. Urine normal. July 16: Distinct tenderness in right lumbar region, but no palpable tumor. Leucocyte count, 27,000. July 20: Negative puncture of right pleural cavity in eighth interspace, scapular line. July 21: Tenderness above and internally to anterior superior spine of right ilium. The septic condition continuing, it was deemed proper, in view of the possibility of an appendicular process, to make an exploration, which revealed an appendix bound down by many adhesions, but evidently not the cause of the present disorder. All the other abdominal organs appeared also normal. The right kidney appeared enlarged and firmly fixed, but no tumor could be felt in its vicinity. Abdominal incision being closed, a puncture was made in the loin and pus was obtained. A small perinephric abscess, holding one ounce of pus, was incised and drained. Kidney was not involved. Discharged cured, August 18, 1904.

A REPORT OF THE CASES OF BENIGN AND MALIGN DISEASES OF THE STOMACH AND DUODENUM, TREATED IN FIRST SURGICAL DIVISION DURING 1903 AND 1904.

By A. A. BERG, M.D.,
ADJUNCT ATTENDING SURGEON.

The number of patients that are annually treated in the first surgical service of the hospital for gastric and duodenal affections is constantly increasing. During the past two years we have had the following cases of gastric and duodenal disease:

BENIGN DISEASES.

	Total.	Cured.	Improved.	Unimproved.	Died.
Uncomplicated gastric ulcer	5	5			
Gastric ulcer; profuse hematemeses	2	1			1
" " single hematemesis*	1	1			
Duodenal ulcer; perforation, diffuse purulent peritinitis; very profuse melena on the ninth day	1	1			
Gastric ulcer; pin-hole perforation; encapsulated intraperitoneal abscess	1	1			
Gastric ulcer; perforation; diffuse purulent peritonitis	1				1
Gastric ulcer; recurrent after gastro-enterostomy	1	1			
Benign stenosis of pylorus from gastric ulcer	3	3			
Peripyloritis, probably from gastric ulcer	1	1			
Gastric succorrhea and pyloric stenosis from ulcer of stomach	1	1			
Acute dilatation of stomach from adhesions with pyloric stenosis, due to chronic perforation of gastric ulcer	1				1
Gastric ulcer with thickened edges, simulating carcinoma	1			..	1
Cholecystitis calculous, with pyloric stenosis from pericholecystitis	1				1

*Not operated.

MALIGNANT DISEASES.

	Total.	Cured.	Improved.	Unimproved.	Died.
Lympho-sarcoma of stomach	1	..	..	..	1
Carcinoma of cardiac end of stomach	2	..	1	..	1
" " " " and lesser curvature	1	..	..	..	1
" " " " " " and pyloric stenosis	1	..	1	..	..
Carcinoma of body of stomach†	2	..	..	2	..
" " anterior wall of stomach	1	..	..	1	..
" " pylorus	12	1	8	1	2
Toxic gastro-enteritis*	1	1	..	..	..

In the following remarks each one of these groups of cases will be considered.

Firstly, as to the indication for operation;
Secondly, as to the nature of the operation that is employed;
Thirdly, as to the treatment after operation; and
Fourthly, as to the results of our operative therapy.

BENIGN DISEASES OF THE STOMACH.

A.—The indications for operation.

It is but proper that we precede our remarks on the indications for operation by a few words in reference to the diagnosis. Our main difficulty in this regard has been encountered in those uncomplicated cases of gastric ulcer that have given, as the only indication of their presence, a most annoying and distressing pain in the epigastric and right hyponchondriac regions. The pain commenced insidiously and grew gradually worse, was not influenced by taking food, and did not come on in attacks. Very slight subconjunctival icterus was present or had been noticed by some of the patients. Repeated and carefully made analyses of the gastric contents in these cases did not throw any light upon the diagnosis. In most instances the gastric juice was normal, occasionally it was hyacid and only rarely was it hyperacid. A diligent and systematic employment of the X-ray, cystoscope, and ureteral catheter, with analyses of the separated urines, enabled us to exclude affections of the kidney as a cause of the patient's

*Not operated.
†1 case not operated; 1 case exploratory laparotomy.

complaint, but only by exploratory laparotomy were we enabled in some of the cases to decide between affections of the gall bladder, vermiform appendix, stomach and duodenum.

As instances of the difficulty in making the diagnosis in this class of cases the following histories are quoted:

1902-1903, Vol. i., page 105.—Max L., a barber, 27 years old, with an entirely negative family and previous personal history, was suddenly taken with pain in the right iliac region. The pain was severe, and a few days after its onset it moved upward into the liver region. Subsequently it came on in attacks, starting in the region of the liver and passing upward to the sternum and around the side to the back, and to the left shoulder. With the pain there was nausea, but no vomiting. The conjunctivæ were said to be yellow at times. The patient had lost ten pounds in weight and considerable strength during the nine weeks of his illness. On physical examination, there was slight subconjunctival icterus. The lungs, heart and liver were normal; there was no abdominal rigidity, and no abdominal tenderness, except on deep palpation in the right iliac region. There was no tumor in the gall-bladder region. The only complaint was the pain which completely incapacitated the man from doing his work, and in spite of a careful and somewhat extended observation the cause of the pain remained in doubt. Exploratory laparotomy was proposed to the patient, and readily accepted by him. An open pyloric ulcer, about the size of a twenty-five cent piece, was found. The gall passages and appendix were normal. The head of the pancreas was normal. A posterior gastro-enterostomy, with Murphy's button, was established. The patient made an uninterrupted convalescence, and the pain was never felt after the operation.

1902-1903, Vol. i., page 107.—Samuel L., clerk, 23 years old, had suffered for ten months with inconstant, dull pain in the right hypochondrium, radiating into the lumbar region. The pain was not influenced by meals; there was no vomiting, no marked indigestion, and no jaundice. His previous history was negative, except for the infectious diseases of childhood. Three months prior to his admission to the hospital he had been operated upon in another hospital for chronic appendicitis. His lungs, heart, liver, spleen and kidneys appeared to be normal; the abdominal wall was lax, and there was no abdominal tenderness. The gastric secretion and the size of the stomach were entirely normal. The pain was severe and distressing, enough to interfere with the patient's occupation, and, as a careful internal treatment had failed to relieve him, he sought surgical aid. The case impressed us as one of cholelithiasis, and we advised exploratory laparotomy. On exploration through a vertical incision in the right hypochondriac region, the liver, bile passages, duodenum, and pancreas were found to be normal. The pylorus was surrounded by a few adhesions, and was decidedly thickened; the tip of the little finger could scarcely be invaginated through it. A posterior gastroenterostomy (Carle-Fantino method) was done. Convalescence uninterrupted; the button was not recovered. The pain was very much less at the time of his discharge from the hospital.

The comparative frequency with which errors in diagnoses are made in this class of ulcer cases has not discouraged us, however, and we still continue to exercise all our efforts toward a correct determination of the patients' malady. In this we are considerably aided where the patient's symptoms permit of it, by continued observation and repeated examination. Diagnosis by exclusion will be found especially valuable in these cases.

Before proceeding to operation in these cases of gastric ulcer, we invariably refer the patients to the internist for dietary and local treatment. Only when this proves of no avail do we advise and resort to laparotomy.

Pyloric stenosis from the cicatrization of an ulcer has usually been readily diagnosed from the presence of a dilated stomach and from the evidences of disturbed gastric motility, i.e., stagnation within the stomach and prolongation of the time the stomach should normally require to empty itself after a meal. In one of our cases during the present year the disturbed gastric motility and dilated stomach were due to stenosis of the duodenum, which, in turn, was dependent upon a compression of this viscus by omental bands and adhesions that had resulted from a previous operation for chronic appendicitis.

In another case the chief complaint was gastric succorrhea. His history was as follows:

1903-1904, Vol. ii., page 120. *Gastric ulcer; gastric succorrhea; gastro-enterostomy posterior; cured.*—A. H., 30 years old, had suffered with gastric pain, vomiting, hematemeses for nine years, during a large part of which time he was under expert and careful dietary and internal treatment. He had lost considerable weight and strength. On admission to the hospital, February 23, 1904, he was pale and poorly nourished. His lungs, heart, liver, spleen and kidneys were normal. His stomach was dilated; there was marked clapottage; there was some pain and tenderness in the epigastrium. His stomach contents, after a test meal, contained total acids, 80; free HCl, 35, and combined HCl, 15. His stomach, at two successive washings, could hold 1900 and 2170 ccm., respectively.

February 26, 1904.—Posterior gastro-enterostomy; Murphy's button. The pylorus was considerably thickened: on the posterior walls, just to the left of the pylorus, there was an indurated area about the size of a half dollar, with thickened edges. The post operative course was uneventful, except for a slight infection in the outer wound. The button was passed on the ninth day. Entire relief of the symptoms. April 19: Discharged cured.

We have had no cases in this series in which, with benign stenosis of the pylorus, there was an anacidity of the gastric juice, though, as will be mentioned later on, there was one case of cancer with a marked hyperacidity of the gastric secretion.

The indications for operation in our cases of benign gastric affections have been urgent in five; in the other sixteen operation has been done at a time of our selection, and only after careful deliberation. Of the urgent operations two were for acute sudden perforation of the ulcer with extravasation of gastric and duodenal contents into the free peritoneal cavity and consequent diffuse purulent peritonitis, two were for repeated profuse hematemeses, and one for acute dilatation of the stomach.

Of the two cases of perforating ulcer with diffuse peritonitis one recovered and one died. The diagnosis of perforation in these, as well as in four other cases that were operated upon in previous years, was readily made from the symptoms of sudden tearing pain in the epigastric region, vomiting, abdominal rigidity, and gradually rising pulse rate, following upon a history of gastric disturbances. We have not noticed, nor has there been recorded in the anamnesis of our cases, much shock at the time of perforation, nor has there been, in most of the cases, a diminution or disappearance of liver or splenic dullness.

In the cases which we have seen shortly after the perforation has occurred, we have proceeded to immediate laparotomy, because we have not been able to decide whether the extravasation of intestinal contents following upon the perforation would be confined by peritoneal adhesions to a local region around the ulcer, or whether this septic material would be spread throughout the peritoneal cavity. In our six cases of perforating ulcer of the anterior gastric and duodenal wall the extravasated material was not confined by adhesions to a local area; but when the perforations were situated on the posterior wall of these viscera, the extravasated material was, for a time at least, confined to the bursa omentalis and retroduodenal tissues, respectively, a localized abscess forming in these regions.

With pin-hole perforations of the anterior wall of the stomach or duodenum, there may be no extravasation, and, consequently, no immediate consequences from the accident, or there may be a very slight amount of extravasation with a secondary formation of an intraperitoneal abscess, an illustration of which was afforded by the following case of the past year:

1903-1904, Vol. ii., page 124.—Minnie K., 28 years old, housewife, was admitted May 1, 1904. Was always well up to two weeks before her admission to the hospital, when she was seized with cramp-like pains in the abdomen, vomiting, chilly sensations, and fever. The pain continued on and off, cramp-like in character, and one day before her admission it became especially severe at the free border of the ribs.

Physical examination showed normal internal organs. The abdominal wall was moderately rigid and tense. The abdomen was tympanitic, and tender in the left hypochondriac region. Temperature was 103.4°; pulse, 116; leukocyte count, 15,200. Under anesthesia there was rigidity of the left rectus muscle, and a mass with indefinite outlines could be palpated in the left hypochondriac region. On May 5, 1904, the abdomen was opened over the mass. There were numerous adhesions of the omentum to the anterior abdominal wall and underlying intestines. The anterior gastric wall was especially adherent to the under surface of the left lobe of the liver, and between them was a small encapsulated abscess. No perforation of the stomach could be identified, though at one spot the peritoneal coat of this viscus was very much roughened. This area was inverted by two rows of Lembert sutures, the abscess was drained by gauze, and the abdominal wound closed down to the emergence of the drain. Uninterrupted convalescence. Gradual closure of the drainage opening. Discharged cured, June 16, 1904.

Our reasons for immediate laparotomy in the cases of acute perforation seen shortly after the perforation has occurred, is to avoid or prevent the spread of the extravasated septic material throughout the peritoneal cavity. Such action will often bring us to operate upon cases in which the extravasated material is well encapsulated by adhesions that have previously formed around the ulcer.* but,

*It may be safely assumed that if no adhesions are present prior to the perforation which will confine the extravasated material to a local region,

inasmuch as we cannot foretell in which cases such adhesions are present, nor determine the exact anatomical site of the ulcer prior to opening the abdomen, it seems best in our opinion to proceed to immediate laparotomy in all cases. Even if it were possible to determine the situation of the ulcer on the gastric or duodenal wall, and the presence of limiting adhesions, it would be very doubtful whether it would be desirable to delay operation. For such delay would expose the patient to the grave risks of intraperitoneal sepsis, would render it much more difficult to close the perforation, would endanger the integrity of the surrounding organs, such as pancreas, spleen, kidneys, etc., and would materially weaken the patient, for during the period of waiting no nutrition can be given by the stomach. As an example of delay in operating for encapsulated abscess following perforating ulcer of the posterior wall of the stomach, see Mt. Sinai Hospital Reports, 1898.

The histories of the two cases of perforating ulcer operated upon during the past year are as follows:

1902-1903, Vol. i., page 106. *Perforated gastric ulcer, diffuse purulent peritonitis; suture of perforation sixteen hours after its occurrence; death thirty-six hours later.*—John M., a Russian tailor, 22 years old, was admitted to the hospital, at 5 P. M., on February 9, 1903. He was absolutely well until sixteen hours before admission, when he was suddenly seized with severe cramps around the umbilicus; the pain soon localized itself in the right iliac fossa. He vomited repeatedly, the ejected material being brownish in color; it did not contain blood. There was no fever and no chills.

On admission he was apathetic and restless, his heart, lungs, liver and spleen were normal to percussion, palpation and auscultation. The abdominal wall was very rigid; the abdomen was distended and markedly tender, especially so in the right iliac fossa. There was a shifting dullness in the flanks. No tumor was to be felt. Rectal examination was negative. The temperature was 101.4°; the pulse rate, 132. The preoperative diagnosis of acute perforative appendicitis with diffuse peritonitis was made and immediate laparotomy proceeded with. On opening the abdomen in the right iliac region,

---

that none will form subsequently which will effectively prevent the spread of the infected material in the peritoneal cavity.

It is well known to surgeons that successful closure of the perforation depends chiefly upon the adhesive quality of the peritoneum adjacent to it. If this has been lost or if the whole peritoneum has become altered or destroyed by the suppurative process not much hope can be entertained for a successful closure of the perforated ulcer.

there was a gush of non-odorous purulent fluid from the free peritoneal cavity. The intestines were covered with lymph. The appendix was normal. Suspecting then a perforation of the intestine or stomach, these organs were exposed, and on the anterior wall of the stomach, about one inch from the pylorus, a perforation about the size of a split pea was found. This was closed by several rows of Lembert sutures, the peritoneal cavity was flushed with saline solution and drained. Closure of the abdominal wound down to the emergence of the drains. The patient reacted poorly, and in spite of free stimulation he succumbed thirty-six hours after operation.

NOTE.—This is a case in which the first evidence of the ulcer was its perforation. It is all the more strange in this particular case that no symptoms of gastric ulceration were afforded prior to the perforation, because the ulcer was situated on the anterior wall near the pylorus.

1903-1904, Vol. i., page 123. *Perforated duodenal ulcer; diffuse purulent peritonitis; suture of perforation thirty-two hours after its occurrence; severe repeated hemorrhages on the tenth day after operation; recovery.*—Samuel H., secretary, 46 years old, was admitted to the hospital on the evening of the 6th of August, 1904. He had been somewhat indisposed for a week before the present illness, and during this time he had vague abdominal pains. Thirty-two hours before his admission, while riding in a cab, he was suddenly seized with severe cramp-like, tearing pains in the umbilical and lower abdominal region. He felt faint and was taken to a neighboring physician, who injected a dose of morphine and advised him to go home. On his arrival home he was seen by his family physician, who found his pulse and temperature normal; his abdomen was rigid and everywhere tender. During the following twenty-four hours his pulse gradually rose to 120, his temperature to 100.8°. His abdomen became distended and very tender and rigid. When he was seen by the writer his pulse rate was 125 to 130, his temperature 101°; his abdomen was very rigid, moderately distended, everywhere tender, but especially so in the right hypochondriac region. There was shifting dullness in the flanks. The diagnosis of perforated gastric or duodenal ulcer, with advancing peritonitis, was made by his family physician and the writer, and immediate operation advised. He was at once removed to the hospital, and under chloroform the abdomen was opened by a longitudinal incision in the right hypochondrium.

On incising the peritoneum there was a gush of non-odorous purulent fluid. The omentum was adherent to the liver and stomach and covered with fibrin. On separating the adhesions and exposing the stomach and duodenum, a perforation about three-quarters inch in diameter, in the first portion of the duodenum, partly closed by fibrin, was found. This was closed by three layers of Lembert silk sutures,

The pus and fibrin were carefully sponged away, and the whole infected region drained with gauze, the omentum being deflected upward to cover the site of perforation and infection. Closure of the abdominal wound down to emergence of the drain.

The reaction from the operation was good. During the subsequent three days the patient showed evidences of intense poisoning; he was jaundiced, his pulse rate rose to 148, his temperature to 102.8°. Gradually his general condition improved, the pulse rate and temperature approached the normal, and from small doses of water by the mouth on the third day he had gradually come to take about forty ounces of general fluids by mouth per day. On the ninth day the patient seemed to be on the road to recovery, when suddenly in the early morning of the tenth day, after a little gastric pain and distress he went into collapse: pulse, 148, weak and thready, and passed an enormous, tarry stool. Large doses of ergot and morphine were at once administered subcutaneously. Within an hour another large, tarry stool was passed: the patient was exceedingly pale, his respirations were sighing, and he looked as if he might expire at any moment. Stypticin by mouth was administered in one grain doses every hour. His wretched condition absolutely contraindicated any surgical procedure that aimed to control the bleedings; had such been undertaken the patient would surely have died. The following morning his hemoglobin count was 19 per cent. His pulse was a little better in quality and its rate was between 110 and 120. During the day he had another very large, tarry movement, but did not show any signs of renewed bleeding. The stomach was kept absolutely at rest. Large doses of bismuth (30 to 40 grains every two hours, with just enough water to enable the patient to swallow it) were given by mouth. Rectal alimentation was resorted to and occasionally a subcutaneous saline infusion, to relieve thirst. Several further large, tarry evacuations occurred during the following three days, but they were not accompanied by any signs of fresh bleeding. Gradually the pulse became less rapid, and of better quality, and the hemoglobin commenced to rise. On the fifth day after the first hemorrhage, ten drops of the Tr. ferri chloridi, well diluted, were given three times a day; the stypticin being discontinued. On the tenth day after the bleeding, fluid nourishment by mouth was cautiously administered. From then on gradual improvement took place. The wound healed kindly, the patient gained in weight and in strength, and was discharged cured, September 10, 1904.

Of the two cases of gastric ulcer complicated by sudden profuse hemorrhage, one recovered and one died; in both a rapid gastro-enterostomy posterior with Murphy's button was done. In neither case was there any evidence of fresh bleeding from the ulcer after the gastro-enterostomy had been established.

We have heretofore been guided in making a decision for operation in the face of bleeding from gastric ulcer, by the rules which were formulated by Mikulicz and Leube (Langenbeck's archiv), as the result of their observation and study of a very large number of cases of this malady. These rules, which have been accepted by most surgeons and internists, are as follows:

Operation is indicated,

(1.) In the presence of acute, profuse, uncontrollable bleeding, which places the life of the patient in grave jeopardy.

(2.) In the presence of frequently repeated bleedings, even if they are not very profuse, that undermine the patient's strength and lead to a chronic anemia.

We have not had occasion in our service to interfere surgically for frequently repeated small hemorrhages from gastric ulcers, but in the past few years we have had upon our service four cases of gastric and duodenal ulcer that were suddenly complicated with several times repeated profuse hemorrhages. In three of these cases gastroenterostomy was done, and in one the expectant plan of treatment was pursued. In two the operation was done as a "dernier ressort" in enfeebled and exsanguinated patients, after internal treatment had failed to check the bleeding; both patients died shortly after operation. In one the operation was done while the patient was still in comparitively good condition. This patient recovered. The patient who was treated expectantly likewise recovered. He was the man whose history has already been cited under perforating duodenal ulcers (Samuel H.). As will be seen from his history, he had commenced to convalesce from the diffuse peritonitis to which the perforation had given rise and our minds were commencing to be at ease as to the ultimate outcome, when suddenly there were, in rapid succession, three enormous, bloody (tarry) evacuations from the lower bowel. His pulse rate jumped from 92 to 148, became thin and compressible, his respirations were sighing, his color was extremely pallid, and his heart sounds feeble. The hemoglobin of his blood was 19 per cent. The experience I had gained from the two other cases in which, in the face of such a desperate general condition, a gastroenterostomy had been established under cocaine anesthesia, led me to refrain from and advise against operating in this patient. I preferred to trust to internal remedies, such as morphine, stypticin, and tinct. of the chloride of iron, to check the bleeding and prevent its recurrence; the decision turned out to be a wise one, for the patient did not have a recurrence of the bleeding and thereafter made an uninterrupted convalescence.

Only in the first one of these three cases was an attempt made by opening the stomach to locate the bleeding point and directly control it. When the stomach was opened the bleeding had ceased; the ulcer was readily located; it was on the posterior wall, immediately over the celiac axis. Its base was cauterized with the Paquelin cautery, and then an anterior gastro-enterostomy was established. In this patient the search for the ulcer somewhat prolonged the operation, which was done under cocaine anesthesia. In the other two cases no attempt was made to find the bleeding point; we contented ourselves with rapidly establishing a posterior gastro-enterostomy. As stated above, in none of the three cases that were operated upon was there any evidence of further bleeding.

The method in which a gastro-enterostomy checks the bleeding is not quite clear, but probably by putting the stomach at rest it permits the bleeding vessels to contract and retract within their sheath, and the clot which forms over them is not constantly displaced by the peristaltic movements of the viscus.

The number of the cases with sudden profuse bleeding from gastric and duodenal ulcers that we have had is still much too small to permit us to form any decided rules for future guidance in such cases. A review of the cases we have had may, however, afford a hint that may help in the successful management of patients whose lives have suddenly been placed in the gravest jeopardy by the occurrence of this complication.

Of our four patients three were in a most desperate condition, as a result of the bleeding; one (1901, Vol. iii., page 142, Mt. Sinai Hospital Reports) had had repeated hemorrhages (hematemeses and melena) for six days, and just before operation had a pulse of 156, soft and thready in character, and a hemoglobin percentage of 30; one had had repeated hemorrhages for twelve days; her hemoglobin was less than 25 per cent., her pulse was 140 to the minute, soft and scarcely perceptible, and her sensorium was clouded. In both of these cases the attending physicians had called upon the surgeons to stop the bleeding, only after all internal measures had failed to accomplish this, and as a dernier ressort gastro-enterostomy was done. Neither patient reacted from the laparotomy. Death occurred in one case fourteen hours after the operation, and in the other about ten hours after. These two experiences would seem to show the futility of operating when the patients are in such desperate conditions. They are scarcely able to withstand any operative shock and rapidly succumb to it, and that whether a general anesthesia has been administered or not. When the patient is in such desperate condition it seems to the writer that it is better to continue with internal measures than to do any operation, no matter how simple it is, nor how rapidly executed it may be. This view would seem to be borne out by the result in our fourth case, in which the hemorrhage occurred on the tenth day after a successful operation for the closure of a perforating duodenal ulcer, and for which no operation was done.

The brilliant influence of gastro-enterostomy in instantly checking the bleeding that was noticed in one of our cases, and the uninterrupted convalescence that followed the operation, shows what can be accomplished when the operation is done at a time when the patient is still in fair condition. Her hemoglobin was 45 per cent., and her pulse rate, though 120, was good in quality.*

If we sum up the impressions made upon us by the observation of these four cases, we would say that operation is not advisable when the patient's general condition is bad, the hemoglobin very low (19 or 20 per cent.), and the pulse rate very rapid.

In such a condition the operative shock, no matter how slight it may be, whether or not it is combined with the added depressing and hemolytic influence of a general anesthetic, is sufficient to cause the death of the patient. It is far better in such cases to trust to internal remedies and complete rest, induced by morphine, to check the bleeding. When, however, the patient's general condition is still good, and the hemoglobin count is above 35 to 40 per cent., we would strongly advise immediate operation. This will have a double effect; it will check the bleeding and so remove the immediate threatening complication to life, and it will further favor the rapid healing of the ulcer.

*The previous clinical history of this patient (Vol. I., 1903-1904) was that of an ordinary case of gastric ulcer. She had never vomited blood until the evening prior to her admission to the hospital, when she suddenly vomited about one quart of fluid and clotted blood. Within the following twelve hours she twice vomited considerable fresh blood, and when seen by the writer she was in the condition above described.

Immediate laparotomy was also proceeded with in one case of acute dilatation of the stomach, secondary to pyloric stenosis from chronic perforated ulcer with peripyloritis. His history was as follows:

1903-1904, Vol. ii., page 125.—*Acute dilatation of the stomach; secondary to chronic perforated ulcer of the pylorus, with extensive peripyloritis and pyloric stenosis; gastro-enterostomy; death.*—Fred S., 32 years old, a brass worker, had suffered with gastro-intestinal symptoms for seven or eight years. Six years before he had been in a hospital for abdominal pain and intestinal distention. His present illness was of indefinite duration. There had been a gradual increase in the severity of the gastric symptoms. There was more pain in the epigastric and umbilical regions, and occasional vomiting.

His bowels were constipated, and he had lost considerable flesh and strength. On the day before his admission, he vomited some blackish material. Physical examination on admission, December 7, 1903, showed his lungs, heart and kidneys to be normal. The liver dullness was absent at the lower border. The stomach was somewhat dilated, reaching to one finger breadth above the umbilicus.

In the night of December 8 the patient had severe, cramp-like abdominal pain, referred chiefly to the umbilical region. The abdominal wall was very rigid. A dose of morphine was administered, and the pain was somewhat relieved. The following morning the pain returned; it was very intense; the abdomen was somewhat distended, and the pulse was accelerated. A high oxgall enema was ineffectual. By the afternoon the abdomen was very much distended, the pain was very severe and came on in paroxysms; the pulse was rapid (120), and its quality was not so good. In the early afternoon the patient commenced to fail rapidly; his pulse became progressively more and more rapid and feeble, and his abdomen more distended; the pain was somewhat less. Another high enema was ineffectual. The attending physician was suspicious of an acute intestinal obstruction and, therefore, withheld morphine.

When the writer was asked to see the patient, he found him in collapse. The upper part of the abdomen was much distended and entirely dull. No tumor and no fixed coil of intestine could be made out on abdominal palpation. The patient's condition was too wretched to permit of immediate operation; free stimulation was, therefore, ordered. Two hours later the pulse had become somewhat better and, though not much was hoped for from operation, this was, nevertheless, undertaken as a last hope of saving an apparently lost life. Just prior to operation a stomach tube was passed, and about six quarts of highly acid, brownish-black, watery material was evacuated; this caused a partial subsidence of the epigastric swelling. The abdomen was opened under sleich and gas anesthesia. There was a moderate amount of cloudy fluid in the peritoneal cavity, the intestines were distended in some places, and collapsed in others; the stomach was considerably enlarged, its walls were somewhat thickened, and its pyloric end and lesser curvature were imbedded in dense, hard, firm adhesions. The pylorus was firmly adherent to the pancreas and under surface of the right lobe of the liver. The gall bladder and ducts were normal, and the pancreas was apparently healthy. A posterior gastro-enterostomy with Murphy's button was rapidly established and the abdominal incision closed with through and through sutures. During the operation, which lasted about three-quarters of an hour, an intravenous saline infusion and free hypodermic stimulation had to be employed. The patient did not react from the operation and died about four hours later.

Post-mortem examination through the wound showed a much dilated stomach, with a large ulcer in the posterior wall of the pyloric portion; the ulcer had perforated through the stomach wall and its base was formed by the pancreas and left lobe of the liver.

We have considered this case to be one of acute gastric dilatation, though we have not been able to dismiss the thought that the adhesion of the ulcer to the pancreas with the involvement of this organ in the ulcerative process may have had a close connection with the collapse symptoms. The cardiac collapse was, perhaps, the most striking feature of the case. Within twelve hours the pulse rate increased from 80 to 140, and in quality became almost imperceptible. The question of the advisability of operation under the circumstances was carefully considered by the writer, and only a recent report by Moynihan of a successful result from gastro-enterostomy in a somewhat similar case induced him to proceed to operation. In a future case it would seem preferable to first try the effect of frequently repeated gastric lavage.

Few, if any, will question the advisability of operation in the acute complications of gastric and duodenal ulceration. In the uncomplicated cases of ulcer, however, and in the condition of benign pyloric stenosis, arising from the cicatrization of pyloric ulcers, there is no such unanimity of opinion as to the necessity for surgical interference. The surgeon who sees and has to operate for the complications of these ulcers, who has witnessed the distress and wretched existence of patients who have a benign pyloric stenosis, and who has observed the marvelous beneficial effects which are produced in them by a gastro-enterostomy, is led more and more to the belief that gastric and duodenal ulcers that are not healed by dietary and local treatment should be treated surgically, and that stenotic conditions of the pylorus severe enough to occasion disturbances of gastric motility should be relieved by some one or other of the operations of gastro-duodenostomy or jejunostomy. He recognizes the fact that an open gastric or duodenal ulcer, no matter how mild its manifestations may be, has in itself the potentiality of grave and life threatening complications, and that if these are to be avoided an operation must be done. By this is not meant that every patient who manifests the symptoms of gastric ulceration should be immediately operated upon, but what is demanded is that every patient who is not entirely cured of the symptoms of ulcer by a properly instituted and carefully maintained dietary and local treatment should be referred to the surgeon for operation.

It is claimed by some that in conditions of benign pyloric stenosis, comparative comfort can be maintained by systematic gastric lavage and proper dietary regulations. That this is so in a proportion of the cases cannot be denied, but such practice condemns the patient to the daily use of the stomach tube, and to existence on a limited diet for the rest of his life. Not even the strongest advocates of this method of treatment claim to be able to cure the stenosis in this way. In a larger proportion of the cases the stomach tube and dietary regulations finally fail to maintain a condition of comparative well being. In such cases gastro-enterostomy must eventually be done, and then its attendant mortality is naturally considerably higher than is ordinarily the case, because the long continued underfeeding and poor absorptive powers have weakened the constitution of the patient.

In twelve unselected cases of gastric ulcer and benign pyloric stenosis that have been operated upon in our service during the past two years there has been one death. In this case (1903-1904, Vol. ii., page 131) a pylorectomy had been done, because the very much thickened edges of the ulcer and the enlarged celiac glands gave the surgeon the impression that he had to deal with a malignant tumor. A typical pylorectomy with a posterior gastro jejunostomy (Murphy button) had been done. An infection of the omentum took place, with the formation of an intraperitoneal abscess, and though this was incised and drained new abscesses formed in the omentum and between the intestinal coils. After several months, death occurred from exhaustion and sepsis; one of the abscesses had perforated into the stomach. With this exception, all of our patients made a smooth recovery and were exceedingly grateful that they had been relieved of their distressing and annoying symptoms.

We have to record one other case (1903-1904, Vol. ii., page 130) in which, from a long-standing calculus cholecystitis, a benign pyloric stenosis had taken place. In this patient the removal of the gall-bladder was combined with a Finney gastro-duodenostomy. On the third day, when all was apparently well, one of the anterior sutures gave way; extravasation of duodenal contents followed and from the shock of the operation that was immediately performed for the repair of the perforated intestine death occurred. In this case it would have been wiser to have selected some other method of gastro-enterostomy, for the brittleness of the walls and lack of adhesive quality of the peritoneal covering of the pyloric portion of the stomach and first portion of the duodenum, which were occasioned by the long continued pericholecystitis, materially contributed to the giving way of the suture line.*

This case, however, though she succumbed from a gastric operation, should not be classed with the cases of gastric and duodenal ulceration. We have then to record one death in twelve cases, i.e., a mortality of $8\frac{1}{2}$ per cent., and this death followed a pylorectomy, an operation that is not ordinarily practiced for benign affections of the stomach, and one that is attended with a much higher mortality rate than is simple gastro-enterostomy. Can the internal methods of treatment achieve equally good results? Further, it must not be considered that these figures are unusually good, for the Mayos, in a much larger material, report a smaller mortality. With such results from operative curative treatment, can there be any doubt as to which course we are to advise our patients with these maladies to pursue?

B.—THE OPERATIONS THAT HAVE BEEN EMPLOYED FOR THE BENIGN GASTRIC AND DUODENAL AFFECTIONS.

During the past two years the following operations† have been done in our cases:

*In similar cases the writer would advise not to do the Finney operation.
†Twenty-one operations upon nineteen patients.

	Total	Cured	Died
Posterior gastro-enterostomy	10	8	2†
Finney's gastro-duodenostomy	3	2	1*
Suture of perforated ulcers	2	1	1‡
Division of peripyloritic adhesions due to ulcer which had since healed	1	1	
Exploratory laparotomy for peripyloritis due probably to gastric ulcer	1	1	
Incision and drainage of intra-peritoneal abscess due to pinhole perforation of ulcer on anterior gastric wall	1	1	..
Pylorectomy	1	..	1
Posterior gastro-enterostomy and secondary entero-enterostomy for vicious circle vomiting	1§	1	

Gastro-enterostomy.—This has been and still is the operation of our choice. Whenever possible, the posterior operation of VonHacker is performed. The anastomosis is made between the lowest point of the stomach, i.e., just above its greater curvature and near to the pyloric end, and a loop of the jejunum at a point about 12 to 14 inches from the duodeno-jejunal junction, the viscera being united in an isoperistaltic direction. No entero-enteric anastomosis is established. The anastomosis is always made with the Murphy button, the segments of which are held in place with a purse-string silk suture that includes all the coats but the mucosa. If the retaining suture is passed in this way there will be no irregular puckering of the gastric wall around the shank of the button to interfere with a smooth, flat apposition of the intestinal and gastric walls. We find, furthermore, that the button is not retained at the site of the anastomosis quite so long if the suture is passed in this way. The method is a modification of that of Carle-Fantino; it is more rapidly carried out than the procedure of the latter.

Profiting by our past experience, with imperfectly manufactured buttons, and their retention in the anastomotic orifice, we have made it an invariable rule to carefully test the spring and the closure of the segments of each button, before it is employed, and since we have adopted this precautionary measure we have not had any evidence of retention of the button in the anastomotic orifice. There does not

*This case was one of calculus cholecystitis with extensive peripyloritis and benign pyloric stenosis; death was due to the giving way of the anterior suture line on the third day after operation.
†Case of acute dilatation of the stomach.
‡Death due to diffuse purulent peritonitis.
§Two operations on this patient.

seem to be any regularity as to when the button is passed, nor as to whether it will be passed. In the nine cases in which a simple posterior gastro-enterostomy was done, and in which recovery took place, the button was passed in the stools in six, and on the 8th, 10th, 27th, 15th, 25th, and 9th day, respectively. In one other case the patient thought he felt the button pass though the anus. Though the button was not recovered in the two remaining cases, we are not at all sure that it was not passed and escaped the attention of the nurse, for the X-ray did not show, in either instance, the presence of the button in the stomach or intestine, nor were there any evil symptoms to suggest its retention.

In this series of cases we have experienced our first instance of vicious circle anastomosis. The vomiting was not incessant, but its persistence, in spite of gastric lavage and upright posture of the patient, led us to reopen the abdomen on the eighth day after the gastro-enterostomy. The proximal loop of the anastomosing coil of jejunum was not much distended and no explanation for the condition could be found. An enter-anastomosis was established with Murphy's button. The vomiting ceased at once, and the patient subsequently made an uninterrupted recovery. (1903-1904. Vol. ii., page 128.)

Finney operation. Gastro-duodenostomy.—During the past year we have done the Finney operation three times, once for recurrent symptoms of ulcer after gastro-enterostomy, once for pyloric ulcer, and once for benign pyloric stenosis from pericholecystitic adhesions. The first two cases made an excellent recovery; the recurrent case has not suffered any annoyance since the last operation, which is now almost eight months ago. The third patient succumbed on the third day from the shock of reopening the abdomen for leakage from the duodenum. The leakage was due to the parting of one of the anterior row of sutures. In this case the walls of the stomach and duodenum were quite brittle and their peritoneal covering had been materially altered by the long continued pericholecystitic inflammation, and to these conditions was probably due the tearing out or giving way of the suture line. In similar cases it would be better to employ some form of gastro-enterostomy.

Operations for perforating ulcer.—In the case of perforating ulcers, situated on the anterior wall of the stomach and duodenum, or along the greater and lesser curvatures of the stomach, i.e., in an accessible position, we have confined our efforts to closure of the perforation by inverting the entire ulcerated area into the stomach by two or three rows of Lembert silk sutures. Several years ago we had to deal with a case of perforating ulcer situated on the posterior duodenal wall. The writer was asked to see the case seven days after perforation had occurred, when a large retrocolic abscess had formed. The wretched physical condition of the patient at that time precluded any further procedure than simple evacuation and drainage of the abscess cavity; the patient succumbed several days later from exhaustion and sepsis (see Mt. Sinai Hospital Reports, Vol. iii., page 102).

As the closure of ulcers on the posterior duodenal wall is not very likely to succeed because of the lack of peritoneal covering to this portion of the bowel, the writer has proposed (see *Medical Record and Central. f. Chirurgie*) to simply drain the site of perforation, and to unilaterally exclude it from the rest of the gastro-duodenal tract by closing the pylorus with purse-string suture, and establishing a gastro-enterostomy. In this way leakage of duodenal contents through the perforated ulcer will be prevented and the danger of death from inanition and sepsis will be rendered much more unlikely. (The purse-string suture is to be passed around the pylorus without opening into its lumen.)

In a recent article (*Medical Record*, 1903) the writer expressed his opinion against the advisability of establishing a gastro-enterostomy at the same time that the perforating ulcer was repaired. It seemed to him that the carrying out of such a procedure would be likely to spread the infection of the peritoneum from the site of the perforation to the rest of the peritoneal cavity and, furthermore, the experience that was gained in the previous cases of perforating ulcer seemed to render gastro-enterostomy unnecessary; for the two patients that recovered were not subsequently (in a period of two years after the perforation) bothered by the symptoms of ulceration. In other words the ulcers seemed to heal spontaneously after their perforation. During the past summer, however, the writer has had one experience that would seem to speak in favor of establishing such a primary gastro-enterostomy. The history of the case has already been detailed on page 185, under perforating ulcer. In this patient there was a profuse hemorrhage from the ulcerated area on the tenth day after a successful operation for closure of its perforation. The question, naturally, at once arises, could this life-threatening complication have been avoided by a gastro-enterostomy at the time of the primary operation? This case of profuse bleeding from an ulcer, after a successful operation for closure of its perforation had been made, is not at all unique in literature. In the *London Lancet* of 1904, page 886, vol. 2, a similar case in the practice of Allingham & Thorpe is reported; and Lindner and Kutner refer to several such cases in their book "Chirugische Magen Krankheiten." In Allingham and Thorpe's case a gastro-enterostomy had eventually to be done in order to save the life of the patient, and Lindner and Kutner remark that this complication has frequently proved fatal. Nor is such a secondary hemorrhage likely to be an unusual accident; on the contrary, it is what we would be most apt to expect when the gangrenous edges of the perforated ulcer separate from the surrounding tissues. Furthermore, we must not lose sight of the fact that there may be multiple ulcers and that any one of these may occasion bleeding or perforation. As said above, the questions that arise are: can these life-threatening complications be averted by establishing gastro-enterostomy at the same time that the perforation is repaired; and, secondly, does such gastro-enterostomy expose the patient to such great risks of diffuse peritonitis by spreading the infection to previously uninvolved portions of the peritoneum, that it is better to take the risks of these secondary complications occurring, than it is to expose the patient to the dangers of a more diffuse peritonitis? It seems to the writer that gastro-enterostomy would protect, to some extent, against the secondary complications of hemorrhage and perforation, and that it will be possible, as a rule, to establish an anterior gastro-enterostomy without materially spreading the infection in the peritoneal cavity. The writer knows of no case in which a gastro-enterostomy has been done at the time of repair of a perforating ulcer; in the future cases in his own practice he would be inclined, if the patient's condition permitted of it, to carry out this procedure in addition to repairing the ulcers.

C.—After treatment.—The immediate treatment after operations has already been described in previous volumes of these reports. The stomach is kept empty for forty-eight hours, and then fluids in small quantities are given. Rectal nourishment is maintained until the patient is able to sustain himself on the food he takes by mouth. If vomiting occurs and is repeated, gastric lavage is immediately instituted, and repeated every six to eight hours if necessary. We have not experienced any bad results in our cases from gastric lavage, even when it has had to be done within the first twelve to twenty-four hours after operation.

In cases of open ulcer, dietary regulations are prescribed and the patient is requested to report for observation until all the evidences of ulceration have disappeared.

In cases of perforating ulcer we have kept the stomach empty at least three days, and when the patient was not too intractable five days. The bowels are moved by daily enemata; a mild cathartic is usually administered about the fifth or sixth day.

D.—Results.—The immediate results from our operations are stated in the table on page 194.

The late results, as far as we have been able to ascertain them, are that all but two of the cases have remained cured. In one of these cases the symptoms of gastric ulcer returned about three months after a posterior gastro-enterostomy for an open pyloric ulcer had been made. During these three months she had felt so well that she had disregarded all our advice as to dietary regulations. She was readmitted to the medical division of the hospital, where she was placed on rectal feeding and put to bed. Several times she vomited small amounts of blood, and she lost considerable weight. Every time gastric feeding was commenced the symptoms of the ulcer returned. Another laparotomy was, therefore, proposed and accepted by the patient. On opening the abdomen the gastro-enteric orifice was found to be closed, there were numerous adhesions of the anterior gastric wall to the abdominal parieties, and the pylorus was partially patent. A thickened ulcer could be felt on the anterior wall, near to the pylorus. Finney's gastro-duodenostomy was done. The patient made an uninterrupted convalescence and up to the present, about eight months after the last operation, she has remained well. (1903-1904, Vol. ii., page 119.)

In the other case mild recurrent symptoms of ulcer appeared about eight months after a Finney operation. This disappeared at once when the patient's diet was regulated.

MALIGNANT DISEASE.

	Total.	Cured.	Improved.	Unimproved.	Died.
Lympho-sarcoma of stomach	1				1
Carcinoma of cardiac end of stomach	2		1		1
" " " " " and lesser curvature	1				1
Carcinoma of cardiac, and benign stenosis of pylorus	1		1		
Carcinoma of body of stomach	3*			3	
" " pylorus	12	1	8	1†	2

A.—The only hope of patients afflicted with malignant disease of the stomach lies in the radical removal, by the knife, of all the cancerous tissue. For this to be feasible the diagnosis of the malady must be made early, i.e., before metastatic cancerous deposits have appeared in the neighboring glands and liver. Such early diagnosis is not, however, easy, and if it is to be made, the general practitioner who sees the cases first, must completely change his present methods of dealing with them. By many physicians the diagnosis of cancer of the stomach is not made until a tumor becomes palpable; until such a time all sorts of opinions are expressed as to the cause of the gastric symptoms, the most common being chronic dyspepsia, neurasthenia, and anemia. The appearance of a tumor is the first suggestion of the true nature of the malady, and then the patient is sent post-haste to the surgeon for operation. Unfortunately for the patient, however, it is now too late for radical operation, for by this time the malady has advanced so far that a lasting radical cure from surgical efforts is not possible. So great an authority as Czerny has stated that no case of cancer of the stomach should be operated upon radically when its recognition as a tumor has become certain.

The diagnosis of malignant disease of the stomach must, therefore, be made before a tumor becomes palpable if we are to afford the patient the only hope he has for radical cure of his malady.

This can only be possible when patients who are suspected of being afflicted with this malady are advised and urged by their physicians to undergo an exploratory laparotomy, in order to ascertain the exact cause of the gastric disturbances. We advisedly say, "patients

*1 case not operated; 2 cases explored.
†Not operated.

who are suspected of having this malady," because during the early stages of gastric cancer we cannot be certain of the diagnosis until the abdomen has been opened and the parts rendered accessible to direct inspection and palpation. The suspicious signs of cancer of the stomach are:

(a) *Dyspeptic symptoms coming on in a patient beyond 40 years of age*, for which no cause can be found, and which are exceedingly rebellious to treatment. It would be far better to suspect all patients beyond 40 who suddenly manifest rebellious dyspeptic symptoms as afflicted with cancer and devote our efforts to disprove its presence, than it is to disagnosticate some benign affection and let the patient continue to go along until the development of a tumor dispels all doubt as to the diagnosis, and at the same time all hope of radical cure.

(b) *Changes in the chemical composition of the gastric juice.*—Such changes are (1) an absence of free hydrochloric acid and ferment, and (2) the presence of lactic acid. To detect these changes it is necessary to make chemical examinations of the gastric secretion. This should be a part of our routine examination in these cases. The tests are simple, and can be readily and quickly made in the office or laboratory by every physician. To neglect making them is as serious an oversight as is the failure to examine the urine in a case of suspected nephritis. These changes in the chemicity of the gastric secretion are not present in all cases, nor do they invariably indicate that a cancer is present. Thus, when the cancer develops on the base of an old ulcer, the gastric juice may contain HCl, and may even be hyperacid.

Anacidity, again, occurs in all forms of atrophy of the gastric mucosa, no matter what its cause may be.

As regards lactic acid, we find this is present in the gastric contents whenever there is coincident stagnation within the stomach and anacidity of the gastric juice. Both these conditions are not always present in carcinoma of the stomach, e.g., in those cases where the carcinoma is not situated at the pyloric orifice, and, consequently, lactic acid is not invariably present in the gastric contents of patients suffering with carcinoma of stomach. Furthermore, these conditions may be present in benign stenosis of the pylorus, associated with marked atrophy of the gastric mucosa. Consequently lactic acid may be present in the gastric contents of non-malignant disease of the stomach.

No one of the chemical changes in the gastric juice is thus seen to be conclusive evidence of, or an invariable accompaniment of gastric cancer. This does not permit us, however, to ignore them. Positive or negative as they may be, they have a real value in the early diagnosis of cancer, and especially if they are considered in conjunction with the previous clinical history and the other clinical data.

(c) *Disturbances of gastric motility.*—These are present only when the neoplasm is at the pylorus, whose lumen it constricts. Such disturbances are evidenced by stagnation of food within the stomach, and by prolongation of the time that the stomach normally takes to empty itself after a meal. Such symptoms are very significant, when they are combined with the symptoms that have already been mentioned, and especially when they occur in a patient beyond 40 who never has had any gastric malady.

(d) *Secondary anemia.*

The most that can be said of the value of these symptoms for diagnosis, is that they are suspicious. Should they, however, prove rebellious to local and dietary treatment, they demand that we lose no further time in useless observation, but proceed to open the abdomen and ascertain their cause.

It has been said against this argument, that exploratory laparotomy has its dangers, and that patients will not accept the proposition of exploration while they are in the early stages of the malady. As regards the first objection, viz., "that exploration is attended with risk to life," this cannot be denied, but this risk in proper hands is very slight, a small fraction of one per cent., and certainly cannot be compared to the risks to which the patient is exposed when we allow to slip by the only period in which a radical cure can be effected of the cancerous malady from which he may be suffering. In reference to the second objection the writer has found that few patients reject the proposal when the matter is put to them in the proper light, provided they see that all efforts at making a diagnosis in other ways have been resorted to. And if we do find difficulty in persuading patients to early exploratory operation, it is our duty to educate the public to the real importance and life-saving value of such early exploratory operations in cancerous disease of the stomach, and other internal organs.

In the patients that came to the hospital for treatment we had no difficulty in making a diagnosis, for they were all well advanced in the disease, and in all a tumor was palpable. Similarly, in all but one radical cure was impossible, and that one was on the border line. In the cases in which we practiced exploratory laparotomy, this was not done for diagnostic purposes, but to ascertain whether radical operation was still feasible. In all such cases it was found that the malady had advanced too far to permit of our attempting its radical removal. Besides the radical operations, palliative measures have been practiced by us when the neoplasm constricted the pyloric or cardiac orifices of the stomach. We have carried out such palliative operations in spite of their attendant high mortality, because in the surviving cases relief of suffering and some prolongation of life were afforded thereby.

(B.)—OPERATIONS FOR MALIGNANT DISEASE OF THE STOMACH, 18 OPERATIONS, 5 DEATHS.

	Total.	Cured.	Improved.	Unimproved.	Died.
Exploratory laparotomy	2	..	..	2	..
Gastrostomy	3	..	1	..	2
Gastro-enterostomy; anterior	4	..	4	..	..
" " posterior	7	..	4	..	3
" " gastrostomy (Witzel)	1	..	1	..	..
Partial gastrectomy, with resection of the transverse colon and removal of the celiac glands.	1	1			

Gastrostomy is done according to the Kader or Senn method. The fistula that is established in either of these ways has always been tight and easily cared for by the patients.

Our method of doing gastro-enterostomy has already been detailed. We always use the Murphy button. The button has been passed in the stools in three cases, and on the 18th, 23d, and 24th day, respectively. In the other cases it was not recovered, though the X-ray did not show it to be lodged in the gastro-intestinal tract.

Partial gastrectomy with resection of the transverse colon and removal of the celiac glands. 1903-1904, Vol. ii., page 144, *Carcinoma of pylorus and celiac glands.*—Herman H., 49 years old, was admitted June 24, 1904. The first evidences of his malady were manifested fifteen months before, when he began to have cramp-like pains in the epigastrium and vomiting. The pain gradually disappeared, but the vomiting became more frequent. The vomitus consisted of undigested food, and on one occasion of blood. He had lost 30 pounds in weight, and felt too weak to do any work.

On admission physical examination showed the heart, lungs, liver, spleen and genitals to be normal. The patient was much emaciated; in the epigastrium there was a hard, tender, slightly movable mass the size of a lemon. The gastric contents after Ewald's test meal were acid, contained no free HCl, no lactic acid, and had a total acidity of 28.0. There was stagnant food in the stomach sixteen hours after its ingestion.

The diagnosis was very evident, pyloric carcinoma causing stenosis. Gastro-enterostomy was proposed to the patient, with the promise that if radical extirpation of the tumor was feasible this would be attempted. June 27, the abdomen was opened in the median line from the ensiform to the umbilicus. A large annular tumor of the pylorus was found, extending on to the adjacent wall of the stomach, its transverse diameter being one and a half inches. The stomach was perfectly movable and could be brought out of the abdomen. There were numerous hard, but movable glands in the gastro-hepatic omentum, and also a number of glands in the gastro-colic omentum, especially near the pylorus. The mobility of the stomach tumor prompted the writer to attempt the radical operation. The liver was apparently not involved in the malignant disease. The removal of the tumor and of the stomach walls was accordingly proceeded with. The gastric pyloris and gastro-epiploic arteries were first doubly deligated and divided. The gastro-hepatic omentum was then divided close to the liver and the celiac glands all excised, together with their surrounding fat. The duodenum well beyond the tumor was then divided with the Paquelin between two clamps. The gastro-colic omentum was grasped in sections between two clamps and divided. It was fairly closely adherent to the transverse mesacolon and, though especial care was taken to avoid the middle colic artery, this was, nevertheless, included in one of the clamps and divided. The transverse colon, which this artery supplied, immediately became pale, and its excision had to be decided upon. The stomach, well beyond the limits of the last glands in the gastro-colic omentum, was grasped by two large clamps and divided between them with the Paquelin. There was left of the stomach a little less than one-third. The duodenum was now closed by three rows of sutures, the inner of which (catgut) was a Connell suture of all the coats. The stump of the stomach was similarly closed. The compromised portion of the transverse colon (about 8 inches) with its mesocolon was excised and its ends brought together with Murphy's button. A posterior gastrojejunostomy with the button was finally established, and the abdominal wound closed, with drainage down to the duodenal stump.

The operation lasted about two and a half hours, and at its end the patient was in good condition. The pathological report of the tumor and glands was adeno-carcinoma. The reaction from the operation was prompt and good. The removal of the colon precluded our using rectal stimulation and alimentation, and compelled us to give fluids by mouth much earlier than we usually do. Water, in drachm doses, by mouth were given after twenty-four hours. There was no vomiting. Liquid peptonoids were given by mouth on the third day, and gradually other forms of fluid nourishment were added. He vomited once on the fifth day. His bowels were moved by enema on the fifth day, and thereafter daily enemata were given. The first dressing of the wound was made on the eighth day after operation. The rubber tissue gauze drain was removed. It was slightly bile stained. It was replaced by a strip of gauze.

Soft diet (farina, etc.) was given on the ninth day. The drainage opening discharged a little bile which seemed to come from the duodenal stump. This discharge of bile continued with intermissions of few days for about eight weeks. The patient gained gradually in weight, and by November 21 he had gained 31 pounds; on this day he returned to his home in Texas, feeling perfectly well, with no evidence of recurrence. The intestinal button was passed on the sixteenth day. The stomach button was not recovered, but could not be seen with the X-ray.

COMMENTS.—Although in this case the greatest care was exercised to avoid injuring the middle colic artery, nevertheless, on account of the adhesion of the posterior surface of the stomach to the upper layer of the transverse mesocolon, this vessel was included in one of the mass ligatures and divided.

In a similar experience in Körte practice, in which the division of this vessel was, however, not noticed at the time of the operation, a second laparotomy had to be done and the gangrenous colon removed. In our case an immediate removal of the portion of the transverse colon, whose blood supply had been compromised, was made.

Although but less than one-third of the stomach remained, the patient was able to take and thoroughly digest enormous quantities of food at one sitting. His usual dinner was about three times as much as the ordinary working man takes.

Our department of physiological chemistry will, at a future time, report the results of their investigations on the assimilation and excretion of this patient.

The immediate results of our operation for malignant disease of the stomach are given in the table. In the only case in which radical cure was attempted no recurrence was noted at the time of his discharge from the hospital, i.e., five months after operation. No news has since been obtained from him.

Patients in whom a palliative operation was done, were relieved of much of their suffering. They were able, in most instances, to get about, they gained in weight and could digest food. Their life was undoubtedly considerably prolonged.

DRY IODINE CATGUT.

By Alexis V. Moschcowitz, M.D.,
ADJUNCT ATTENDING SURGEON.

We have used, in the first surgical division of Mount Sinai Hospital, catgut sterilized after the method of Claudius, since the publication of his first article on the subject in August, 1902. The catgut thus prepared had many advantages over the von Bergmann catgut, which had been in use at the hospital prior to that time; but it had one disadvantage, namely, that in time it has lost considerable of its tensile strength. Its advantages were, however, so preponderating that, instead of abandoning it, I set myself the task to find and, if possible, to eliminate the causes of this deterioration. It soon became evident that this was due solely to the long-continued immersion of the catgut in the aqueous iodine solution; I have, therefore, modified the original method of Claudius in so far, that after exposing the catgut to the action of the iodine solution for a time, sufficiently long to render it absolutely sterile, I remove it from the solution, and thereafter preserve it dry in a sterile container. Be this modification ever so slight, it was, nevertheless, an important departure from Claudius' method; it was necessary, therefore, to subject the catgut prepared according to the modified method to a strict scrutiny regarding its qualities. The requisite experimental work I was enabled to do, through the courtesy of Dr. T. Mitchell Prudden, at the Pathological Laboratory of the College of Physicians and Surgeons, Columbia University, and a detailed account of it will shortly appear in the *Annals of Surgery*. The following is merely a condensed abstract from it, in order to call attention to the method of sterilizing catgut, now in use at the hospital.

A perfect catgut should have the following attributes:

(*a*) It should be absolutely sterile.
(*b*) It should not loose any of its tensile strength.
(*c*) It should be readily, simply and cheaply prepared.
(*d*) It should be absorbed, but only after it has served the purpose for which it was intended.

(*a*) *Sterility.*—On the first surgical division of Mount Sinai Hospital we have used the catgut prepared according to the modified method since July, 1904, on every occasion where the use of catgut was at all indicated, both as ligature and suture material, and in no instance did we have occasion to regret our confidence in it. This much for the clinical evidence of its sterility; but as this would hardly be sufficient to convince the skeptic, it was also necessary to determine its sterility from a bacteriological point of view.

Three sets of experiments were carried out in the following manner:

I. Experiments to prove the sterility of the catgut.

II. Experiments to show the behavior of bacteria in the presence of the catgut.

III. Experiments to show the effects of infected catgut.

At the outset I would state that all of the experiments were carried out with No. 1 iodine catgut, and that in every instance control tests were made with von Bergmann catgut of similar size.

I. Experiments to prove the sterility of the catgut.

These experiments were carried out in the following manner: Pieces of iodine and von Bergmann catgut, about one inch in length, were planted in the following media: bouillon, gelatine (previously liquified and poured into Petri dishes), agar-agar (previously liquified and poured into Petri dishes), and mixtures of hydrocele serum and bouillon. The gelatine cultures were kept at room temperature, the remainder were kept in the thermostat, and all were observed daily for about two weeks.

The result of these experiments was the following. None of the experiments made with iodine catgut was followed by a growth, while some of those made with the von Bergmann gut, notably those in liquid media, were followed by a growth.

In refutal of the possible argument, that the iodine contained in one inch of No. 1 iodine catgut was sufficient to render antiseptic the entire, though comparatively small, amount of medium used, I also planted one-inch pieces of iodine catgut in large amounts (60 c.c.) of media, but in no instance did I obtain a growth.

The conclusion arrived at by these experiments was, that the iodine catgut is positively sterile.

II. Experiments to show the behavior of bacteria in the presence of Iodine catgut.

These were carried out in the following manner. Gelatine and agar-

agar were liquified, and inoculated with one of following bacteria, Bac. coli communis, Staphyl. aureus, Strepto. pyogenes, Bac. anthracis and Bac. subtilis; they were then poured into Petri dishes, and after solidification a piece of iodine catgut was placed upon them. Control plates were made with von Bergmann catgut. The gelatine plates were kept at room temperature, while the agar plates were kept in the thermostat. Daily observations were taken for about two weeks, and the state of growth noted.

It was seen that numberless colonies developed upon all the plates, with the exception of a clear space immediately surrounding the catgut. This clear space surrounding the iodine catgut was at least four times as large as that surrounding the von Bergmann gut, and in no case was there subsequently noted an encroachment of the colonies upon the clear space surrounding the iodine catgut, but some was noted in the experiments made with von Bergmann catgut.

Another series of experiments was carried out in the following manner. Agar-agar was liquified and poured into Petri dishes; after solidification a number of streaks were made upon the surface with one of the following bacteria, Bac. coli communis, Staphl. aureus, Strepto. pyogenes, Bac. anthracis and Bac. subtilis. Upon these a piece of iodine catgut was placed; control plates were made with von Bergmann catgut. All were kept in the thermostat, and daily observations were taken for about two weeks.

It was seen that colonies developed upon the ends of the streaks furthest away from the iodine catgut, while upon the plates made with the von Bergmann catgut colonies developed and extended toward the gut, so as to be in some instances in actual contact with it.

This duplicate set of experiments shows the powerful action of the iodine gut, in preventing the development of colonies, not only in its immediate vicinity, but also at some distance from it. I assumed *a priori* that in the von Bergmann catgut we are dealing with an aseptic, and not with an antiseptic catgut, and, in consequence, I was at first unable to explain the clear space surrounding this catgut. The explanation of this phenomenon was forthcoming only after Dr. Bookman, physiological chemist to Mount Sinai Hospital, was kind enough to undertake for me a chemical analysis of the catgut in question; he found that one yard of No. 1 von Bergmann catgut contained an amount of mercury which would be equivalent to

0.008825 of HgCl2. This will readily explain the relatively small sterile area upon the plates.

With a certain amount of justice, it might be argued that in these experiments the iodine exerts merely an inhibitory action, and that there are still numerous active and living bacteria in the clear space surrounding the iodine catgut, which are only temporarily prevented from developing, but which would still develop if placed under more favorable surroundings. The assumption of this theory was disproven by making cultures from this clear area, which were, however, never followed by a growth. This was also corroborated by implanting a liberal piece of the clear agar surrounding the iodine gut on an anthrax plate under the skin of a guinea-pig, which the animal survived without the slightest disturbance, despite the high virulence of the particular anthrax culture used. This, and other additional factors, too numerous to mention, are sufficient to prove that the iodine not only inhibits the growth of the bacteria, but completely destroys them.

The conclusions arrived at by these experiments were that the iodine catgut will at least in a measure assist in neutralizing accidental infections in wounds.

III. Experiments to show the effect of infected catgut.

These were carried out in the following manner. Bouillon cultures were made of the following actively growing bacteria, Bac. coli communis, Staphylo. aureus, Strepto. pyogenes, Bac. anthracis and Bac. subtilis, and were allowed to grow in the thermostat for twenty-four hours. In every instance an abundant growth was obtained. At this time the culture medium was divided into two halves; into one there were placed about one dozen pieces of iodine catgut, about one inch in length, and into the other an equal number of pieces of von Bergmann gut, of similar size. They were then replaced for a further twenty-four hours into the thermostat. At this time pieces of the various kinds of catgut, still wet, were taken out and planted in bouillon, or placed on agar, previously liquified and poured into a Petri dish. The supernatant culture was then poured off and the container was replaced for a further twenty-four hours into the thermostat, by which time the catgut had become perfectly dry. With this dry catgut another series of experiments was carried out. All the cultures were kept in the thermostat, and daily observations were made for about two weeks.

The result of all these experiments was, that in no instance was the infected iodine catgut followed by a growth, while on the other hand every experiment made with the infected von Bergmann catgut was followed by an abundant growth.

In addition to the above experiments I have also infected both iodine and von Bergmann catgut with pus obtained from various sources, and in which various micro-organisms were found, either by slides or cultures, and in no instance did I obtain a growth in the experiments made with iodine catgut, but a growth was obtained in every instance in the experiments made with von Bergmann catgut.

All of the experiments just related show, at least as far as the bacteriological test is concerned, that not only is the iodine catgut absolutely sterile, but also that it is impossible to infect it, either with cultures of known activity, or with resistant spores, or with ordinary pus.

I know full well that the human organism is not a bacteriological test tube, and it would be entirely erroneous to transfer these bacteriological experiments to the operating room; but this much at least may be taken for granted, that with the precautions ordinarily taken at an operation, it ought to be impossible to introduce infections into a wound with iodine catgut.

(*b*) *Tensile strength.*—As already stated, the only reason for modifying Claudius' original method was, that it was followed by an appreciable loss of tensile strength. I was compelled, therefore, to prove that the catgut prepared by the modified method is a real improvement over the older method also in this respect.

It is not sufficient for me to state that in actual use we have found that the catgut is sufficiently strong for all the requirements or demands made upon it; nor should much credence be put upon the statements of others, who have perhaps found that it was too brittle. A great deal depends upon the personal equation of the individual who is using or testing it. If "A" wishes to prove that a given catgut is strong he does not pull quite as hard as "B," who wishes to prove the contrary, and vice versa. The only way to prove or disprove anything of this nature is by actually and accurately determining the breaking point.

With catgut this is particularly difficult on account of many qualities inherent in it, of which I would call attention merely to the following: (1) the variations in so-called and presumably true standard sizes; (2) the variations in size in different parts of the same roll; (3) the variations in texture, and (4) the variations in the method of manufacture. In addition I also had some difficulty, because I had no accurate apparatus to use in my measurements; but, finally, Dr. Forbes, of the Physical Laboratory of Columbia University, very kindly constructed one for me, which I believe to be devoid of gross errors. Its principle is that a given piece of catgut is accurately weighted until it breaks. As an average of a great many measurements I have found that No. 0 iodine catgut broke at 3665 grammes, No. 0 von Bergmann catgut at 3180 grammes, and No. 0 raw catgut at 3081 grammes. No. 1 iodine catgut broke at 5446 grammes, No. 1 von Bergmann catgut at 4592 grammes, and No. 1 raw catgut at 4961 grammes. No. 2 iodine catgut broke at 7320 grammes, No. 2 von Bergmann catgut at 7132 grammes, and No. 2 raw catgut at 6526 grammes. This gives us an excellent and very fair estimate of the tensile strength of the three varieties of catgut, as used as suture material, but if used for ligatures there enters the additional and very important element of the knot. It was necessary, therefore, to repeat the measurements with the addition of a knot. Following were the findings obtained: No. 0 iodine catgut broke at 2220 grammes, No. 0 von Bergmann catgut broke at 2244 grammes, and No. 0 raw catgut at 1984 grammes; No. 1 iodine catgut broke at 3557 grammes, No. 1 von Bergmann catgut at 3446 grammes, and No. 1 raw catgut at 2996 grammes; No. 2 iodine catgut broke at 4678 grammes, No. 2 von Bergmann catgut at 5217 grammes, and No. 2 raw catgut at 3800 grammes.

These tests show that with one exception the iodine catgut, both with and without knots, is not only equal to the other varieties, but that in most instances it is far superior to raw catgut or von Bergmann catgut. The only exception to be noted is with the No. 2 catgut, which, if used as ligature material, shows a slight inferiority; but I believe this to be due to a particularly poor lot of catgut; and it is not impossible that more extensive measurements will equalize the values here also.

(c) *Method of preparation.*—The preparation and subsequent preservation of this catgut is simplicity itself. The raw catgut, just as it is bought from the dealers and without any previous preparation, is loosely wound on a glass spool, preferably in a single layer, and fastened at both ends, in order to prevent unraveling. It is then immersed for eight days in a solution containing one part of iodine, one part of iodide of potassium in one hundred parts of distilled water. (The solution is prepared by dissolving the iodide of potassium in a small quantity of the water, to which the iodine, previously finely pulverized, is added, and the whole diluted up to one hundred parts.)

After an immersion of eight days in this solution the catgut is removed therefrom and kept merely in a sterile container, preferably protected from the light. Any unused catgut may be resterilized on a subsequent occasion.

It is used dry, just as it is cut from the spool, without any previous immersion in carbolic solution or distilled water.

That this method of preparation is simple, no one can deny; that it is extremely cheap, itself no mean item, particularly in hospitals where large quantities are used, is also self evident; one gallon of the solution requiring 608 grains each of iodine and iodide of potassium, costing only 42 cents.

It is important to keep the solution in well-stoppered bottles or jars, because the iodine is volatile and in time it deteriorates. Solutions good enough to use should have in bulk a deep-brown, almost black color.

The catgut itself is also of a deep-brown, almost black color, and still retains the characteristic odor of iodine; it is perfectly smooth, not swollen, as one might be inclined to expect from its immersion in an aqueous solution. It has no tendency to kink, like catgut used from alcohol, but it is somewhat stiff, like a very fine wire; should it at any time prove too stiff, immersion for a few minutes in sterile water will render it perfectly smooth and pliable.

(*d*) *Absorption.*—Regarding this point we can only assert from a practical experience that the knots stay tight, and do not tend to untie or loosen, and we have never seen any untoward symptoms which could be traced to a too early or too late absorption.

Disadvantages.—Of these I know none, but in order to prevent any misconception, it will perhaps not be amiss if I briefly mention those possibilities which might be raised against it.

The toxic effects of the iodine might cause some apprehension: there need be no fear on this account, because (1) even in the most extensive operations, e.g., radical operation for carcinoma of the breast, the toxic dose can never be reached; (2) the iodine is divided so minutely that it quickly enters into a chemical combination with the salts of the body fluids, and forms only the innocuous iodides, etc., and (3) because of late, after being so astonished at the almost marvelous antiseptic properties of the iodine solution, I have in a large number of cases used iodine solutions for dressing wounds, using at each dressing large quantities of gauze dipped in the iodine solution, but in no instance did I find even the slightest trace of irritation, either in the wound or on the part of the excretory organs. (I may mention here that I am now carrying on extensive experiments with iodine gauze as a dressing, and with iodine for the purpose of sterilizing chromicized catgut, etc., which will be published at an early date.) For the reasons stated, I may also allay the apprehension that the iodine may act as an irritant upon the tissues.

The odor of the catgut and the staining of the linens, through the formation of iodide of starch, are so trivial that they do not even merit discussion; particularly is this true of the latter, as by experience we have found, that the stains are not permanent and readily disappear in the laundrying process.

I believe our clinical experience and the experimental work carried out in connection with this research fully justify the following conclusions:

1. Dry iodine catgut is absolutely sterile.
2. It is impossible to infect it either with ordinary germs, or with spores, or with pus.
3. Its tensile strength fully equals, and in most instances is superior to that of raw catgut, or von Bergmann's catgut.
4. It is readily and cheaply prepared.
5. It is absorbed only after it has served the purposes intended for.
6. It is very agreeable to use, and
7. It is absolutely safe in every respect.

DISEASES TREATED IN THE SECOND SURGICAL DIVISION,

From December 1, 1902, to December 1, 1903.

HOWARD LILIENTHAL, M.D.,
ATTENDING SURGEON.

JOSEPH WIENER, JR., M.D., CHARLES A. ELSBERG, M.D.,
ADJUNCT ATTENDING SURGEONS.

TOTAL, 632.

	Total	No operation	Died
Cranium—8.			
Scalp—4.			
Abscess of	1	..	..
Wound of	3	3	..
Skull and Contents—4.			
Fracture of base	1	1	..
Cerebellar tumor	1	1	..
Arterio-venous aneurysm, intracranial	1	..	..
Thrombosis of cavernous sinus	1	..	1
Face and Mouth—23.			
Infected wound of forehead	1	1	..
Contusion of face	1	1	..
Lacerated wound of mouth and chin	1	1	..
Epithelioma of lip	1	..	..
Facial palsy	1	1	..
Adenoids	1	..	..
Sarcoma of parotid	1	..	..
Alveolar abscess	1	..	..
Hare lip	2	..	..
Abscess of tongue	1	..	..
Cicatricial contraction of face following burns	2	1	..
Burns of face and arms	1	1	..
" " head and chest	1	1	..
Erysipelas and otitis media	1	..	..
Sarcoma of tonsil	1	..	1
Necrosis of superior maxilla, empyema of antrum	1	..	..
Osteomyelitis of inferior maxilla	4	..	..
Sarcoma of inferior maxilla	1	1	..

	Total	No operation	Died
Neck—21.			
Abscess of	1	..	..
Chronic phlegmon of	1	..	..
Actinomycotic abscess of	1	..	..
Cellulitis of	1	..	..
Tubercular abscess of	2	..	..
Carbuncle of	2	..	..
Lipoma of	1	..	..
Tubercular adenitis of	5	..	..
Arterio-venous aneurysm of	1	..	1
Retropharyngeal abscess	1	1	..
Parenchymatous goitre	1	..	..
" cystic goitre	1	..	..
Persistent thyro-glossal duct	1	..	..
Suppurating glands of neck, mediastinal tumor	1	..	1
Angina Ludovici	1	..	..
Upper Extremity—30.			
Shoulder—5.			
Lipoma	1	..	..
Scapula, sarcoma of	2	..	..
Clavicle, osteomyelitis	1	..	..
" " tubercular	1	..	..
Axilla—3.			
Adenitis	1	..	..
Cyst	1	..	1
Carcinoma, recurrent, of glands	1	..	..
Arm—4.			
Cellulitis	1	1	1
Wounds of arm, acute osteomyelitis of humerus	1	..	1
Humerus, osteomyelitis, chronic	1	..	..
Tuberculosis of fascia	1	..	..
Forearm—9.			
Cellulitis, and of ankle, pyemia	1	..	1
"	1	..	..
Radius and ulna, osteomyelitis, acute	1	..	..
" " " compound fracture	2	..	..
" tubercular ostitis	1	..	..
Elbow joint, tubercular arthritis	1	..	..
" " " " and of ankle, sepsis	1	..	1
Contusion of musculo-spinal nerve	1	1	..

Hand—9.

	Total.	No operation.	Died.
Sinus of wrist, tubercular	1	..	..
Cellulitis, of hand and arm	1	..	..
Infected wound, hand	1	..	..
Traumatic amputation of hand	1	..	..
" " " fingers	2	..	..
Lacerated wounds of fingers	1	..	..
Gangrene of fingers	1	1	..
Cicatricial deformity of thumb	1	..	..

Breast—8.

Abscess of breast	1	..	..
Chronic mastitis	1	..	..
Carcinoma of breast	6	1	..

Thorax—21.

Necrosis of sternum	1	..	..
Osteomyelitis of rib	2	..	..
Fracture of ribs	1	1	..
Traumatic pleurisy	1	..	..
Empyema	1	..	..
" sinus	11	..	..
Tumor of thorax, suppurating glands of neck	1	..	1
Lipoma of back	2	..	..
Carbuncle of back	1	..	..

Spine—2.

Cyst of sacral region	1	..	..
Infected lumbar meningocele	1	..	..

Abdominal Wall—5.

Abscess of	2	..	..
Sinus of	2	..	..
Diastasis of recti muscles	1	1	..

General Abdominal Cavity—13.

Intra-abdominal abscess	1	..	..
Peritonitis, diffuse, purulent	2	..	1
" " " pneumococcus	1	..	1
" " " gonorrheal	1	..	..
" chronic adhesive	1	..	..
" tubercular	2	..	..
Omental adhesions causing symptoms after laparotomy	4	2	..
Intra-abdominal omental torsion	1	..	..

Esophagus and Stomach—13.

	Total	No operation	Died
Esophageal stenosis	2	2	..
" " malignant	1	..	..
Pyloric stenosis, benign	2	..	..
Carcinoma of pylorus	4	..	..
" " stomach	3	..	1
" " " hour-glass contraction	1	..	..

Pancreas—3.

Acute pancreatitis, chronic appendicitis	1	1	..
" " hemorrhagic	1	..	1
Carcinoma	1	..	..

Liver—6.

Abscess	1	..	..
Echinococcus cyst	2	..	..
Suppurating gumma	1	..	..
Carcinoma	2	..	1

Gall Bladder and Ducts—32.

Acute cholecystitis	1	1	..
" " and cholelithiasis	5	1	..
" ulcerative cholecystitis and cholelithiasis	1	..	..
" " " cholelithiasis, diffuse peritonitis	1	..	1
Post-typhoid cholecystitis	1	..	..
Pericholecystitis	2	..	..
Gangrenous cholecystitis and fracture of femur	1	..	1
" "	2	..	..
Empyema of gall bladder and cholelithiasis	1	..	..
Cholelithiasis	10	2	..
Chronic cholecystitis	1	..	..
" " and cholelithiasis	6	..	..

Intestines—21.

Constipation	4	4	..
Entero-colitis	3	3	..
Colitis, chronic	1	..	..
Perforation of intestine, typhoid	5	..	3
Ileo-colic intussusception	2	..	1
Volvulus of small intestine	1	..	1
Intestinal obstruction, due to band	2	..	1
" " " " cholecystitis and peritonitis	1	..	1
Fecal fistula	1	..	..
Carcinoma of sigmoid flexure	1	..	1

	Total.	No operation.	Died.
Appendicitis—143.			
Acute catarrhal	15	3	..
" ulcerative	3	..	..
Empyema of appendix	5	..	..
Gangrenous appendicitis	27	..	..
" perforative	6	..	..
" " with abscess	18	..	1
" " " serous peritonitis	2	..	..
" " abscess, serous peritonitis	2	..	..
" " diffuse peritonitis	6	..	2
" " purulent "	7	1	4
" " abscess, diffuse peritonitis	2	..	..
Acute perforative, general purulent peritonitis	1	..	1
Gangrenous, omental thrombosis	1	..	..
Appendicitis abscess	1	..	..
Chronic catarrhal	43	3	..
" " chronic intestinal obstruction	1	..	..
Adhesions after appendicectomy	1	..	..
Sinus after appendicitis	2	..	..
Hernia—60.			
Inguinal	33	5	..
" strangulated	5	..	..
" congenital	4	..	..
" recurrent	2	..	..
" following Alexander operation	1	..	..
" with hydrocele of canal of Nuck	1	..	..
" incarcerated congenital	1	..	..
" strangulated "	1	..	..
" infantile	1	..	..
Femoral, strangulated	1	..	..
Ventral	7	1	..
Umbilical, strangulated	1	..	..
Epigastric	1	..	..
Diastasis of recti abdominis	1	1	..
Genito-Urinary Diseases—59.			
Kidney—15.			
Cyst of kidney	1	..	1
Calculus in one ureter	1	..	..
" hydronephrosis, stones in both ureters	1	..	1
Pyonephrosis	3	..	2
Abscesses of kidney, multiple	1	..	..
Sinus after removal of calculus	1	..	..
Torsion of pedicle of kidney	1	..	..
Hypernephroma	2	..	1
Perinephric abscess	1	..	..
Surgical kidney, uremia	1	1	1
Pyelonephritis, gonorrheal	1	1	..
Renal colic	1	1	..

	Total	No operation	Died
Bladder—5			
Cystitis	1	..	..
Vesical hemorrhage	1	..	..
Papilloma	1	..	..
Calculus	1	..	..
Vesical fistula	1	..	..
Urethra—9.			
Stricture	5	..	1
Periurethral abscess	3	..	..
Phagedenic chancre	1	..	..
Prostate—8.			
Hypertrophy of prostate	8	2	2
Penis—4.			
Hypospadias	4	..	..
Scrotum and Testes—15.			
Varicocele	3	..	..
Tuberculosis of testes	1	..	..
Suppuration " "	1	..	..
Undescended testis	1	..	..
Tumor of undescended testicle	1	..	1
Hydrocele	2	..	..
Spermatocele	2	..	..
Gangrene of scrotum and perineum from ischio-rectal abscess	1	..	..
Chronic epididymitis	1	1	..
Gonorrheal orchitis	1	1	..
Orchitis following prostatectomy	1	1	..
Miscellaneous—3.			
Gonorrhea	1	1	..
Pyuria	1	1	..
Genito-urinary tuberculosis, with advanced pulmonary tuberculosis	1	1	..
Rectum and Anus—77.			
Hemorrhoids	41	..	..
Fissure in ano	6	..	..
Fistula " "	16	..	..
Carcinoma of rectum	1	..	..
Ischio-rectal abscess	7	..	..
Ulcer of rectum	1	..	..
Tumor of rectum	1	..	..
Stricture of rectum	1	..	..
Prolapse of rectum	2	..	..
Imperforate anus	1	..	..

Lower Extremity—72.

Pelvis and Hip Joint—11.

Abscess of hip..
Contusion of hip..
Groin, abscess of...
" adenitis of ....
" epithelioma of ....
Buttock, tuberculosis of skin of................................
" abscess of ....
Hip joint, tubercular coxitis, psoas abscess....................
" " chronic arthritis ....

Thigh—14.

Abscess, tubercular ....
Cellulitis ....
Hematoma, infected ....
Sarcoma, recurrent ....
Femur, metastatic carcinoma.....................................
" fracture of shaft................................
" " " ununited ....
" " " neck ....
" osteomyelitis, acute ....
" " tubercular ....
" acute, staphylococcemia ....

Knee—7.

Foreign body ....
Hemarthros ....
Arthritis, acute suppurative....................................
" tubercular ....
" " general tuberculosis ....
Gummata of knee..

Leg—21.

Abrasion of ....
Burns of ....
Phlebitis, suppurating ....
Phlegmon ....
Ulcer ....
" varicose ....
Varicose veins ....
Tibia, compound fracture.......................................
" necrosis ....
" osteomyelitis ....
" " tubercular ....
Fibula, fracture ....
Genu valgum ....
" extrorsum ....
Painful stump after amputation of leg..........................

Foot—19.

	Total	No operation	Died
Cellulitis	2		
" diabetic	1		
Foreign body in foot	1		
Gangrene, arterio-sclerotic	2		
" diabetic	3		1
" Raynaud's disease	2		
Persistent sinus	1		
Phlegmon	1		
Ankle joint, tuberculosis	2		
" " abscess, periarticular	1		
Calcaneo-astragaloid joint, tuberculosis	1		
Toe, gangrene, arterio-sclerotic	1		
Hallux valgus	1	1	

Female Genitals—6.

	Total	No operation	Died
Endometritis	2		
Uterine fibroids	1		
Pelvic cellulitis, gonorrheal (?)	1	1	
Tuberculosis of parovarian region	1		
Carcinoma of vulva and vagina and kraurosis vulvæ	1		

Miscellaneous—9.

	Total	No operation	Died
Broncho-pneumonia, empyema	1	1	1
Coprostasis	4	4	
Lead colic	1	1	
Endocarditis, malignant	1	1	
Neurasthenia	1	1	
Tuberculosis, general miliary	1	1	

OPERATIONS PERFORMED IN THE SECOND SURGICAL DIVISION FROM DECEMBER 1, 1902, TO DECEMBER 1, 1903.

TOTAL, 550; 44 DEATHS.

Cranium—3.

	Total	Died
Incision and drainage, abscess of scalp	1	
Exploratory craniotomy, thrombosis cavernous sinus	1	1
Ligature both common carotids, arterio-venous aneurysm at base of skull	1	

Face and Mouth—15.

	Total / Died
Excision of lip for epithelioma	1 / ..
Incision and drainage for empyema antrum of Highmore	1 / ..
" " " " osteomyelitis inferior maxilla	1 / ..
Osteotomy for osteomyelitis inferior maxilla	3 / ..
Excision of adenoids	1 / ..
" " parotid for sarcoma	1 / ..
" " tonsil " "	1 / 1
Incision and drainage for alveolar abscess	1 / ..
" " " " abscess of tongue	1 / ..
Plastic for hare lip	2 / ..
" " contracture due to burns of face	1 / ..
Paracentesis for otitis media	1 / ..

Neck—20.

Incision and drainage for abscess of	1 / ..
" " " " chronic phlegmon of	1 / ..
" " " " actinomycotic abscess of	1 / ..
" " " " cellulitis of	1 / ..
" " " " tubercular abscess of	2 / ..
" " " " carbuncle of	2 / ..
Excision of lipoma	1 / ..
" " parenchymatous goitre	1 / ..
" " cystic goitre	1 / ..
" " tubercular glands	5 / ..
" " arterio-venous aneurysm of	1 / ..
" " thyro-glossal duct	1 / ..
Tracheotomy for suppurating glands of neck, mediastinal tumor	1 / 1
" and incision and drainage for Angina Ludovici	1 / 1

Upper Extremity—37.

Amputation of arm for septic osteomyelitis	1 / 1
Excision, glands of axilla	1 / ..
" " " " carcinomatous	1 / ..
" cyst " "	1 / 1
" lipoma of shoulder	1 / ..
" sarcoma of scapula	2 / ..
" cicatrices of thumb	1 / ..
Incision and drainage, tubercular osteomyelitis of clavicle	1 / ..
" " " infected wounds of arm	2 / ..
" " " abscess of arm	1 / ..
" " " " " forearm	10 / 1
" " " sinus of elbow	1 / ..
" " " " " wrist	1 / ..
" " " phlegmon of hand	5 / ..
Osteotomy and drainage, osteomyelitis of clavicle	1 / ..
" " " " " humerus	2 / ..
" " " " " radius	1 / ..
" " suture, compound fracture of radius and ulna	1 / ..

	Total.	Died.
Upper Extremity—*Continued.*		
Osteotomy and drainage, arthritis of elbow and ankle...............	1	1
Skin plastic, traumatic amputation of hand........................	1	..
" " " " " fingers	1	..
Thorax—19.		
Thoracoplasty, empyema...	8	2
" thoracic sinus	2	..
Thoracotomy, empyema	2	..
Aspiration, traumatic pleurisy	1	..
Resection, osteomyelitis of rib...................................	2	..
Osteotomy, " " clavicle	1	..
Incision and drainage, tuberculosis...............................	1	..
" " " abscess infraclavicular region..................	1	..
Osteotomy, necrosis of sternum....................................	1	..
Breast—7.		
Amputation of breast, chronic mastitis............................	1	..
Incision and drainage, abscess of breast..........................	1	..
Radical amputation, carcinoma of breast...........................	5	..
Abdominal Wall—4.		
Incision and drainage abscess.....................................	2	..
" " " for sinus	1	..
Excision for sinus..	1	..
General Abdominal Cavity—11.		
Laparotomy and drainage, intra-abdominal abscess..................	1	..
" " " diffuse purulent peritonitis.............	2	1
" " " " " pneumococcus..	1	1
" " " " " gonorrheal peritonitis	1	..
" and breaking up of adhesions, chronic adhesive peritonitis.	1	..
" " " " " " tubercular peritonitis......	2	..
" division of omental adhesions after laparotomy............	2	..
" resection of omentum, intra-abdominal omental torsion.....	1	..
Esophagus and Stomach—12.		
Gastrostomy (Hall), for malignant stricture of esophagus...........	1	..
Gastroenterostomy, anterior (McGraw), for malignant stricture of pylorus	1	..
Gastroenterostomy, posterior (McGraw), for malignant stricture of pylorus	4	1
Gastroenterostomy, posterior (Kocher), stricture of pylorus.......	1	..
" " " (McGraw), for carcinoma of stomach.....	1	..
Gastrogastrostomy (McGraw), hour-glass contraction due to carcinoma	1	..
Gastroduodenostomy (Finney), for benign stenosis of pylorus.......	2	..
Exploratory laparotomy, carcinoma of stomach, inoperable..........	1	..

	Total	Died
Pancreas—3.		
Laparotomy and drainage, acute hemorrhagic pancreatitis	1	1
" " " " pancreatitis	1	..
" " " carcinoma of pancreas	1	..
Liver—6.		
Laparotomy and drainage, echinococcus cyst	1	..
" " " broken-down gumma	1	..
" " extirpation echinococcus cyst	1	..
Transpleural hepatotomy and drainage, for abscess	1	..
Exploratory laparotomy, carcinoma	2	1
Gall Bladder and Ducts—28.		
Cholecystectomy for acute ulcerative cholecystitis, cholelithiasis	1	
" " " " " diffuse peritonitis	1	1
" " " cholecystitis, cholelithiasis	4	..
" " empyema of gall bladder, cholelithiasis	1	..
" " gangrenous cholecystitis	2	..
" " " " suture of old fracture of femur	1	1
" " post-typhoid cholecystitis	1	..
" " chronic cholecystitis	1	..
" " " " cholelithiasis	4	..
" " cholelithiasis	6	..
" " and choledochotomy for chronic cholecystitis, cholelithiasis	4	
Incision and drainage for pericholecystitis	1	
" " " " " perforation of duodenum	1	
Intestines—14.		
Laparotomy, suture of typhoid perforation	5	3
" reduction, ileo-colic intussusception	1	..
" resection of gangrenous intussusception	1	1
" reduction, volvulus of small intestine	1	1
" division of bands causing acute obstruction	1	1
" drainage, peritonitis and intestinal obstruction	1	1
" appendicostomy for chronic colitis	1	..
" resection of sigmoid flexure for carcinoma	1	1
Plastic operation for fecal fistula	1	..
Appendicitis—136.		
Appendicectomy for acute catarrhal	12	..
" " " ulcerative	3	..
" " empyema of appendix	5	..
" " gangrenous appendicitis	27	..
" " " perforative	6	..

Appendicitis—Continued.

	Total	Died
Appendicectomy for gangrenous perforative with abscess	18	1
" " " " " serous peritonitis	2	..
" " " " abscess and serous peritonitis	2	..
" " " " diffuse peritonitis	6	2
" " " " general purulent peritonitis	6	3
" " " " abscess and diffuse peritonitis	2	..
" " acute perforative, general purulent peritonitis	1	1
" " gangrenous, omental thrombosis	1	..
" " chronic catarrhal	40	..
" and entero-enterostomy for chronic appendicitis and chronic intestinal obstruction	1	..
Incision and drainage for appendicitis abscess	1	..
Appendicectomy for persistent sinus after appendicitis abscess	2	..
Laparotomy for adhesions after appendicectomy	1	..

Herniotomies—53.

	Total	Died
Inguinal hernia, Bassini's operation	28	..
" " hydrocele of canal of Nuck; Bassini	1	..
" " congenital, Bassini	5	..
" " strangulated "	3	..
" " " herniotomy, Bassini	2	..
" " incarcerated, Bassini	2	..
" " " hernia of bladder, Bassini	1	..
" " after Alexander	1	..
" " recurrent, Bassini	2	..
Femoral hernia, strangulated, Bassini	1	..
Umbilical hernia, strangulated, herniotomy and colostomy	1	..
Ventral hernia, plastic	4	..
" " recurrent, plastic	1	..
Epigastric hernia, herniotomy	1	..

Genito-Urinary Diseases—50.

Kidney.

	Total	Died
Nephrotomy, transperitoneal, for cyst of the kidney	1	1
" for calculus in one ureter	1	..
" " " hydronephrosis, stones in both ureters	1	1
Nephrectomy for pyonephrosis	3	2
" " abscesses of kidney, multiple	1	..
" " sinus after removal of calculus	1	..
" " torsion of pedicle of kidney	1	..
" " hypernephroma	2	1
Incision and drainage for perinephric abscess	1	..

Bladder.

	Total	Died
Suprapubic cystotomy for cystitis	1	..
" " " vesical hemorrhage	1	..
" " " papilloma	1	..
" " " calculus	1	..
Cauterization for vesical fistula	1	..

Prostate.

	Total	Died
Suprapubic prostatectomy for hypertrophy of prostate	6	...

Urethra.

	Total	Died
Urethrotomy, external, for stricture	5	1
" and cauterization for phagadenic chancre	1	..
Incision and drainage for periurethral abscess	3	..

Penis.

	Total	Died
Meatotomy for hypospadias	1	..
Urethroplasty for hypospadias	3	..

Scrotum and Testes.

	Total	Died
Aspiration of hematocele of tunica vaginalis	1	..
Extirpation for varicocele	3	..
Orchidectomy for tuberculosis of testis	1	..
" " suppuration of testis	1	..
Plastic on epididymis for undescended testis	1	..
Exploratory celiotomy for tumor of undescended testicle	2	1
Excision of tunica, Bergmann, for hydrocele	2	..
" " for spermatocele	1	..
Incision and drainage for spermatocele	1	..
" " " " gangrene of scrotum and perineum from ischio-rectal abscess	1	..

Operations on Rectum and Anus—71.

	Total	Died
Hemorrhoids, clamp and cautery	39	..
" excision and clamp and cautery	1	..
" Whitehead	5	1
" and prolapse of rectum, Whitehead	5	..
" thrombosed, incision	1	..
Fistula in ano	1	..
Fissure in ano divulsion	2	..

Operations on Rectum and Anus—*Continued.*

	Total	Died
Fissure in ano and polyp of rectum, divulsion and excision	1	..
Ischio-rectal abscess, incision and drainage	10	..
Periproctitic " " " "	1	..
Insufficiency of sphincter ani, plastic	1	..
Polyp of rectum, excision	1	..
Adenoid of rectum, avulsion	1	..
Adenomata of rectum, cauterization	1	..
Condyloma of anus, excision	1	..

Pelvis and Spine—2.

	Total	Died
Excision of cyst of sacral region	1	..
Partial excision of meningocele	1	..

Lower Extremity—59.

	Total	Died
Amputation, of thigh (Bier), for osteomyelitis of tibia	1	..
" " " for diabetic gangrene	3	1
" " " " Raynaud's disease	1	..
" " leg " " "	2	..
" at knee, for Raynaud's disease	1	..
" " " " arterio-sclerotic gangrene	1	..
" of leg " " " "	1	..
" " toe " " " "	1	..
Arthrotomy, for tuberculosis of ankle	2	..
Arthrectomy " " " calcaneo-astragaloid articulation	1	..
Excision, carcinoma of inguinal glands	1	..
" foreign body in foot	1	..
" " " about knee	1	..
" skin of buttock for tuberculosis	1	..
" varicose ulcer of leg	1	..
" " veins " "	2	..
Incision and drainage, abscess of buttock	2	..
" " " inguinal abscess	2	..
" " " abscess of thigh	1	..
" " " infected hematoma of thigh	1	..
" " " tubercular abscess " "	1	..
" " " suppurative tubercular arthritis of knee	2	1
" " " (Mayo) suppurative " " "	2	..
" " " abscess of leg	1	..
" " " " " ankle	1	..
" " " persistent sinus of foot	1	..
" " " phlegmon of foot	2	..
" " " " " " diabetic	1	..
Osteotomy, of femur, metastatic carcinoma	1	1
" " " acute osteomyelitis	1	..

Lower Extremity—*Continued.*

	Total	Died
Osteotomy, of femur, tubercular osteomyelitis.	2	..
" " " acute " staphylococcemia	1	1
" " " mal-union after fracture	1	..
" " tibia, for chronic osteomyelitis.	5	..
" " " " tubercular "	1	..
" " " " compound fracture	1	..
" " " " genu valgum	1	..
" " " " " extrorsum	2	..
" for hallux valgus.	1	..
Skin-grafting (Thiersch), for varicose ulcer of leg.	1	..
" " for burns	3	..

DISEASES TREATED IN THE SECOND SURGICAL DIVISION.

From December 1, 1903, to December 1, 1904.

HOWARD LILIENTHAL, M.D.,
ATTENDING SURGEON.

JOSEPH WIENER, JR., M.D., CHARLES A. ELSBERG, M.D.,
ADJUNCT ATTENDING SURGEONS.

TOTAL, 690.

	Total	No operation	Died
Cranium—12.			
Scalp—3.			
Incised wound of	1		
Sebaceous cyst of	1		
Metastatic perithelioma frontal region	1		
Skull and Contents—9.			
Fracture of vault	1		
" " " depressed	1		1
" " base, streptococcus meningitis	1		1
" " " intradural abscess	1		
" " " "	1		1
Extradural abscess	1		
Cortical cerebral cyst, Jacksonian epilepsy	2		
Cerebellar tumor	1		
Face and Mouth—20.			
Epithelioma of	1		
Myxo-endothelioma of parotid region	1		
Salivary calculus	1		
Facial palsy	1		
Cellulitis of face	1		
Hare lip	4	1	
Cleft palate	3	3	
Tongue, carcinoma of	3		
Superior maxilla, necrosis of	1	1	
" " osteomyelitis of	1		
" " periostitis and infection of antrum	1		
" " antrum infection and chronic suppurative ethmoiditis	1		
Inferior maxilla, acute necrosis of	1		

Neck—30.

	Total	No operation	Died
Abscess of	2	..	..
Submaxillary abscess	1	..	..
Carbuncle of	1	..	..
" gangrenous, diabetes	1	1	1
Infected gunshot wound of	1	1	..
Foreign body, bullet	1	..	..
Adenitis of	1	..	..
" syphilitic	1	..	..
" tuberculous	4	1	..
" " with sinus	1	..	..
" carcinomatous	1	..	..
Lipoma of	1	..	..
Nevus of	1	..	..
Lympho-sarcoma	2	1	..
Carcinoma of glands	1	1	..
Cyst	1	..	..
Thyroid gland, adenoma	1	..	..
" " colloid goitre	3	..	..
" " cystic "	2	..	..
Prethyroid cyst	1	..	..
Carcinoma of parathyroid	1	..	..
Exophthalmic goitre	1	..	1

Pharynx—2.

	Total	No operation	Died
Carcinoma	1	..	..
Peritonsillar abscess	1	..	..

Larynx—1.

	Total	No operation	Died
Laryngeal fistula	1	..	..

Upper Extremity—27.

Shoulder—5.

	Total	No operation	Died
Abscess	1	..	..
Lipoma	2	..	..
Fibrous anchylosis, shoulder, elbow, wrist, after fracture	1	1	..
Scapula, sarcoma of	1	..	..

Axilla—5.

	Total	No operation	Died
Cyst of	1	..	..
Sinus of	2	..	..
Tubercular glands of	1	..	..
Brachial plexus, neuritis after dislocation of humerus	1	1	..

	Total	No operation	Died
Arm—4.			
Cellulitis of, and forearm	1	..	..
Lacerated wounds of	1	..	..
Humerus, osteomyelitis	1	..	..
" fracture of greater tuberosity	1	..	..
Forearm—6.			
Elbow joint, tuberculous arthritis	1	..	..
" " sinus after tuberculous arthritis	1	..	..
Ulna, deformity of	1	..	..
" chronic osteomyelitis	1	..	..
" and radius, ununited fracture	1	..	..
Radius, osteomyelitis of	1	1	..
Hand—7.			
Osteomyelitis, tuberculous, and of ankle	1	..	..
Dactylitis, tuberculous	2	..	..
Finger, infected wound	1	..	..
" necrosis of phalanx	1	..	..
" contracture of	1	..	..
Fingers, fracture, with gangrene of thumb and index finger	1	..	..
Breast—25.			
Acute suppurative mastitis	1	..	..
Abscess of	4	..	..
Chronic mastitis	2	..	..
Intracanalicular fibroma of	1	..	..
Fibroma of	2	..	..
Adenoma of	1	..	..
Cysts of	1	..	..
Papillary cyst of	1	..	..
Fibro-adenoma of	1	..	..
" carcinoma of	1	..	..
Carcinoma of	7	2	..
" " recurrent	1	..	..
" " ulcerating	1	1	..
Chronic mastitis, diabetes	1	..	..
Thorax—22.			
Fracture of ribs, broncho-pneumonia	1	..	..
Foreign body in chest	1	..	..
Tuberculosis of ribs	1	..	..
" " sternum	1	..	..
Arthritis, sterno-clavicular	1	..	..
Empyema of	7	1	..
" " pneumonia	2	..	..

Thorax—*Continued.*

	Total	No operation	Died
Empyema of, interlobar	1	..	..
Sinus after thoracotomy	5	..	..
Pulmonary abscess	1	..	..
Ulcer of chest	1	..	..

Spine—11.

	Total	No operation	Died
Chronic coccygitis	1	..	..
Transverse myelitis	1	..	..
Meningocele	1	..	..
Lumbar abscess	2	..	..
Psoas "	2	..	..
Dermoid cyst over coccyx	1	..	..
" infected, with hemorrhoids	1	..	..
" with ischio-rectal abscess	1	..	..
Fibro-cyst over sacrum	1	..	..

Abdominal Wall—2.

	Total	No operation	Died
Contusion of	1	1	..
Lipoma of	1	..	..

Esophagus and Stomach—19.

	Total	No operation	Died
Spasmodic stricture of esophagus	1	1	..
Benign " " "	1	1	..
Malignant " " "	4	..	..
Stomach, ulcer of	1	1	..
" benign stenosis of pylorus	7	1	1
" malignant " " "	1	1	..
" carcinoma	1	..	1
" " and of gall bladder	1	..	..
" dilatation and gastroptosis	2	..	..

Pancreas—2.

	Total	No operation	Died
Pancreatitis, acute hemorrhagic	1	..	1
" " general peritonitis	1	..	1

Liver—4.

	Total	No operation	Died
Abscess	2	..	1
" amebic	1	..	1
Acute fatty degeneration	1	..	1

	Total	No operation	Died
General Abdominal Cavity—8.			
Visceral carcinomatosis	1		
Retroperitoneal exudate	1		
Extraperitoneal abscess	1		1
Pneumococcus peritonitis	1		1
Tubercular peritonitis	1		
Foreign body, catheter, in retroperitoneal tissue	1		
" " in abdominal wound	1	1	
Multiple abscesses of spleen, pseudoleukemia	1		1
Gall Bladder and Ducts—44.			
Acute cholecystitis and cholelithiasis	4		
" " " pericholecystic abscess	1		
" ulcerative cholecystitis and cholelithiasis	1		
" " perforative cholecystitis, cholelithiasis, serous peritonitis	1		1
" perforative cholecystitis, pericholecystic abscess, cholelithiasis	1		
Perforative cholecystitis, bile peritonitis, irreducible inguinal hernia	1		1
Gangrenous cholecystitis and cholelithiasis	3		
" " cholelithiasis and pericholecystic abscess	1		
Post-typhoid gangrenous cholecystitis and cholelithiasis	2		
Suppurative cholecystitis and pericholecystitis	1		
Cholelithiasis	7	1	
" multiple neuritis	1		
" pericholecystitis and pneumonia	1		1
Empyema of gall bladder and cholelithiasis	3		
" " " " multiple abscesses of liver	1		1
Suppurative choleangitis	1	1	1
" " cholelithiasis and colitis	1		
Chronic cholecystitis	1		
" " and cholelithiasis	5	1	1
" " " " and colitis	1		
Obstructive jaundice	3		3
Stenosis of cystic duct	1		
Biliary fistula	2	2	
Fistula between gall bladder and duodenum, pericholecystitis	1		
Intestines—13.*			
Intestinal colic	1	1	
" perforation by foreign body†	1		1
" " typhoid fever	1		1
Sarcoma	1		
Intussusception, acute, ileo-colic	1		

*See also Hernia, Rectum, Stomach.
†See Pelvic Abscess, operation.

Intestines—*Continued.*	Total	No operation	Died
Intestinal obstruction (see also strangulated hernia)	1	1	1
" " chronic, stricture of ileum	1	..	..
Fecal fistula	1	..	..
Jejunal fistula, general peritonitis	1	..	1
Ulcerative colitis	2	1	..
Typhoid fever	1	1	..
Constipation	1	1	..

Appendicitis—129.

	Total	No operation	Died
Acute catarrhal	15	2	..
" " with ovarian dermoid	1	..	..
" " serous peritonitis	1	..	1
" " pyosalpinx, diffuse peritonitis	1	..	..
" ulcerative	2	..	..
Gangrenous	20	..	..
" with abscess	9	..	..
" perforative with abscess	7	..	1
" with thrombosis of mesenteriolum	1	..	..
" " pyelitis	1	..	..
" perforative, pyelitis and general purulent peritonitis	1	..	..
" with pyosalpinx	1	..	..
" perforative abscess, sero-purulent peritonitis	3	..	1
" serous peritonitis	2	..	..
" sero-purulent peritonitis	5	..	1
" perforative, with sero-purulent peritonitis	3	..	1
" general purulent peritonitis	5	1	3
Empyema of appendix	5	..	..
Subacute	4	..	..
Chronic catarrhal	25	4	..
" with cystic ovaries	2	..	..
" " ovarian cyst	1	..	..
" " fibro-adenoma of ovary	1	..	..
" hypertrophy of cervix	1	..	..
" with endometritis	1	..	..
" " ventral hernia	1	..	..
Adeno-carcinoma	2	..	..
Appendicitis abscess	5	..	..
" sinus	2	..	..
Adhesions after appendicectomy	1	..	..

Hernia—65.

	Total	No operation	Died
Inguinal, indirect, reducible	12	1	..
" " " nephritis	1	..	1
" " " recurrent	2	..	..
" " " hydrocele	1	..	..
" " " congenital	1	..	..
" " irreducible; acute mania	1	..	..
" " strangulated	5	..	..

Hernia—Continued.	Total	No operation	Died
Inguinal, indirect, strangulated, fecal fistula	1	..	1
" " " acute catarrhal appendicitis	2	..	..
" " reducible, double	19	..	..
" " " " hydrocele	1	..	..
" " " " hemorrhoids	1	..	..
Femoral, reducible	3	..	..
" strangulated	1	..	..
" double	2	..	..
Umbilical	4	..	..
" with hemorrhoids	1	..	..
Ventral	2	..	..
" with inflamed omentum	1	1	..
" " post-operative adhesions	1	..	..
" after appendicectomy	1	..	..
" with chronic appendicitis	2	..	..

Genito-Urinary—54.

Kidney—22.

	Total	No operation	Died
Movable kidney	3	..	..
" " with chronic appendicitis	1	..	..
Renal calculus	2	..	1
" colic	4	3	..
Cystic kidney with pneumonia	1	..	1
Abscess of kidney	1	..	..
Tuberculosis of kidney	1	..	..
Hypernephroma	1	..	..
Sarcoma of kidney	1	..	..
Pyonephrosis	2	..	1
Post-operative kidney sinus with abscess	1	..	..
Perinephritic abscess	3	..	..
Hemorrhagic nephritis	1	1	..

Prostate—13.

	Total	No operation	Died
Hypertrophy of prostate	9	..	..
" " " with vesical calculus	1	..	..
" " " " cystitis and pyelonephritis	1	..	1
Adenoma of prostate, rectum and bladder	1	..	1
Adeno-carcinoma of prostate	1	..	1

Bladder—5.

	Total	No operation	Died
Sarcoma of bladder	1	..	..
Vesical fistula	3	2	..
Retention of urine	1	1	..

	Total	No operation	Died

Urethra—5.

Urethral fistula	1		
" " perineal fistula with hemorrhoids	1		
" stricture with inguinal abscess	1		
" " perineal fistula with hemorrhoids	1		
Perineal hypospadias	1		

Testicle and Scrotum—7.

Hydrocele and hemorrhoids	1		
Traumatic hydrocele	1	1	
Tuberculous testicle	1		
Chronic inflammation of testicle	1		
Epididymo-orchitis	1	1	
Varicocele	2		

Penis—2.

Tuberculosis of penis and inguinal glands	1		
Redundant prepuce	1		

Female Genitals—38.

Vulva—7.

Bartholinian abscess	1		
Congenital malformation	2	2	
Lacerated perineum	4		

Uterus—12.

Prolapsus	1		
" cystic ovaries	1		
Fibromata	2		
" chronic appendicitis	1		
Perforation, traumatic, laceration of intestines	1		1
Lacerated cervix	2		
Endometritis, thrombosis of femoral vein	1		
" retroversion, cystic ovary	1		
Metrorrhagia	2		

Tubes and Ovaries—19.

Salpingitis	1	1	
Salpingo-oöphoritis	1		
" " pelvic abscess	1		
Ectopic gestation, ruptured	5	1	1
" " " septicemia	1		1
Ovarian cyst, twisted pedicle	4		
" " " " purulent peritonitis	1		1
" abscess, general peritonitis	1		1
Pelvic abscess	4		

Rectum and Anus—76.

	Total	No operation	Died
Hemorrhoids	41	1	..
" and fistula in ano	1	..	..
Stricture of rectum, syphilitic	1	..	..
Prolapse " "	1	..	..
Malformation "	1	..	..
Carcinoma of "	4	1	..
Ulcer " "	1	..	..
Fissure in ano	1	..	..
Fistula " "	17	..	..
Ischio-rectal abscess	7	2	..
Periproctitis	1	..	..

Lower Extremity—79.

Pelvis and Hip Joint—11.

	Total	No operation	Died
Gluteal fistula	1	..	..
Subgluteal gumma	1	..	..
Tuber ischii, osteomyelitis	1	..	..
Groin, abscess of	2	..	..
" tuberculous adenitis	1	..	..
Hip joint, contusion	1	1	..
" " congenital dislocation	1	1	..
" " osteo-arthritis	1	..	1
" " " " tuberculous	1	..	1
" " " " chronic, of pelvis	1	..	1

Thigh—26.

	Total	No operation	Died
Abscess	2	1	..
Cellulitis	2	..	..
Phlebitis with fat necrosis	1	..	..
Hematoma	1	..	..
" infected	1	..	..
Lipoma	1	..	..
Femur, fracture of neck	2	2	..
" " " " diabetes	1	1	..
" " " " shaft	2	1	..
" " " " mal-union	1	..	..
" chronic osteomyelitis	8	..	..
" " " sinus	1	..	..
" " " " tubercular	1	..	..
" sarcoma	1	..	1
Phlegmon, periarticular, of thigh	1	..	..

Knee—10.

	Total	No operation	Died
Prepatellar bursitis	1	1	..
Patella, fracture of	3	..	..
Knee joint, tuberculous arthritis	1	1	..
" " chronic "	1	1	..
" " suppurative "	1	..	..
" " gonorrheal "	1	..	..
" " anchylosis	2	..	..

Leg—18.

	Total.	No operation.	Died.
Abscess	1	..	..
Cellulitis	2	..	1
Granulating wounds	1	1	..
Varicose veins	2	2	..
" " ulcer	2	..	..
Ulcer	1	..	..
" embolic	1	..	..
Gangrene, embolic	1	..	..
Genu valgum	1	..	..
Tibia, acute osteomyelitis, path. fracture	1	..	..
" chronic "	3	..	..
" fracture	1	1	..
Fibula "	1	1	..

Foot—14.

	Total.	No operation.	Died.
Os calcis, osteomyelitis of	2	..	..
Gangrene, due to ruptured aneurism	1	..	..
Cellulitis	1	1	..
Gangrene, Raynaud's disease	2	..	..
" arterio-sclerotic	3	..	1
" diabetic	1	1	..
Infected wound	1	..	..
Hallux valgus, double	1	..	..
Toe, ulcer	1	..	..
" osteomyelitis of phalanx	1	..	..

Miscellaneous—3.

	Total.	No operation.	Died.
Burns, second degree	2	1	..
" " " pneumonia	1	1	1

Infectious Diseases—1.

	Total.	No operation.	Died.
Diphtheria	1	1	..

Constitutional Diseases—3.

	Total.	No operation.	Died.
Scurvy	1	..	..
Pseudoleukemia	1	..	..
" multiple splenic abscesses, cholelithiasis	1	..	..

OPERATIONS PERFORMED IN THE SECOND SURGICAL DIVISION FROM DECEMBER 1, 1903, TO DECEMBER 1, 1904.

TOTAL, 627.   DEATHS, 53.

Cranium—10.

	Total	Died
Craniotomy, extra dural abscess	1	1
Osteotomy, fract. int. table of skull	1	1
Craniotomy, depressed fracture	2	..
" meningeal hemorrhage	1	1
Excision sebaceous cyst of scalp	1	..
Craniotomy, cyst of brain	1	..
" cerebellar tumor, relief of intracranial pressure	3	1

Face and Mouth—18.

Plastic, hare lip	4	..
Osteotomy, necrosis of inferior maxilla	1	..
Incision and drainage for alveolar abscess	1	..
Partial removal tumor of gums and tonsils	1	..
Incision and drainage, acute necrotic parotitis	1	1
Excision, epithelioma of face	1	..
" carcinoma of tongue	4	..
Anastomosis of spinal accessory with facial nerve for facial paralysis	1	..
Osteotomy and drainage for osteomyelitis of antrum of Highmore	2	..
Extirpation of salivary sinus	1	..
Plastic on soft palate	1	..

Neck—29.

Excision lipoma of neck	1	..
Ligation com. carotid for pulsating tumor of scalp	1	..
Extirpation of cyst of neck	2	..
Ligat. com. carotid for sarcoma of tonsil	1	..
Excision tuberculous glands of neck	4	..
" sup. clavic. metastatic carcin. glands of neck	2	..
Removal foreign body, bullet, from neck	1	..
Incision and drainage, abscess of neck	1	..
Excision nerves of neck	1	..
Plastic, closure thyro-hyoid sinus	1	..
Excision, hemorrhagic thyroid cyst	2	..
" thyroid cyst	1	..
" parathyroid tumor	1	..
" syphilitic glands of neck	1	..
Thyroidectomy, exophthalmic goitre	1	..
" colloid goitre	2	..
Excision and drainage, suppurative glands of neck	1	..
" carcinomatous glands of neck	1	..
Curetting tuberculous glands of neck	1	..
Ligation of lingual artery	1	..
" " both lingual arteries	1	..
Excision of carcinoma of thyroid	1	..

Upper Extremity—23.

	Total	Died
Amputation of arm for osteomyelitis of humerus	1	..
" " finger for diabetic gangrene	1	..
" " " " dry gangrene	2	..
Excision cyst of axilla	1	..
" sinus "	1	..
" of axillary glands	2	..
" " ulna for deformity	1	..
" " lipoma of shoulder	1	..
" " head of scapula for sarcoma	1	..
Incision and drainage, abscess of shoulder	1	..
" " " cellulitis of forearm	2	..
" " " arthritis sterno-clavic. joint	1	..
" " " osteomyelitis of humerus	1	..
Osteotomy, for dactylitis, tubercular	1	..
" " chronic osteomyelitis of ulna, iodoform wax filling	2	..
" " ununited fracture of radius and ulna	1	..
" and suture of fracture of humerus	1	..
Tenoplasty, for contracture of finger	1	..
Resection of elbow for tuberculous arthritis	1	..

Thorax—17.

	Total	Died
Thoracoplasty for chronic empyema with sinus	5	..
Thoracotomy for acute empyema	9	3
Plastic for persistent ulcer of chest wall	1	..
Exploratory thoracotomy for pulmonary abscess	1	1
For gun-shot wound of chest and abdomen	1	..

Breast—17.

	Total	Died
Amputation, radical, for carcinoma	9	..
Extirpation of tumor	3	..
Excision of fibro cyst	1	..
Incision and drainage for acute suppurative mastitis	3	..
" " " " chronic " "	1	..

Spine—1.

	Total	Died
Incision and drainage of spinal canal for suppurative cerebro-spinal meningitis	1	1

Abdominal Wall—1.

	Total	Died
Excision of lipoma	1	..

General Abdominal Cavity—10.

	Total	Died
Incision and drainage, abscess of spleen	1	1
Exploratory laparotomy, retro-peritoneal exudate	1	..
Laparotomy for tubercular peritonitis	2	..

General Abdominal Cavity—*Continued.*

	Total.	Died.
Laparotomy for general pneumococcus peritonitis．	1	..
" " intra-abdominal abscess	3	..
" " foreign body in retro-peritoneal region	1	..
" drainage, extra-peritoneal abscess	1	1

Esophagus and Stomach—13.

Gastrostomy (Kader) for malignant stricture of esophagus	2	..
" (Hall) " " " "	2	..
Gastro-duodenostomy (Finney) for benign stenosis of pylorus	3	1
Gastroenterostomy, posterior	..	..
" button, for carcinoma of stomach	1	1
" suture, for benign stenosis of pylorus	2	..
" " " dilatation of stomach and gastroptosis	2	..
Exploratory laparotomy for carcinoma of stomach	1	..

Pancreas—2.

Laparotomy and drainage, acute pancreatitis	1	1
" " " " " general peritonitis	1	1

Liver—4.

Laparotomy and drainage of abscess	1	..
Transpleural hepatotomy for abscess	2	2
Exploratory laparotomy, acute fatty degeneration of liver	1	1

Gall Bladder and Ducts—38.

Cholecystectomy for acute cholecystitis, cholelithiasis	4	..
" " " ulcerative cholecystitis, cholelithiasis	1	..
" " " " perforative cholecystitis, cholelithiasis, serous peritonitis	1	1
" " empyema of gall bladder, cholelithiasis	3	..
" " " " " " multiple abscesses of liver	1	1
" " chronic cholecystitis, cholelithiasis	3	..
" " " "	1	..
" " cholelithiasis	4	..
" " " multiple neuritis	1	..
" " chronic cholecystitis, cholelithiasis, colitis	1	..
" " cholelithiasis, pericholecystitis, pneumonia	1	1
" " gangrenous cholecystitis, cholelithiasis	3	..
" " " " " pericholecystic abscess	1	..
" " post-typhoid gangrenous cholecystitis, cholelithiasis	2	..
" " stenosis of cystic duct	1	..
" and pyloroplasty for fistula between gall bladder and duodenum, pericholecystitis	1	..
" " choledochotomy for cholelithiasis	2	..

Gall Bladder and Ducts—*Continued.*

	Total	Died
Cholecyst-enterostomy for obstructive jaundice	1	1
Choledochotomy and hepaticotomy for obstructive jaundice	1	1
Incision and drainage for acute cholecystitis, pericholecystic abscess	1	..
Incision and drainage for acute perforative cholecystitis, pericholecystitis and cholelithiasis	1	..
" " " " suppurative cholecystitis, pericholecystitis	1	..
Exploratory laparotomy for perforative cholecystitis, bile peritonitis	1	1
" " " obstructive jaundice	1	1

Intestines—10.

	Total	Died
Exploratory laparotomy for carcinoma of colon	1	..
" " " sarcoma of intestine	1	..
Laparotomy and suture of typhoid perforation	1	1
" " reduction of acute intussusception	1	..
" " resection of intestine, entero-anastomosis, Murphy button, for stricture of small intestine	1	..
" resection of intestine, entero-anastomosis for jejunal fistula	1	1
Appendicostomy for mucous colitis	1	..
Colostomy for ulcerative colitis	1	..
Enterorrhaphy for fecal fistula	1	..
Incision and drainage of abscess from perforation of intestine by foreign body	1	1

Appendicitis—122.

	Total	Died
Appendicectomy for acute catarrhal	13	..
" and salpingo-oöphorectomy for acute catarrhal appendicitis and ovarian dermoid	1	..
" for acute catarrhal appendicitis with serous peritonitis	1	1
" " " ulcerative	2	..
" " " catarrhal, pyosalpinx and diffuse peritonitis	1	..
" " gangrenous	20	..
" " " appendicitis with abscess	9	..
" " " perforative appendicitis with abscess	7	1
" " " appendicitis with thrombosis of mesenteriolum	1	..
" " " " " pyelitis	1	..
" " " perforative appendicitis, pyelitis, general sero-purulent peritonitis	1	..
" and salpingo-oöphorectomy for gangrenous appendicitis and pyosalpinx	1	..
" for gangrenous, perforative, appendicular abscess and sero-purulent peritonitis	3	1
" " " appendicitis with serous peritonitis	2	..
" " " " " sero-purulent peritonitis	5	1
" " " perforative appendicitis with sero-purulent peritonitis	3	1
" " " appendicitis with general purulent peritonitis	4	2

Appendicitis—Continued.

	Total	Died
Appendicectomy for empyema of appendix	5	..
" " subacute appendicitis	4	..
" " chronic catarrhal appendicitis	21	..
" and salpingo-oöphorectomy for chronic appendicitis and cystic ovary	1	..
" " plastic on ovary for chronic appendicitis and cystic ovary	1	..
" salpingo-oöphorectomy and ventro-fixation for chronic catarrhal appendicitis and ovarian cyst	1	..
" and excision of fibro-adenoma for chronic catarrhal appendicitis and fibro-adenoma of ovary	1	..
" " amputation of cervix for chronic catarrhal appendicitis and hypertrophy and prolapse of cervix	1	..
" " curettage for chronic appendicitis and endometritis	1	..
" " herniotomy for chronic appendicitis with ventral hernia	1	..
" for adeno-carcinoma of appendix	2	..
Incision and drainage for appendicitis abscess	5	..
Appendicectomy and drainage for appendicitis sinus after abscess	1	..
Excision and suture for sinus after appendicectomy	1	..
Laparotomy and division of adhesions for adhesions after appendicectomy	1	..

Hernia—63.

	Total	Died
Radical for ventral	5	..
" " umbilical	6	..
Herniotomy for strangulated umbilical	1	..
" " " " with resection	1	..
Bassini for unilateral inguinal	14	1
" " double "	20	..
" " congenital "	1	..
Herniotomy for strangulated inguinal	6	..
" " recurrent "	1	..
" " incarcerated "	3	1
" " unilateral femoral	1	..
" " strangulated "	1	..
" " double "	2	..
" " incarcerated "	1	..

Genito-Urinary Diseases—46.

Kidney—18.

	Total	Died
Nephrotomy for renal calculus	1	..
" " pyonephrosis	2	1
" " renal colic	1	..
Nephrectomy for cystic kidney, pneumonia	1	1
" " abscess of kidney	1	..

Genito-Urinary Diseases—*Continued.*

	Total	Died
Nephrectomy for hypernephroma	1	..
" " tuberculosis of kidney	1	..
Nephropexy for movable kidney	3	..
" and appendicectomy for movable kidney and chronic appendicitis	1	..
Excision of post-operative kidney sinus with abscess	1	..
Incision and drainage perinephric abscess	3	..
Exploratory laparotomy for sarcoma of kidney	1	..
" " " suspected stone of ureter, renal colic	1	..

Bladder and Prostate—15.

	Total	Died
Suprapubic prostatectomy for hypertrophied prostate	9	..
" " " " " with stone in bladder	1	..
" cystotomy for hypertrophied prostate, cystitis, pyelonephritis	1	1
" prostatectomy for adeno-carcinoma of prostate	1	1
Suture suprapubic vesical fistula	1	..
Extirpation of bladder, adenoma	1	1
Partial extirpation for sarcoma of bladder	1	..

Urethra—5.

	Total	Died
Plastic, perineal hypospadias	1	..
Excision perineal-urethral fistula	1	..
Internal urethrotomy, stricture urethra	2	..
Plastic, perineal-urethral fistula	1	..

Testicle and Cord—7.

	Total	Died
Eversion of tunica, hydrocele	1	..
Orchidectomy for tuberculosis of testicle	1	..
" " chronic inflammation	1	..
Excision for varicocele	2	..
Circumcision, elongated prepuce	1	..
Actual cauterization for tuberculosis of penis	1	..

Rectum and Anus—77.

	Total	Died
Excision for rectal ulcer	1	..
Incision for examination of rectal tumor	1	..
Resection for carcinoma of rectum	1	..
Preparatory enterorrhaphy for stricture of rectum	1	..
Incision for ischio-rectal abscess	7	..
" and drainage for blind fistula in ano	1	..
Excision of prolapsed rectum	1	..
Plastic for imperforate anus	1	..
Clamp and cautery for prolapsus ani	1	..
Incision of fistula in ano	14	..
Excision " " " "	2	..

Rectum and Anus—*Continued.*

	Total.	Died.
Clamp and cautery for hemorrhoids	41	..
Dilatation of fissure in ano	4	..
" " sphincter ani	1	..

Female Genital Organs—37.

Aspiration of left pelvic abscess	1	..
Laparotomy for pelvic abscess	3	1
Excision of Bartholinian gland for abscess	1	..
Posterior vaginal section for pelvic abscess	1	..
Plastic for recto and cystocele	4	..
Curettage for chronic endometritis	3	..
" " incomplete abortion	1	..
" " metrorrhagia	1	..
Amputation of cervix for laceration	1	..
" " " " elongation	1	..
Oöphorectomy for simple cyst	1	..
" " twisted dermoid	2	..
Laparotomy for twisted ovarian cyst	1	..
Salpingectomy for ectopic pregnancy	1	..
Salpingo-oöphorectomy for twisted cyst	2	1
" " " diseased appendages	4	..
" " " ectopic	2	1
Ventral fixation for prolapsus uteri	4	..
Vaginal hysterectomy for fibromata uteri	1	..
Pan-hysterectomy	1	..
Laparotomy for ruptured uterus and perforated intestines	1	1

Lower Extremity—89.

Amputation of thigh for arterio-sclerotic gangrene	3	1
" " " " ruptured aneurism	1	..
" " " " sarcoma of femur	1	1
" " leg for arterio-sclerotic gangrene	4	..
" " " " " " gangrene	1	..
" " " " " " Raynaud's disease	1	..
" " foot, Lisfranc, for Raynaud's disease	3	..
" " toes for arterio-sclerotic gangrene	1	..
" " " " " " osteomyelitis	1	..
" " " " " " supernumerary	1	..
Aspiration, irrigation, for suppurative gonorrheal gonitis	1	..
Brisement forcé, of knee joint	3	..
Excision, inguinal glands	1	..
" " " and pelvic glands	1	..
" " " sinus	1	..
" lipoma of thigh	1	..
" dermoid cyst near coccyx	1	..
" multilocular cyst near sacrum	2	..
" varicose ulcer of leg	1	..
Incision and drainage, lumbar abscess	2	..

Lower Extremity—*Continued.*

	Total	Died
Incision and drainage, psoas abscess	3	..
" " " periarticular abscess of hip	1	..
" " " abscess of thigh	5	..
" " " " " leg	2	..
" " " cellulitis of leg	2	1
" " " suppurative gonitis	1	..
" sarcoma of thigh	1	..
" tenosynovitis of ankle	2	..
Osteotomy and drainage, osteomyelitis of femur	5	..
" " " " " os calcis	1	..
" " " near sacrum	1	..
" " " osteomyelitis of tibia	5	..
" for genu varum	1	..
" " hallux valgus	3	..
" and suture, fracture of femur and malunion	1	..
" osteoplastic for osteomyelitis of tibia	1	..
" iodoform wax filling, for chronic osteomyelitis of femur	9	..
" " " " chronic osteomyelitis of tibia	1	..
Resection of hip joint for tuberculous osteomyelitis	6	3
" " " " " perithelioma	1	..
" " phalangeal joint	1	..
Suture for fracture of patella	5	..

REPORT OF THE DEPARTMENT OF GENERAL SURGERY.

REPORT OF THE SECOND SURGICAL DIVISION.

December 1, 1902, to December 1, 1904.

HOWARD LILIENTHAL, M.D.,
ATTENDING SURGEON.

JOSEPH WIENER, JR., M.D., CHARLES A. ELSBERG, M.D.,
ADJUNCT ATTENDING SURGEONS.

The following report of the work of the Second Surgical Division covers the period between December 1, 1902, and December 1, 1904. For purposes of comparison the statistics of each year are given separately.

In March, 1904, Mt. Sinai Hospital took possession of its new buildings, and during the troublesome time of removal, a period of about six weeks, the service suffered considerably in the amount of work which it was possible to do. Then, too, it was several months before the division was running to its full capacity of fifty-two beds. It will, therefore, be noted that the number of cases treated during the second year, or from December, 1903, to December, 1904, is comparatively small. For the seven months preceding December 1, 1904, the Second Surgical Division consisted of a female ward of twenty-five beds, a male ward of sixteen beds, and a half ward for the surgical diseases of children, seven beds. Several beds in the reception wards are also usually occupied by surgical patients. The list of cases is further increased because of the fact that the attending and adjunct surgeons usually have a number of patients in the private pavilion, and this clinical material is reported as part of the Second Division.

It is too soon to draw comparisons between results now obtained and those of former years before we had the advantages of the beautiful new buildings with their full modern aseptic equipment. But, whether the improvement in statistics is marked or not, the economy of time and strength is surely to be considered. It is a pleasure to work with perfect tools in a beautiful and stimulating environment. The new hospital has given us something to live up to.

Very few changes in method have been made within the past two years. Rubber gloves are now worn at nearly every surgical manipulation—at dressings, at examinations, and at all operations, excepting that of suprapubic prostatectomy, when nothing can replace the naked finger. In certain operations when the tissues must be considerably handled, cotton gloves are worn over the rubber ones so as to do away with troublesome slipping. This has been found of special value in major amputations, in amputations of the breast, and in certain cases of hernioplasty with particularly bulky sac and contents. Sterile gowns with long sleeves, covered at the wrist by the rubber gauntlets, have replaced the old-fashioned short-sleeved garments, and the absurdity of sterile gown and boiled glove at either end of a naked, hairy forearm and elbow is a thing of the past.

An operating-table, with a device of great value in work about the gall-bladder, the pancreas and the kidney, has given us satisfaction. This table has a transverse, enameled iron piece, about six inches wide, which may be raised or lowered by means of a crank, so as to serve instead of a sandbag or pad under the patient's back or loins. The device permits any degree of lordosis, and the gain in accessibility is remarkable. When the work in the depths has been completed this support may be gradually lowered, while the wound is exposed with the aid of blunt retractors; injured vessels which may not have bled on account of the tension may be easily secured, as their location is made evident when the return to the normal posture permits the occurrence of hemorrhage. Should dangerous bleeding occur, it may be instantly checked by once more raising the patient.

Cigarette drains are now rarely made with gutta-percha tissue, the more reliable rubber dam being generally used for this purpose. The method of tube drainage devised by the Mayos for clean wounds has been found admirable. A stout piece of silk is fixed to the outer end of the drain and carried under the dressings next to the patient's skin to a point just beyond the bandage where it is fastened by a bit of adhesive plaster. By traction on this ligature the drain may be removed without disturbing the rest of the dressing.

Bichloride solutions have been practically abandoned in the preparation of the operative field, and the sterilization of the surgeon's hands. It probably does more harm as an irritant than good as an antiseptic.

Subcutaneous infusion has largely taken the place of intravenous, the later being employed only in acute anemia following hemorrhage.

Tuberculin is being used diagnostically with increasing frequency.

Catgut prepared with iodine after the method of Claudius has given us a sense of security as to the asepsis and even antisepsis of this rather troublesome but necessary material. (See paper in this volume, by Dr. A. V. Moscheowitz.)

As usual, abstracts are here given of most of the cases ending fatally or unsuccessfully. When the patient's condition was practically hopeless before operation these abstracts have been condensed as much as possible. The report of an unsuccessful case is most instructive when the death or failure was unexpected.

HEAD AND NECK.

In operations upon the skull we still employ the De Vilbiss drill. This instrument is safe and accurate either with electric or hand power.

We can highly recommend the method of Heidenhain for avoiding hemorrhage from the scalp by the insertion of a preliminary row of deep sutures around the operative field.

The first case here recorded is in many ways unusual. The ligation of both common carotids within fourteen days was not followed by any ill effect. The patient is still under observation.

Arterio-venous aneurysm of cavernous sinus; ligation of both common carotid arteries; secondary craniotomy; improvement.—Jette O., 18 years old, admitted November 6, 1902. Nine years before admission, without any trauma or pre-existing disease, the patient became deaf on the left side, and at the same time she began to notice buzzing in the left side of the head. The buzzing and deafness on the left side persisted. Two years before admission bilateral pulsating exophthalmos developed, more marked on the left side. Of late this had become pronounced, and the buzzing had become so loud that sleep was interfered with. The tongue deviated slightly to the right. The left tonsil was pushed forward, and behind it a large artery was felt. The left eyelid could not be closed, and there was facial palsy on the same side. Behind and below the left ear there was an elongated pulsating tumor. Over it there was a systolic thrill, and a loud systolic murmur. By compressing the left carotid and jugular the size of the tumor was diminished. There was a faint systolic murmur at the apex of the heart, and over the aortic valve. On November 11, 1902, the left common carotid artery was divided between two ligatures. On November 25 the same procedure was carried out on the right side. On December 14 the patient left the hospital somewhat improved. She was readmitted May 12, 1903. She complained of the same buzzing and headache as before the operation. On May 16, 1903, a Hartley-Krause craniotomy was performed in the left temporofrontal region. There was profuse diploic hemorrhage; the brain and membranes were apparently normal. When the exploring finger was passed between the dura and the base of the brain, a very profuse venous hemorrhage resulted. Toward the apex of the temporal bone marked pulsation was felt. A packing was introduced to control the bleeding, and the bone flap replaced. Three days later the wound was reopened, the packing removed, and exploration again made with the finger. Nothing was gained, and the wound was finally closed. The flap healed, and the patient was able to leave the hospital on August 10, 1903, but very little improved as to buzzing, but with headaches greatly relieved.

Thrombosis of cavernous sinus; exploratory craniotomy; death.—Fanny M., five years old, admitted November 25, 1903. Two weeks before admission a swelling around one of the lower left molars had been incised. On the day before admission the right upper eyelid became edematous. The following morning both upper lids were markedly swollen, and the child was then brought to the hospital, after having had a severe chill. On admission the temperature was 102°F. The child was in a semi-conscious condition. There was marked edema of both upper lids, and conjunctival ecchymosis. There was no deviation of the tongue. Babinski's sign was present, but no Kernig's. There was marked swelling of the gum around the incised wound on the lower jaw. The heart and lungs were normal. A curved supraorbital incision was made on the left side, and with the gouge the frontal bone was penetrated. The dura was exposed, but no pulsation was noticed. Aspiration was negative. More bone was removed and the orbit was exposed, but nothing abnormal was found. Death took place on the following day. No autopsy.

Depressed fracture of the skull; craniotomy; cure.—Morris P., 47 years old, admitted March 31, 1904. Three weeks before admission the man had been struck in the back of the head. On the following day weakness of the right arm set in and became progressively worse. There was no facial palsy. Over the posterior part of the left parietal bone there was a granulating wound leading down to bone. Craniotomy was performed over the right arm centre and a piece of bone the size of a silver dollar was removed from the outer table. A depressed fracture of the inner table of the skull was thus exposed. The depressed bone was removed, and the man was discharged twenty-four days later with almost complete restoration of function of the arm.

Fracture of skull; craniotomy; death.—Richard S., 12 years old, admitted April 24, 1904. Three hours before operation the boy had fallen from a third story window to the sidewalk, striking on the frontal region. There was profuse bleeding from the nose and mouth, with marked infiltration of the tissues with blood. The boy remained conscious and did not vomit. There were no paralyses. On admission the condition was precarious. The pulse was imperceptible, the extremities cold and clammy. There was a depressed fracture of the nasal bones, and a fracture of the hard palate, from which there was free bleeding. The whole frontal region was the site of a hematoma. A transverse incision was made over the hematoma, and disclosed a comminuted depressed fracture of the frontal bone. There was profuse bleeding from the dural veins. The wound was packed, and the scalp partly sutured. Death resulted two hours after operation.

Fracture of skull; exploratory craniotomy; death.—Samuel F., 64 years, admitted June 14, 1904. A few hours before admission the man had been kicked on the right side of the head by a horse. This was followed by convulsions at intervals of a few minutes. He was brought to the hospital in a comatose condition. The reflexes were exaggerated, ankle clonus and Babinski sign were present. An exploratory craniotomy in the right parietal region revealed nothing abnormal. Death occurred two days later. At the autopsy a fracture of the skull was found beginning three-quarters of an inch to the right of the internal occipital protuberance, extending through the occipital bone and over the petrous portion of the temporal to the posterior lacterated foramen. The inferior surface of both frontal lobes and of the right tempero-sphenoidal lobe showed laceration (contre-coup).

Cortical cerebral cyst; Jacksonian epilepsy; cure.—Carmine P., 33 years old, admitted April 21, 1904. Six years before admission the patient had been shot in the head with a revolver. Four years later epileptic attacks developed, recurring every two or three months. The aura was regularly in the right hand. Four days before admission patient had a severe convulsion, followed by the status epilepticus.

On admission one convulsion followed the other at intervals of a few minutes; the right arm was totally paralyzed and there was paresis of the right side of the face. On opening the skull in front of the fissure of Rolando a small cyst was found at the site of an old depressed fracture of the skull. Part of the cyst and the depressed bone were removed, and the wound closed with drainage. A month later the use of the right arm was almost fully restored, the facial paresis had disappeared, and there had been no return of the convulsions.

Cerebellar tumor; exploratory craniotomy; death.—Esther S., 10 years old, admitted September 9, 1904. The child had the symptoms of a cerebellar tumor, but its exact location could not be diagnosed. Pressure symptoms became so marked that on October 12, 1904, craniotomy was performed and the cerebellum exposed, but no tumor was found and no search was made. Death took place on November 23, 1904.

Endothelial sarcoma of tonsil; enucleation; death.—Abraham L., 63 years old, admitted March 23, 1903. Speech was thick and muffled, and there was a stridor on deep inspiration. Occupying the site of the left tonsil was a mass of the size of a small peach. No glands were felt. Operation March 24, 1904. Left common carotid exposed, and a ligature placed loosely around it. Then, in Rose's position, with the mouth held widely open, the capsule of the tumor was incised and the tumor removed bluntly piecemeal. The ligature around the common carotid was then tightened. Throughout the operation the man was deeply cyanosed. He remained cyanosed after the operation, and three hours later respiration suddenly became very slow. The pulse remained good for several minutes, but the cyanosis became more marked, and death took place in a few minutes. The cause was thought to be one of cerebral embolism. No autopsy.

Exophthalmic goitre; partial thyroidectomy; death.—Sarah W., 21 years old, admitted August 14, 1904. The symptoms of the disease had been present for five years, and in spite of long periods of rest in bed and hospital treatment, the patient had been going from bad to worse. She was very weak and nervous; there was palpitation and marked exophthalmos. The thyroid had grown to such a size that pressure symptoms had begun to manifest themselves. There were two distinct tumors, extending almost to the clavicle, with the narrow isthmus between. The right lobe was shelled out without much difficulty, and with little bleeding. On attempting to remove the left lobe, severe hemorrhage was encountered, which necessitated the use of several mass ligatures. The ligatures were passed as close as possible to the thyroid especially at the lower angle, to avoid the laryngeal nerves. The isthmus was not removed. Death took place six hours after operation. At the autopsy it was found that neither recurrent laryngeal nerve had been divided, but that they both were included in mass ligatures.

Facial palsy; nerve anastomosis; improvement. Miss C. H., 30 years old, admitted May 9, 1904. After an attack of convulsions at the age of six months there were complete facial paralysis and loss of hearing on the left side. Medical treatment had been of no avail. On admission, the muscles of the left side of the face contracted feebly to strong galvanic and faradic currents. An incision was made from the mastoid process along the edge of the sterno-mastoid to the cornu of the hyoid bone. The spinal accessory nerve was exposed as it emerged from under the posterior belly of the digastric muscle. Two inches of the nerve were isolated and it was tested with the faradic current. The parotid gland was turned forward, and along the upper border of the posterior belly of the digastric the facial nerve was isolated as it emerged from under the mastoid process. On applying faradism the facial muscles contracted. The spinal accessory was split longitudinally and the upper inner half divided at the upper limit. By means of two fine silk sutures this was sutured to the facial at a point where it had been nicked. The wound healed by primary union. When the patient was discharged on May 17 there had been no change in the facial muscles.

Arterio-venous aneurysm of internal jugular and external carotid; extirpation of sac; death.—Sebastian E., 28 years old, admitted August 3, 1903. Seven months before the man had been struck in the right side of the neck by a splinter of iron. There was an immediate profuse hemorrhage, the blood spurting several feet. By a compression dressing the bleeding had been arrested, but a pulsating swelling persisted at the site of injury. This tumor remained about the same size until two weeks before admission. Since that time it had been gradually increasing in size; the pulsation became more pronounced and there was constant buzzing in the right ear. The man had been hoarse for six and a half months before operation. On examination, a fusiform swelling was seen on the right side of the neck, extending to beyond the angle of the jaw. There was pronounced expansile pulsation, and a loud bruit transmitted along the great vessels. Under chloroform, the common carotid was cut between two ligatures. The pulsation was then still present, though less marked. On cutting down on the sac it was found to consist of the external carotid and the internal jugular. The internal jugular was divided between two ligatures low down in the neck. The inferior thyroid, lingual and facial arteries and veins were then ligated and divided. After ligating several other small vessels the arterial part of the tumor was removed. The venous portion of the sac was then attacked, and a profuse hemorrhage resulted. Several clamps had to be applied and the man lost a good deal of blood before the bleeding was controlled. Death took place two days later. No autopsy.

Perithelioma of frontal region; ligation of common carotid; improvement.—Springe H., 51 years old, had been discharged from the hospital in 1902, after a left-sided nephrectomy for hypernephroma. On readmission there was a pulsating tumor the size of an apricot over the left frontal bone. The tumor showed expansile pulsation. On incising the frontal bone it was found to have been eroded by the tumor. Five weeks later the left common carotid was ligated. The pulsation in the tumor disappeared and patient left hospital improved. Pathological examination of a specimen removed showed perithelioma.

Angina ludovici; tracheotomy; incision and drainage; death.—James F., 51 years, admitted May 24, 1903. The man had a great deal of dyspnea, and swallowing was difficult. The mouth could not be opened sufficiently to allow a laryngoscopic examination to be made. A small incision had been made in the neck a few days before admission, but drainage was insufficient. Temperature, 102.4°F.; pulse, 140. Under local anesthesia, a low tracheotomy was performed, and the abscess was then freely incised. Death took place two hours later.

THORAX.

Eleven cases of acute empyema were operated upon with three deaths, and fifteen cases of chronic empyema with sinus, of which two died. Most of the chronic cases had been operated on elsewhere, and were admitted to the surgical service with a thoracic sinus, often of long standing. Several of these cases required repeated plastic operations on the chest before a final cure was attained. In one case, Rebecca M., 3 years old, admitted May 4, 1903, six plastic operations were performed, and then the child was discharged with a small sinus still remaining. This finally healed, and she is now well.

Empyema; resection of rib; broncho-pneumonia; death.—Samuel M., 2½ years old, admitted June 8, 1903. Seven weeks before admission the child had had pneumonia of four weeks' duration. He had then been well for two weeks. A week before admission the temperature rose to 104°F. There was flatness over the left side of the chest, bronchial voice and breathing, and absence of fremitus. On June 9, under chloroform, after aspirating and finding pus, Dr. Koplik resected a rib and evacuated a few drams of pus. The pus contained pneumococci. A week later the child was sent home because the ward nurse had contracted scarlatina. On June 28 the boy was admitted to the surgical division. There was a profuse foul discharge from the sinus in the chest. Temperature, 104°F.; pulse, 140. Five days later a swelling was noticed in the right submaxillary region and over the inferior maxillary bone. There was also marked resistance in the right supraclavicular region, but no enlarged glands were felt. Venous congestion developed over the right half of the chest anteriorly. Dyspnea set in, and the general condition became worse. Accordingly, on July 5, under ethyl chloride, an incision was made over the swelling in the neck, but no pus was found. Death took place a few hours later. No autopsy.

Empyema; thoracoplasty; gonorrheal peritonitis; celiotomy; death. —Sarah K., 3 years old, admitted November 9, 1902. A year before admission the child had been operated on for empyema following pneumonia. Four weeks later measles had developed, together with swelling of the right knee, which had been incised and pus evacuated. The child had then been well for ten months, when an abscess opened spontaneously on the anterior part of the chest on the left side. On admission, the child had this discharging sinus, and there were signs of pneumonia on the left side. On November 25 several ribs were resected and considerable pus evacuated. On January 1 gonococci were found in the vaginal discharge. On January 10 a modified Schede's thoracoplasty was done. Two days later the abdomen became distended and painful, and there were signs of free fluid. Vomiting set in, and the bowels could not be moved with enemata or cathartics. The abdomen was opened through a right rectus incision. There was free fluid, and the intestines were covered with fibrin. After free saline irrigation, the abdomen was closed with sutures, and a drain left in the lower angle. Culture from the peritoneal fluid showed gonococci. Death took place on the following day.

Empyema; thoracotomy; pneumonia; death.—Rosie L., 2½ years old, admitted May 16, 1904. Five weeks before admission she had had a pneumonia on the right side. On admission, pus found in the right chest. Under gas and ether the eighth rib was resected and considerable pus evacuated. Eight days later a broncho-pneumonia developed at the right apex, and death took place ten days after operation.

Empyema; thoracotomy; pneumonia; death.—Annie L., 3 years old, admitted June 18, 1904. She was admitted with a right-sided empyema, probably following a pneumonia. There was also a swelling of the right forearm. This was incised, and a subperiosteal abscess of the radius opened. The right fifth rib was resected and considerable creamy pus evacuated from the chest. The pus from both incisions contained staphylococci. Sixteen days after operation the abdomen became greatly distended and tender. On aspiration in the right lumbar region bloody fluid was obtained. Examination of the chest showed a double broncho-pneumonia, and death resulted seventeen days after operation.

Empyema; thoracotomy; hemoptysis; death.—Samuel S., 17 years old, admitted November 21, 1903. Eighteen weeks before operation the boy had had a chill, followed by pain in the left side of the chest. There had been slight fever, but no cough and no sweats. Two weeks before operation he began to have a profuse purulent expectoration with some dyspnea. On aspiration, pus obtained from the left chest, and the seventh rib was then resected, and twenty ounces of thin, yellow pus evacuated. No tubercle bacilli were found in the sputum. The general condition gradually became worse, and on March 9 a hemoptysis set in which in a few minutes resulted fatally.

Pulmonary abscess (?); exploratory thoracotomy; death.—Abraham C., 36 years old, admitted December 1, 1903. The patient was transferred from the medical division with signs of a cavity in the left infrascapular region. The seventh and eighth ribs were resected in the axillary line, and the pulmonary and parietal pleura were sewn together. The lung was aspirated in several directions, but no pus was found. However, as the needle seemed to enter a cavity, a hole was burned into the lung with the Paquelin for the distance of an inch. Owing to profuse hemorrhage from the lung, a packing had to be introduced, which controlled the bleeding. Death took place a few hours later.

Tuberculosis of sternum; osteotomy and drainage; cure.—Rose S., 25 years old, admitted August 10, 1904. Eight months before admission the patient noticed a swelling over the left third costal cartilage. There was pain radiating to the left arm, more marked at night. The patient was admitted with a sinus over the sternum, where an incision had been made. Axillary, inguinal and epitrochlear glands were enlarged. There was dullness and harsh breathing at the apices of both lungs. Two sinuses were found leading down to the sternum. The sinuses were lined with necrotic material and considerable diseased bone was removed. Tubercle bacilli were found in the scrapings from the sinuses. On September 17 the patient was discharged cured with a superficial granulating wound.

CARCINOMA OF THE BREAST.

The radical operation for cancer of the breast was done fourteen times. All of the patients recovered from the operation. In all cases the complete operation of removing the breast, axillary contents and both pectoral muscles was carried out. The dissection was generally begun at the tendinous insertion of the pectoralis major, then carried to the axilla, and lastly the breast itself and the origins of the pectoral muscles. Tension sutures and superficial sutures of silk were employed; sometimes zinc oxide plaster was used in place of the superficial silk sutures. In no case was primary skin grafting necessary, although a large amount of skin was regularly sacrificed. The wound was always drained posteriorly with a large tube, and the first dressing was generally changed on the sixth day.

SPINAL CANAL.

Incision and drainage of the spinal canal for cerebro-spinal meningitis; death.—The patient was on the medical service and had been admitted with a well marked cerebro-spinal meningitis. A large trocar and canula were introduced into the spinal canal at the fourth lumbar space, after a preliminary incision of the soft parts. Through the canula a drainage tube was introduced in the spinal canal and allowed to remain there. Death took place two days later, although a temporary improvement gave rise to hopes of recovery. A considerable quantity of pus later becoming sero-purulent drained from the canal. It was a case of meningococcus infection.

This operation is an extremely rare one. In this case it certainly did no harm, and it is probable that in selected cases the drainage may be of great benefit. The operation was performed at the suggestion of Dr. Rudisch, in whose service the case was treated.

ESOPHAGUS AND STOMACH.

During the past two years, from December 1, 1902, to December 1, 1904, twenty-five operations were done on the stomach, for disease of that organ or of the esophagus, with a mortality of three, or 12 per cent. Fifteen operations were done for malignant disease with two deaths, ten for benign disease with one death. Of the twenty-two patients that recovered, the disease was benign in character in eight and all eight were cured by the operative interference; the disease was malignant in twelve, and as radical removal was impossible, palliative operations were performed. In two patients, exploratory laparotomy revealed the malignant disease to be so far advanced that not even a palliative operation was considered justifiable.

It is an unfortunate fact that the large majority of patients with carcinoma of the stomach come to the surgeon too late for radical treatment; by the time that a tumor is plainly palpable or the changes in the gastric juice are well marked, the hope of a radical cure by operation is, in most cases, a forlorn one. The poor results that surgery can show in the treatment of malignant disease of the stomach are due, to a great extent, to the lateness with which the patients come to the surgeon. We can only hope for decided advance in this branch of surgery when we have learned to differentiate more clearly between benign and malignant disease, and to make the diagnosis of malignant disease earlier. As our diagnostic methods are still far from satisfactory, exploratory laparotomy is often justified, although it should be recognized that exploratory operations in malignant disease are attended with not a little danger.

In five of the operations here reported, the laparotomy was an exploratory one. In three patients the disease was found to be benign in character and by the appropriate surgical procedures the patients were cured. In the two other patients the operation revealed hopeless malignant disease.

Gastrostomy for the relief of malignant stricture of the cardia was done five times with five recoveries. The gastric fistula was made three times by the method of Hall, once each by that of Kader and that of Witzel. Local anesthesia was made use of four times and chloroform once. In none of the cases was there any leakage from the fistula after the patients were up and about, although in one case (done by Hall's method) there was slight temporary leakage for about two weeks after the operation.

There is no more deplorable condition than that of a patient with malignant stricture of the esophagus, and there is considerable doubt in our mind how much we really benefit most of the patients by the gastrostomy. After gastro-enterostomy for carcinoma of the pylorus, the patients often gain much in weight and strength, and they are quite comfortable for six months to a year, but after gastrostomy for carcinoma of the cardia the patients rarely gain, and the fatal outcome of the disease is not much delayed.

Gastro-enterostomy was done twelve times, eight times for malignant disease with two deaths, and four times for benign disease with no deaths. The posterior operation of von Hacker was performed eleven times and the anterior operation once—but in the latter case posterior gastro-enterostomy had to be done two weeks later on account of persistent pain and vomiting.

In six of the patients the anastomosis was made with the McGraw ligature, once with the Murphy button, once with the Weir's modified button and four times by the suture method of Kocher. The operation was done under general anesthesia in all but one of the patients. Although in six of the patients we made the anastomosis with the McGraw ligature, we do not consider the method an ideal one. The main advantages are the cleanliness of the procedure and the rapidity with which the ligature can be inserted. The stoma is, however, a slit into which it is possible for the mucous membrane of the stomach to prolapse and thereby interfere with the free passage of the food. In this respect the twine triangular stitch, recently proposed by Maury, is far superior, and in our next report we shall speak of a number of cases in which Maury's method was used.

In all of the cases the anastomosis was made in the most dependent portion of the stomach and near the fixed part of the duodenum. We have had no case of vicious circle.

The average length of stay in the hospital after gastro-enterostomy was twenty-two days. While in the hospital the majority of the patients—whether they were suffering from benign or malignant disease—steadily gained in weight. In the benign cases the gain was not more rapid than in the malignant ones.

In the four patients with benign disease, two with pyloric stenosis and two with gastroptosis and dilatation, posterior gastro-enterostomy was done by suture according to the method of Kocher, because a large opening was considered of primary importance. All four of the patients were cured and gained from 28 to 60 pounds in weight in six months. Three of the patients are entirely free from symptoms, the fourth still has slight gastric disturbances. Synopses of the histories of two of the cases follow:

Benign pyloric stenosis; posterior gastro-enterostomy (Kocher); cure.—Rachel R., 46 years old, gave a history of pain in the region of the stomach and vomiting for three years. At first the attacks were mild, infrequent and relieved by drugs and dieting, but for one year the pain had been almost continuous unless relieved by vomiting, and had been accompanied by nausea, eructations of gas and constipation.

She had lost 25 pounds in weight during the previous six months. Physical examination was entirely negative except for some epigastric tenderness and a slight excess of free hydrochloric acid. Operation on May 20, 1904: Posterior gastro-enterostomy by suture under gas and ether anesthesia; recovery uninterrupted and uneventful. Discharged from the hospital four weeks after operation, entirely relieved of all of her symptoms, gained 60 pounds in weight in six months, and could take all food without discomfort.

Chronic gastric ulcer; gastroptosis; posterior gastro-enterostomy (Kocher); cure.—Rosie R., 24 years of age, was admitted to the medical service with the history of frequent pain in the hypogastrium and left hypochondrium after eating, with vomiting, for five years. For three months she had had constant soreness in the epigastrium, with severe pain after taking food, only relieved by vomiting. Two months before admission she vomited about one pint of blood. One year before she had weighed 106 pounds. On admission, July 9, 1904, she weighed 94 pounds. She was very weak and much emaciated; examination of the stomach contents after a test meal showed nothing abnormal except an excess of free hydrochloric acid; the stomach was markedly prolapsed. The patient was placed upon rectal alimentation, but did not improve; she had continual severe epigastric pain, vomited frequently, and after two weeks weighed only 90 pounds. Posterior gastro-enterostomy was done on July 27, 1904, under gas and ether anesthesia. The stomach was found so much prolapsed that the pancreas could be seen above the lesser curvature; the pylorus was not stenosed or thickened. Convalescence was absolutely uneventful. The patient did not vomit from the time of the operation and, except for occasional discomfort after taking food, has remained well. She gained 28 pounds in weight in six months.

The following are the histories of the two patients upon whom gastro-enterostomy was performed with a fatal outcome:

Carcinoma of pylorus; posterior gastro-enterostomy with McGraw ligature; death from shock.—Henry H., 56 years of age, was admitted to the hospital on December 8, 1903, with a four months' history of stomach trouble—pain in the epigastrium, vomiting, and weakness. The patient had taken no food at all for four days. He was much emaciated, very anemic, and had a large tumor in the pyloric region. Gastro-enterostomy with the McGraw ligature was done under ether anesthesia on December 9, 1903. The operation was easy, and took only twenty-five minutes. Just as the abdomen was being closed the patient, whose condition had been poor during the entire operation, collapsed and died within a few minutes, in spite of energetic stimulation. Permission for a post-mortem examination was not obtained.

Carcinoma of pylorus; posterior gastro-enterostomy with Weir button; death.—Samuel W., 53 years of age, admitted November 23, operated upon December 1, died December 4, 1903. The patient stated that he had been treated for about one year for tuberculosis of the lungs. For one month before admission he had had indefinite gastric symptoms, and during that time lost 16 pounds in weight. He was considerably emaciated and had a large tumor in the epigastrium and right hypochondrium. The operation consisted of posterior gastro-enterostomy by means of the Weir button. The procedure was easy, and lasted only twenty-five minutes. On the second day the patient developed high fever and vomited frequently. The wound was opened but nothing could be found. Death occurred in collapse on the third day after operation. No autopsy.

Gastro-duodenostomy (Finney's operation) was done five times with one death. According to our experience, the Finney operation is a little more complicated than ordinary gastro-enterostomy. It occupies more time, the danger of infection of the peritoneum with stomach or duodenal contents is a little greater, and hence the mortality from the operation is bound to be larger than from the ordinary gastro-enterostomy. The operation is, however, an excellent one in selected cases. The advantages of the Finney operation are: First, that it reproduces normal conditions as nearly as possible, and, second, that it does not, as does gastro-enterostomy, cause a too rapid entry of the acid stomach contents into the jejunum with the resulting danger of peptic ulcer. The disadvantages of the method have been mentioned above. It only needs to be added that where there are dense adhesions around the pylorus, so that this part of the stomach cannot be sufficiently exposed, Finney's operation should not be attempted.

Case I.—Rose L., 44 years old, symptoms referable to the stomach for four years; gastro-duodenostomy under chloroform, April 7, 1903. Pylorus found thickened with visible constriction; duration of operation, 55 minutes; fluids third day, soft diet seventh day, full diet thirtieth day; gained steadily in weight; free from all symptoms when discharged on thirty-sixth day after operation.

Case II.—Max S., 40 years of age, three years' history of pain and vomiting; gastro-duodenostomy under chloroform on May 23, 1903. Stomach dilated with thickening of pylorus; duodenum mobilized by incising peritoneum along its outer border; duration of operation, 90 minutes; convalescence uneventful; discharged cured 21 days after operation.

CASE III.—Samuel C., 40 years of age, admitted October 31, discharged December 16, 1903. One year's history of stomach symptoms. Gastro-duodenostomy November 14. Stomach dilated; pylorus stenosed and thickened; duration of operation, 60 minutes; convalescence uneventful; discharged relieved of all symptoms 31 days after operation. (This patient had been operated upon four days before the operation here reported—a band attached to the liver and hepatic flexure of the colon and compressing the latter having been divided—but as the patient's symptoms were not relieved, the second operation was done.)

CASE IV.—Henry Z., 33 years of age, admitted February 10, operated upon February 13, discharged cured March 5, 1904. Three years' history of stomach symptoms. Gastro-duodenostomy on February 13; stomach found dilated with greater curvature at level of navel; pylorus thickened; convalescence uneventful; discharged 23 days after operation. (Has remained well to date of this writing, March, 1905.)

CASE V.—Frances M., admitted May 5, died May 11, 1904. The patient had been operated upon for chronic appendicitis one year before. There was an old history of pain in the epigastrium and vomiting after meals; the patient had lost 20 pounds in weight. Gastro-duodenostomy was done on May 6, 1904, and at the operation the pylorus was found much thickened. The operation was easily performed. On the first day after the operation, the patient developed tonsilitis with high temperatures; on the second day there were some signs of consolidation in the upper lobe of the right lung; on the third day she complained of pain in the wound. When the wound was examined on the fourth day it was found that there was some sero-purulent discharge through the drain, and that the abdomen was slightly distended and tender. The patient's general condition became gradually worse, so that by the morning of the fifth day after the operation she was in poor condition, with a rapid pulse and high temperature, but she had not vomited and her bowels had moved every day after enemata. The entire wound was reopened under chloroform anesthesia and the abdomen found partly filled with sero-purulent fluid. The peritoneal cavity was washed out with saline solution and the abdominal wound widely drained; the gastro-duodenal anastomosis seemed in perfect condition. The patient grew steadily weaker, death occurred a few hours later. No post-mortem examination was permitted, but the culture from the fluid from the peritoneal cavity yielded a pure growth of the streptococcus pyogenes.

PANCREAS.

During the last few years we have learned much about acute pancreatitis but even now, in the majority of the cases, the correct diagnosis is not made before operation. In many, if not most, of the cases the disease is ushered in by a sudden attack of severe pain in the abdomen, vomiting and constipation, so that the case is supposed to be one of intestinal obstruction. The following is an example:

Acute pancreatitis; exploratory laparotomy; death.—Bernard R., 45 years old, was admitted on September 21, 1903, with the history that two and one half days before he was suddenly attacked with excruciating pain in the upper part of the abdomen, persistent vomiting and absolute constipation, which symptoms had remained up to the time of admission. The patient was very fat, his abdomen was distended, rigid and everywhere tender. On the suspicion that he had intestinal obstruction exploratory laparotomy was done. There were serous fluid in the cavity, a large hematoma around the pancreas, and numerous areas of fat necrosis in the omentum. The hematoma was drained, but the patient never rallied from the operation. The autopsy showed that in addition to the pancreatic hemorrhage, the gall-bladder was filled with stones, the pancreatic duct emptied into the dilated common duct, and both contained numerous small stones. The walls of the pancreatic duct were bile stained.

This case is of especial interest because of the presence of gall-stones and bile in the pancreatic duct. In the following case the onset of symptoms was also acute, and the diagnosis of peritonitis in the upper part of the abdomen, possibly due to gall-stones, was made.

Acute pancreatitis; cholelithiasis; cholecystitis; appendicectomy; cholecystectomy; cure.—Julia M., 41 years old, admitted January 31, discharged February 21, 1903. Two days before admission, sudden violent pain in the epigastrium, tenderness over the entire abdomen, fever, prostration. The symptoms persisted unabated until the operation, when there was tenderness in the epigastrium and right hypochondrium, and abdominal rigidity. At the operation there was found clear fluid in the peritoneal cavity, a distended gall-bladder filled with stones, numerous areas of fat necrosis in the omentum. The appendix and the gall-bladder were removed. Except for a pneumonia of moderate severity, the patient made an uneventful recovery.

This case is interesting from many aspects, but the recovery after removal of the gall-bladder is of especial interest. If the statement first made by Opie is true—and there is little doubt of it—that acute pancreatitis and fat necrosis are in most cases due to the retrojection of bile into the pancreatic duct through the presence and mechanical effects of gall-stones in the common duct, then we believe that the proper course to pursue is to drain the gall-bladder so as to prevent further entrance of bile into the pancreas. We have been waiting for an appropriate case to follow out this idea, but as yet none has presented itself. Recently we have had another case of pancreatitis in which the symptoms became acute after four weeks. The patient was in very poor condition when she was admitted to the hospital, and pancreatitis was suspected. At the operation there was sanguineous fluid in the peritoneal cavity, the omentum and parietal peritoneum very thickly studded with fat necroses, and the pancreas found enormously enlarged. The patient's condition became so poor as soon as the abdomen had been opened, that the operation had to be stopped, the region of the pancreas simply being drained. The patient succumbed a few hours later and the post-mortem examination showed that the left half of the pancreas was gangrenous and infiltrated with blood and that the gall-bladder was filled with stones.

The fourth case of acute pancreatitis was admitted to the hospital with the diagnosis of general peritonitis from an unknown cause. The history in brief is the following:

C. S., 55 years of age, was admitted on February 2, 1904, with the history of three days of severe abdominal pain, incessant vomiting and high fever. The abdomen was distended, rigid, everywhere tender, there was free fluid, and the patient looked very ill. Laparotomy was done at once; the abdomen was filled with chocolate-colored fluid, there were numerous areas of fat necrosis in the subcutaneous fat, the appendix was surrounded by fresh adhesions. The patient's poor condition allowed only drainage of the abdomen. After the operation the patient's condition remained poor, a fecal fistula formed on the right side, the entire wound became gangrenous, she developed septic parotitis, and died four weeks after the operation. No autopsy was permitted.

The fifth case of pancreatic disease was one of carcinoma of the head of the pancreas, in which only an exploratory operation was done. The patient recovered from the laparotomy, but up to the time he left the hospital lost flesh steadily. The interesting facts in his case were that he had at times free fat in his stools, and at other times small quantities of sugar in his urine. A piece of the tumor was removed for examination.

LIVER.

During the past two years ten operations were done on the liver, with four deaths. Two exploratory operations for tumor of the liver were performed, and in both the condition was found to be one of inoperable carcinoma. One of the patients was discharged unimproved three weeks after the operation, the second died from asthenia five days after the laparotomy and at the post-mortem examination the liver was found to be the site of a large primary tumor, with metastatic deposits in the lungs and kidneys.

Five patients with abscess of the liver were operated upon with three recoveries. In four of the cases the abscess was a single one. Three recovered. In the other case there were multiple abscesses, and the patient succumbed about four weeks after the operation.

Of the three cases that recovered, one was a gumma of the left lobe of the liver which had become necrotic, the second a case of abscess of the right lobe, the pus from which contained the bacterium coli; the third a case of abscess of the right lobe, the pus of which contained an anaerobic bacterium. Our experience during the past five years has shown us that surgery can save at least 75 per cent. of patients with single abscess of the liver, and we may hope for better results in the future.

The abscess is most often situated in the upper part of the right lobe, and has to be approached by the transpleural or transdiaphragmatic subpleural route. If there are adhesions between the diaphragmatic and the costal pleura, the operation is much simplified, but when no such adhesions exist the two layers have to be united by suture before the pleural cavity is opened. This can best be accomplished by making upward pressure on the liver and thus approximating the two layers; by this means it is often possible to unite the two layers without the entry of any air into the pleural cavity. We believe that the dangers from acute pneumothorax are still underestimated. If the pneumatic differentiation chamber of Sauerbruch and Mikulicz will accomplish all that its inventors claim for it, the operation of transpleural hepatotomy will be freed from one of its greatest dangers. The only patient that died from the operation during the past two years succumbed from the acute pneumothorax. It was the patient C. S., male, 30 years of age, with an amebic abscess of the right lobe of the liver, who was operated upon on September 3, 1904, collapsed on the operating table as soon as the pleura was opened, and died 20 hours later.

Two cases of hepatic abscess recovered after operation—in the one case transpleural hepatotomy and drainage, in the other laparotomy and incision and drainage was done. The history of the third case follows:

Broken down gumma of liver; laparotomy, incision and drainage; cure.—Samuel W., 42 years of age, was admitted on March 4, 1903, with the history of abdominal pain for six months, worse for four weeks before admission. The liver was enlarged and on the free edge of the right lobe there was a small tender mass. March 10: Laparotomy, incision of soft tumor of liver and evacuation of small quantity of purulent material; drainage. Convalescence uneventful. Pathological report of tissue from abscess wall—gumma.

The following case is of interest on account of the fact that the diagnosis was made before the operation from the presence of well marked hydatid fremitus.

Echinococcus cyst of right lobe of liver; extirpation; incision and drainage of second cyst; cure.—M. K., male, 39 years of age, was admitted on March 8, 1903, with the history that he had had an abdominal tumor for five years, and that for five weeks he had had pain in the region of the tumor. There was a large mass of the size of a child's head below and attached to the right lobe of the liver, over which was to be felt a marked hydatid thrill. At the operation, on March 10, the tumor was found to be attached to the gall-bladder and right hepatic lobe, with many adhesions to the transverse colon and small intestines. The mass was freed from its adhesions with ease and peeled out of its bed, and a second smaller tumor was then found in the right lumbar region, which originated from the posterior part of the right lobe of the liver. It was considered inadvisable to remove the second tumor at once, so the abdomen was closed. The patient made an uneventful recovery, and was discharged on April 12. He was readmitted on April 25, and the other cyst drained through a lumbar incision. Convalescence was uninterrupted, and he was discharged cured about one month later. (This man succumbed some months afterward following operation for an operative ventral hernia of great size with spontaneous fistula of jejunum. See report in Operations on the Intestines.)

Two other fatal cases of disease of the liver occurred on the second surgical service during the past two years, but in both patients the fatal outcome was due not to the operative interference, but to the nature of the affection. One of the cases was that of S. B., transferred to the surgical service with the diagnosis of abscess of the lung or liver. An interlobar abscess of the lung was opened and drained on September 5, but as the symptoms of the patient improved only temporarily transpleural hepatotomy was done on September 21. At the second operation several abscesses of the liver were drained and it became clear that one of the abscesses of the liver had perforated the diaphragm and caused the interlobar abscess. The patient, as was to be expected, did not improve, but died four days later. Permission for a post-mortem examination could not be obtained.

The second case is of sufficient interest to be reported more in detail.

Acute fatty degeneration of the liver; exploratory laparotomy; death.—Frank B., 14 years of age, was admitted to the hospital and died on January 17, 1904. Twenty-four hours before the little patient had suddenly been attacked with severe cramp-like pain in the upper part of the abdomen, which then became swollen and tender in its upper part. He had continuous fever up to 104°F. He had, however, not vomited and his bowels moved regularly. The patient was a well-nourished boy. His condition on admission was very poor, and he looked profoundly poisoned; the liver was enlarged to below the umbilicus and was everywhere tender. The entire abdomen was slightly distended but not rigid. His condition became rapidly worse, so that by the time the patient was brought to the operating-room he was in collapse. After active stimulation, exploratory laparotomy was done, but nothing was found except an enormously enlarged liver. Death occurred a few hours later. At the post-mortem examination there was found a hemorrhagic gastritis, an acute enteritis with the presence of considerable blood in the bowel, and an advanced fatty degeneration of the liver, kidneys and heart. A careful chemical examination of the contents of the stomach and intestines, and of the organs, failed to reveal any evidences of a poison of any kind.

GALL-BLADDER AND DUCTS.

For a fuller discussion of this subject, together with a number of interesting histories, the reader is referred to a paper by Dr. Lilienthal in the *Annals of Surgery* for 1904.

We find, on further experience, that the method of operation described in the above paper gives excellent results and that it is especially to be recommended because of the accuracy of exploration which it affords. The main points in this operation are the separate ligation of the cystic artery and the free slitting up of the ducts. These procedures are rendered possible by the placing of two stout traction sutures through the walls of the cystic duct, so that this structure may be brought up into the wound and within easy reach after the gall-bladder has been ablated and the hemorrhage checked. Though apparently a graver operation, the almost routine performance of cholecystectomy has been followed by a very great reduction in the percentage of mortality. A glance at the statistical table of operations will demonstrate this point.

Because the entire subject of biliary surgery is still under discussion we publish here a greater number of the successful cases than is our custom, together, of course, with all of the failures.

Pericholecystitis (typhoid); incision and drainage; cure.—Y. K., a woman 64 years old, married, was admitted on June 8, 1903. Thirty years before the patient had had an attack of jaundice, with severe colicky pains and the passage of gall-stones. One year before she had had another attack, accompanied by chills and vomiting and the passage of a number of gall-stones. Her present illness began two weeks previous to admission, when she was seized with a chill and vomiting of dark green fluid, jaundice, clay-colored feces, dark urine, and pain in the upper right quadrant of the abdomen, with swelling and rigidity. There was tympanites, with tenderness over the epigastrium and pain on deep pressure. Owing to the thickness of adipose tissue palpation was unsatisfactory.

The patient continued to run a temperature of 102°, and on June 13 it was decided to operate. Accordingly, an incision five inches long was made through the upper part of the right rectus. A large mass was encountered, and upon opening it about eight ounces of malodorous bile-tinged pus were evacuated. The gall-bladder could not be palpated. The cavity was packed and the wound closed. A culture showed typhoid bacillus. On June 15 the packings were removed and another abscess opened. Widal reaction was positive on June 16, and typhoid bacilli were recovered from the evacuations of pus from the wound. From June 18 to June 30 the discharge continued, but grew less profuse, and on July 11 the patient was discharged cured. Blood, on July 8, showed a positive Widal.

Fracture of femur; acute gangrenous septic cholecystitis; revision and suture of fracture of femur; partial cholecystectomy and drain-

age; death.—John G. T., 39 years old, was admitted on July 24, 1903, giving a history of typhoid five years and pneumonia four years before. Since then he had been in good health.

Thirty days before admission he had sustained a fracture of the middle third of the left thigh, which failed to unite. After an unsuccessful attempt, on July 25, to bring the two ends of the bone together it was decided, on August 1, to suture the bone, which was done by means of silver wire. On August 27 the plaster cast was removed and a starch dressing applied.

The patient was progressing nicely when, on September 4, he was seized with colicky pains in the epigastrium. The next day he was jaundiced and physical examination revealed the liver extending one finger breadth below the free costal border, and the gall-bladder plainly palpable and tender. From that time to September 8 the pains continued, jaundice increased and he also had chills. His temperature was intermittent, rising to 104° in the evening. He was severely constipated in spite of medication and treatment. A blood examination for plasmodia proved negative.

On September 9 the patient had a chill, followed by profuse sweating, the area of tenderness in the region of the gall-bladder had spread and, the diagnosis of acute cholecystitis having been made, it was decided that operation was urgently indicated. He was accordingly operated upon the same day, an incision 12 cm. in length being made through skin and right rectus muscle. When the peritoneal cavity was opened the gall-bladder was found much enlarged and bound down by dense adhesions. On a careful attempt to free the gall-bladder the organ ruptured and about a pint of pus escaped. The gall-bladder was then incised and several stones and considerable pus evacuated. The peripheral third of the organ was gangrenous, but owing to the dense adhesions it was found impossible to remove it entirely or even to peel out the mucous membrane. The gangrenous portion was, however, resected, a drainage tube inserted and a careful toilette of the wound made.

The patient reacted well, and on September 11 his general condition showed considerable improvement. Since operation there had been a free discharge of bile through the tube. From September 11, however, he steadily lost ground, his pulse becoming progressively more intermittent, and he ceased to breathe on September 14.

Post-mortem examination showed the remnants of the gall-bladder to be somewhat necrotic, the liver and spleen very large, the pulp soft and congested. The kidneys showed chronic nephritis.

Microscopic examination of the liver showed parenchymatous degeneration and cholangitis with abscesses.

Pericholecystitis; perforation of duodenum; incision and drainage; cured.—Fanny H., 50 years old, married, was admitted on April 12,

1903. Two years before she had had an attack similar to the one from which she suffered when admitted. This was characterized by pain in the right side, fever, chills and vomiting. She was decidedly jaundiced and had been sick about four weeks. Ten weeks before admission she had another attack. Her present illness was of two and a half weeks' standing, and began with pain in the epigastrium and right hypochondrium, radiating into the back and shoulders. The pain was cramp-like in character and she also had a sense of soreness in the right side. She vomited frequently and had fever, frequent chills and sweating. Her bowels were constipated, the stools being sometimes clay-colored and her urine dark red.

Physical examination showed liver enlargement to a hand's breadth below the free border; there was also tenderness. The abdomen was distended, tympanitic, and there were signs of free fluid.

She was operated upon on April 12, a four-inch incision being made between the fibres of the upper part of the right rectus. A mass was found, consisting of colon below, omentum above and dense exudate. This mass had made the impression on palpation of the free edge of the liver. Above was a smooth, fatty, hard mass about the size of a fist. The liver was probably high up above this mass but could not be determined; the site of the gall-bladder could also not be determined. On separating the adhesions between the smooth, fatty mass and the transverse colon an abscess was opened holding about six ounces of foul-smelling pus. The incision was lengthened two inches above and below in order to explore the gall-bladder, but it could not be found. Another incision at right angles to the first in its upper part was now made, but still the gall-bladder could not be located. The abscess cavity was further explored and two gall-stones extracted, one about the size of a pea, the other the size of a hickory-nut. The abscess cavity had rough, doughy walls, trabeculated, and it was not certain whether the finger entered the gall-bladder itself or whether the abscess was a cavity separate from the gall-bladder and communicating with it. Further exploration being deemed inadvisable a tube was inserted and the wound closed.

Culture from pus and spreads showed streptococci. Following operation the patient's life was despaired of, owing to an idiosyncrasy which she showed toward morphine. A small dose had been administered after the operation, but this was followed by such symptoms of morphine poisoning that vigorous stimulation had to be resorted to, and it was only by special effort and good fortune that she was tided over the crisis.

On April 16 the patient's condition was much improved, and the first dressing was done. The next day it was found that the dressings had a distinct acrid odor similar to vomitus, and a connection with the stomach being suspected the patient was given an aqueous solution of methylene blue by mouth. The blue solution appeared in the wound within five minutes. A duodenal fistula was diagnosticated, but in spite of it the patient made an otherwise uneventful recovery, and was discharged cured on May 9.

Acute cholecystitis; cholelithiasis; cholecystectomy; cure.—M. W., female, 35 years old, single, was admitted on May 13, 1904. This patient had been discharged from the hospital on May 1, 1903, after having been operated upon for appendicitis with abscess, complicated by diffuse peritonitis (Friedländer's bacillus). For six years she had suffered from yearly attacks of sharp pain in the right hypochondrium, radiating through to the back and followed by severe chills. During the year before admission these attacks had been very frequent; her bowels had been constipated and stools clay-colored but she had never been jaundiced. Three days previous to admission she had a severe attack of the cutting pain in the right hypochondrium, which radiated up to the left shoulder; this attack was accompanied by fever, chill, nausea, vomiting and constipation, and on admission there was marked conjunctival icterus.

At operation, on May 13, through a 3½-inch right rectus sagittal incision a large, tense gall-bladder presented, and upon aspiration about six ounces of fluid were obtained, the first three being clear and the remainder turbid. The fundus was then cut into and several stones evacuated; a stone the size of a large almond which plugged the cystic duct was also removed. The gall-bladder was then freed and cut away, and the hepatic duct drained. Culture from the gall-bladder showed streptococci.

The patient's general condition remained excellent, nothing occurred to hinder her convalescence, and on June 7 she left the hospital cured.

Acute cholecystitis; cholelithiasis; cholecystectomy and drainage; cure.—Lena A., 38 years old, married, was admitted on October 10, 1904. One year after the birth of her first child she had been operated upon and a vaginal hysterectomy performed; menopause ten years. Eight weeks before admission to the hospital she had an attack of cramp-like pain in the right hypochondrium which lasted for two or three hours and was accompanied by fever and chilly sensations. Similar attacks came on at intervals of four or five days, and four weeks before coming to the hospital she was seized with very severe abdominal cramps, lasting seven or eight hours, accompanied by fever, vomiting, jaundice and clay-colored stools. Since that time she had five similar attacks, the last one on the day before admission. Rigidity of the right rectus was noted, also tenderness in the right hypochondrium and epigastrium.

Operation was performed on October 11, and an elongated, distended gall-bladder removed, the stones in the cystic duct having first been pushed back into the organ. The gall-bladder was four inches long, its walls about one-half inch thick; its mucous membrane was congested and hemorrhagic, and at the fundus was an ulcerated area about one inch in diameter. It contained three medium-sized mulberry-like stones. After an uninterrupted convalescence the patient left the hospital cured on the 10th of November.

Cholelithiasis; acute cholecystitis; cholecystectomy; cure.—H. F. N., 43 years old, was admitted on March 28, 1904. For ten years previous to admission this patient had been subject to semi-annual attacks of colicky pain in the gall-bladder region, accompanied by vomiting, constipation and sleeplessness, and at such times the gall-bladder was felt enlarged and very tender. For six months before admission the attacks became much more frequent and were accompanied by a rise of temperature to 103°; he also lost considerable flesh and strength, and at time of admission pain and tenderness were present, and he suffered from nausea and vomiting. Physical examination was negative except that in the region of the gall-bladder a small, globular, slightly tender mass was palpable.

On March 29 a four-inch incision was made over the right rectus. The gall-bladder immediately presented and was found quite distended; about six ounces of dark, bile-stained fluid were withdrawn by aspirating needle. Two stones felt in the cystic duct were milked into the gall-bladder. The organ was freed from the liver, the cystic duct and vessels ligatured and the gall-bladder removed. The walls of the gall-bladder were thickened, its mucosa congested and at the fundus were two dark, congested, ulcerated areas about the size of a dime. The two stones were about the size of a cherry and were mulberry-shaped. The patient made an uneventful recovery and was discharged cured on April 18.

Obstructive jaundice; choledochotomy and hepaticotomy; death.— B. D., 18 years old, single, admitted July 13, 1904. This patient had been well up to two months previous to admission when she noticed that her sclera were yellow, and thereafter there was a progressively deepenly jaundice, malaise, loss of flesh and strength and loss of appetite. About five weeks before admission she had cramp-like pains in the right lumbar region, which lasted for two weeks; then pain of a similar character was experienced in the left lumbar region, which persisted and for four days before admission she had left-sided pain on urination; on the day before being admitted she had repeated epistaxis.

Her general condition was fair, skin, sclera and mucous membranes jaundiced. The liver was tender to pressure and extended two and a half inches below the free costal border. Its surface was somewhat uneven and its edges sharp and firm. Right kidney was palpable and tender; left not palpable but the region tender to deep pressure.

She was operated upon on July 20, a vertical incision being made over the right rectus muscle from the free border of the ribs to the level of the umbilicus; gall-bladder very small and empty. Palpation of the cystic duct revealed no stones, but an attempt to pass a probe through the cystic duct into the common duct was unsuccessful. An attempt was now made to expose the common duct but it was found difficult as very large dilated vessels were found in that region; it was finally traced, however, to the junction of hepatic and cystic ducts but there was nothing palpable. The duct was now incised and slit up toward the hepatic duct, about three-quarters of its length being opened. A probe was passed into the duodenum but could not be passed upward into the hepatic as it seemed to meet with an obstruction. A fine probe was passed into it, however, and a small amount of bile exuded. The hepatic duct, which was thickened, was then slit open about one-half inch and a fairly free flow of bile obtained. The remaining portion of the duct was then gradually dilated with probes and a No. 7 French catheter put into the hepatic duct and sutured. Cigarette drain to common duct, gall-bladder closed with catgut and peritoneum sutured. Dry dressing.

The patient's condition was very poor and active stimulation was kept up, in spite of which, however, she died on July 22.

SYNOPSIS OF AUTOPSY ON B. D.

Lungs.—In left pleural cavity about 100 c.c. blood-stained fluid; no adhesions. Both were edematous, containing considerable bile-stained fluid. Otherwise negative.

Bronchial nodes.—One node showed old healed tuberculosis.

Heart.—Small in size, ventricles dilated, valves discolored with bile; mitral and tricuspid showed insufficiency; aortic and pulmonic negative.

Abdomen.—Showed incision for gall-bladder operation, packings and cigarette drain surrounding gall-bladder and ducts; small catheter inserted in hepatic duct; no peritonitis.

Liver.—Size increased, surface smooth, bile capillaries injected and prominent; hepatic ducts dilated. Gall-bladder contained considerable clotted blood. Cystic duct slightly stenosed at entrance to gall-bladder. Common duct negative.

Spleen.—Slightly enlarged; capsule wrinkled; size, 14 x 7 x 3 cm.; weight, 300 gm.

Kidneys.—Left kidney much larger than right; both showed parenchyma bile-stained, cortex somewhat narrowed; Malpighian bodies prominent, slight increase of connective tissue and parenchymatous degeneration. Capsule slightly adherent. Pelvis of right showed recent hemorrhage. Left kidney, 14 x 8 x 4 cm.; right kidney, 12 x 6 x 3 cm.

Pancreas and intestines.—Negative.

Obstructive jaundice; cholecystenterostomy; death.—O. C., 46 years old, was admitted on August 20, 1904. This patient had always been constipated, but beyond that had been well until about a month and a half before admission when he noticed a yellowish discoloration of the conjunctiva; about a week later he became jaundiced over the entire body, and had severe itching. The jaundice continued to increase and he had some nausea but no vomiting, fever or chills. Bowels were moved by cathartics, and the stools were occasionally whitish. Three weeks before admission he began to have a dull pain in the right hypochondrium which persisted. For three or four days before coming to the hospital he had a rise of temperature at night, accompanied by sweating and chilly sensations. He had lost about 15 pounds in weight since the beginning of his illness. On admission he was markedly icteric and the liver extended four finger breadths below the free border.

On August 24 an incision was made over the right rectus muscle from the free border of the ribs to the level of the umbilicus and the peritoneum incised; the liver was enlarged but there were no nodules or new growth; gall-bladder small, shrunken and empty. The head of the pancreas was somewhat hard and enlarged, and a new growth of the head of the pancreas being suspected a Murphy button cholecystenterostomy was done.

The patient reacted fairly well but perspired very profusely. Two days later he complained of pressure in the epigastrium and his condition became worse. He vomited frequently, the vomiting toward evening becoming projectile and fecal. He continued to suffer considerable epigastric pain, sank rapidly and died on August 28, four days after operation.

Obstruction to ductus communis choledochus; exploratory laparotomy and drainage; death.—Mrs. R. W., 40 years old, was admitted July 14, 1904. About one year previous to her readmission she had been operated upon at this hospital for cholelithiasis and cholecystitis, a cholecystectomy having been done. Convalescence was rather slow, and during this time she developed jaundice which was more or less marked at different times. She lost considerable weight and had a persistent biliary fistula with which she was discharged and advised to return later for secondary operation to relieve recurring attacks of icterus believed to be due to stone in the common duct. After her discharge the patient's general condition underwent a considerable improvement, but the jaundice did not disappear and she had two distinct attacks of pain resembling gall-stone colic, followed by increase in icterus.

On July 15 incision was made in old scar with a second at right angles to it, extending into the right flank and running parallel to the ribs. Omentum and gut were found adherent to abdominal wall.

The wall of the sinus was also closely adherent to the stomach and was only freed after considerable effort. Digital and visual examination could determine no obstruction to common bile duct so the tract of the sinus was cut away and a probe introduced into the sinus without detecting any stone. Further exploration being deemed inadvisable a cigarette drain was inserted and the wound closed. The patient reacted fairly well, but her temperature rose to 102° and on July 17 reached 104.2°; her condition became much worse, she complained of pain in the left side and her pulse grew more rapid. There was considerable hemorrhagic oozing from the wound, and the patient also passed some clots of blood per vaginam. Her abdomen became more distended, bowels did not respond well, she became continually weaker and five days after operation, on July 20, in spite of increased stimulation she died.

Cholelithiasis; common duct stone; cholecystectomy; choledochotomy; cure.—Mr. K., 55 years old, was admitted March 28, 1904. He stated that about ten years before admission he had a severe attack of abdominal pain accompanied by vomiting and fever, the attack lasting three or four days. He had six or seven attacks up to eight years before admission, when they ceased to trouble him. Six years previous to admission he suffered with pseudo-anginal attacks, and a year and a half before coming to the hospital had diabetes for four or five months. Five weeks before coming to the hospital the attacks of abdominal pain returned, the first lasting four or five days; this was followed by an interval of two weeks when he had another attack with vomiting, fever and jaundice. For a week previous to admission his stools were clay-colored. He complained of weakness and had lost in weight considerably for two years. On admission there was deep mahogany jaundice. No fever but epigastric pain. Gall-bladder not palpable.

He consented to operation on March 29.* An incision five inches long was made through the right rectus muscle from the free border of the ribs to the level of the umbilicus. The opening of the peritoneum disclosed a small, contracted gall-bladder with many adhesions to duodenum and imbedded for fully half its circumference in the liver. The viscus was incised and nine large, hard, facetted gall-stones removed. The cystic duct was also filled with gall-stones and contracted. The gall-bladder was clamped and removed in the usual manner. A probe introduced into the cystic duct stump could not be passed into the common duct. Choledochotomy was then done, and a stone about the size of a small cherry removed, after which there was an escape of bile and the probe passed readily into the duodenum.

* This operation was the first to be performed in the amphitheatre of the new hospital.

Wound in the common duct was sutured, cigarette drain inserted to stump of cystic duct and abdominal wound closed as usual.

The patient reacted well and, without having experienced any untoward symptoms during his convalescence, was discharged cured on April 19.

At the time of operation this patient was in very poor general condition, and was in a deep mahogany jaundice. It is our belief that choledochotomy without removal of the gall-bladder would have been the more dangerous operation.

Cholelithiasis; pericholecystitis; cholecystectomy; choledochotomy; death (pneumonia).—Annie H., 49 years old, married, was admitted on June 3, 1904. She had eight children; one alive in Colorado with tuberculosis. Six weeks before admission she was awakened at night with a severe attack of cramps in the epigastrium, radiating to the back and right shoulder; she also had fever, chills and vomiting, and four days after the attack of pain jaundice appeared. She remained in bed for four weeks, owing to the pain in back and shoulder, and at time of admission still complained of pain in the right lumbar region and epigastrium. The patient was poorly nourished, and her lungs showed signs of emphysema and tenderness to percussion posteriorly on the right side from the angle of the scapula to free border of the ribs. On examination of the abdomen a long, globular mass, the gall-bladder, was palpable, tense and smooth, extending downward and inward toward the umbilicus from just below the free border of the ribs.

On June 8 a four-inch incision was made through the right rectus. The omentum was densely adherent to the gall-bladder and while palpating under surface of gall-bladder and breaking up adhesions a pus cavity was opened. This communicated with the cystic duct in which a gall-stone two inches long and half an inch in lateral diameter was felt and removed. The gall-bladder was freed to the entrance of the cystic into the common duct and excised; stump cauterized with pure carbolic. The common duct was now incised and a probe introduced; it was found patent and a rubber tube was inserted and sutured; usual closure of wound.

The gall-bladder was covered with dense adhesions, its walls about one inch thick and hard, except at the fundus where the wall was thin and ulcerated; the mucous membrane was thickened and chronically inflamed; bacillus coli found in pus from the gall-bladder.

The patient reacted well but her general condition was poor. The tube had not discharged bile, and on the second day following operation it was removed, and its withdrawal was followed by quite a gush of bile and pus from Morrison's space. Pneumonia ensued, involving both lower lobes posteriorly, and two days after operation, June 10, she died. Autopsy.

Cholelithiasis; chronic appendicitis; cholecystectomy; appendicectomy; cure.—Mrs. J. S., 48 years old, was admitted November 6, 1904. For about 17 years previous to admission the patient had suffered from "nervous dyspepsia" with much distress after eating, nausea, vomiting and heartburn. Three years before admission she had an attack of appendicitis with chills and vomiting, lasting three weeks. Since that time she had been subject to attacks of pain in the right iliac region, some tenderness and considerable gas in the bowel. She was also generally constipated. For six months previous to admission she had frequent seizures of sharp, colicky pain in the region of the gall-bladder, so severe as to require morphine and accompanied by nausea and sweating.

On November 8 she was operated upon during an interval. A right rectus incision three inches long was made below the costal margin; exploration revealed smooth ovoid stone, one-half inch in diameter, in a flaccid gall-bladder; the organ was cut away and the stump carbolized. After considerable manipulation the appendix was delivered into the wound; it was curved around the cecum, owing to the shortness of its mesenteriolum. The appendix was removed in the usual manner and a small drain inserted down to the gall-bladder stump, the wound being closed with the usual layer suture. Pathological examination showed lymphoid hyperplasia of the appendix.

The wound healed quickly, and on December 1 she left the hospital cured.

Acute gangrenous cholecystitis and cholelithiasis; cholecystectomy; cure.—Annie P., 40 years old, married, was admitted October 15, 1904. Fifteen months before her admission to the hospital she had had an attack of severe cramp-like pain in the epigastrium, radiating to the back and accompanied by vomiting, fever and chills. Her stools at the time were clay-colored and she also had conjunctival icterus. Five months after her first attack and two months after the birth of her last child she suffered from the same symptoms, but they were more severe in character; just five months before admission she had another attack much worse than those which preceded it. Three days previous to admission she had a recurrence of the cramp-like pain with fever, chilly sensations, slight jaundice and constipation for four days. She had lost weight steadily and complained of marked weakness. Her abdomen was distended, generally tympanitic, and there was rigidity of the upper right rectus; the gall-bladder was felt as a pear-shaped mass, tense, smooth and tender, extending from just below the free border of the ribs to the level of the umbilicus. On admission the patient's condition was considered very grave. Temperature, 104°; pulse rapid, sensorium rather cloudy.

Operation was performed without delay. The opening of the peritoneum through a right rectus incision was accompanied by a gush of greenish sero-purulent fluid. The gall-bladder, which was found distended, adherent and its inner side presenting a number of small gangrenous areas covered with fibrin, was first emptied by aspiration and then removed. It contained a number of small stones. The cystic duct was patent and a rubber tube was inserted; toilet of the wound was made as usual.

For several days there was a profuse discharge of bile and muco-purulent fluid, but this decreased gradually, the patient's general condition was excellent and she was discharged cured on November 8.

Post-typhoid gangrenous cholecystitis; cholelithiasis; cholecystectomy and drainage to stump; cure.—F. S., 35 years old, was admitted on October 11, 1904. Three weeks before she had been discharged from another hospital after an attack of typhoid fever lasting eight weeks. Eight days before admission she had begun to have severe cramp-like pains in the right hypochondrium, radiating to the back and left shoulder; this was accompanied by vomiting and followed by fever and chills; there was constipation but no jaundice. The character of the pain became dull and persistent. Abdomen was distended, upper right rectus rigid, and in the right hypochondrium was a pear-shaped protruding mass below the free margin of the liver and extending down to the level of the umbilicus, smooth, tense and tender.

The usual incision over the right rectus muscle was made on October 12; the gall-bladder was aspirated, clear yellowish fluid being evacuated, at first followed by thick brownish fluid, mucus and blood. The cystic duct was much dilated and contained a large stone, which was pushed back into the gall-bladder, which was then removed. The gall-bladder was five inches long, its wall about one inch thick, except at the fundus, where it was thin and ulcerated; mucous membrane gangrenous; the stone found in the gall-bladder was of a greenish color about the size of an almond. Culture from pus from gall-bladder demonstrated bacillus typhosus. Cigarette drains were carried to stump of cystic duct and the usual method followed as to suturing and closure.

The patient made a quick and uneventful recovery and was discharged cured on November 5.

Gangrene of gall-bladder; serous peritonitis; cure.—Max L., 31 years old, was admitted June 16, 1904. Nine years previous to admission he had had typhoid fever and two months thereafter had the first attack of gall-stone colic. Since that time he had had no symptoms until two days before he was admitted when he had an attack of pain in the right hypochondrium, radiating to the right shoulder, accompanied by fever, vomiting and constipation. There was marked rigidity over the right rectus and tenderness over the whole right side. On June 16 he was operated upon, a three-inch incision being made through the right rectus. When the peritoneum was entered there was an escape of free, bile-stained, non-odorous fluid. The gall-bladder, which was enlarged and distended and showed several large gangrenous areas on the serosa, was quickly peeled off from the under surface of the liver and removed. Clamps were attached to cystic duct and artery, but as the patient's condition was very poor no attempt was made at ligation. Culture from peritoneal fluid showed typhoid bacilli. The gall-bladder contained about an ounce of bile-stained purulent fluid; its walls were thickened, edematous, hemorrhagic and gangrenous. On June 23 the clamps were removed and drainage tube inserted.

In spite of the fact that his condition had been very poor the man improved rapidly and left the hospital cured on July 16.

Suppurative cholangitis with complicating sepsis; death.—S. S., a woman, 40 years old, was admitted August 26, 1904. One and a half years before this patient had been operated upon at another hospital for cholelithiasis and cholecystostomy performed; three months before admission she had again been operated upon at the same hospital. Biliary fistula persisted, the discharge being profuse, and she had not felt well since operation.

Two weeks before admission the biliary discharge became markedly less and she began to have chills, fever, vomiting and headache; she also became much weaker and developed pain in the right hypochondrium.

The patient's condition on admission was too poor to make operative interference advisable; temperature, 102° to 105°; pulse, 90 to 108, feeble; respiration, 24 to 38. She continued to grow worse, pulse more rapid and feeble, breathing more rapid and shallow, and in spite of vigorous stimulation she died on August 30. No autopsy.

Acute perforative cholecystitis; pericholecystic abscess; cholelithiasis; incision and drainage; cure.—Charles H., 29 years old, admitted May 10, 1904. Six years before admission this man had a severe attack of cramps in the epigastrium, accompanied by nausea and vomiting. Since that time had had several mild attacks, and two years ago had quite a severe one, which lasted two weeks. At that time he was jaundiced and had vomiting, nausea and constipation. Seven days before coming to the hospital he was seized with violent cramps in the epigastrium, followed by nausea and vomiting; the pain became localized in epigastrium and right hypochondrium, and was also referred to the back. The liver was extremely tender to palpation; the abdomen distended and dull in the right hypochondrium, where a large, tender mass the size of a man's fist could be palpated.

Operation was performed on May 13, and the abdomen entered

through a four-inch right rectus incision. The gall-bladder did not present but a mass was felt in that region; this mass was bluntly dissected and about four ounces of purulent fluid evacuated. The cavity was cleaned out and several stones, varying in size from that of a pea to a bean, were removed. A small, ruptured gall-bladder containing many stones was now located; the stones were removed and the cavity cleaned and a drainage tube inserted well into the fundus of the organ. The cystic and common ducts were free. Culture from the evacuated fluid showed bacillus coli.

The patient's general condition was good, the sinus closed rapidly and he was discharged cured on June 8.

Acute cholecystitis; pericholecystic abscess; incision and drainage; cure.—S. F., female, 64 years old, was admitted February 4, 1904. She stated that since her climacteric at her 51st year she had never been strong, but had had no symptoms referable to liver or abdomen with the exception of an attack of gall-stones seven years before, which had not been accompanied by chill, vomiting or fever, and from which she recovered in ten days.

Three weeks previous to admission, during an attack of acute bronchitis, she was seized with a severe lancinating pain in the right hypochondrium which lasted all night; this was accompanied by fever, chilly sensations and nausea. These symptoms subsided, but there was considerable tenderness in the right hypochondrium, and every night the patient suffered with headache and was feverish and chilly; bowels constipated. When examined her abdomen was distended, the liver extending to the umbilicus and there was much tenderness in the right hypochondrium.

Operation was performed on February 6, the intention being to perform cholecystectomy. A three-inch intermuscular incision was made over the gall-bladder region, but when the peritoneum was opened the gall-bladder was found densely surrounded by adhesions. While breaking up the adhesions an 'abscess cavity was entered into and six stones, ranging in size from a lima-bean to a cherry, removed. Whether this cavity was the gall-bladder or an abscess cavity could not be ascertained. Drains were inserted and a wet dressing applied. Pathological report on pus from the abscess cavity demonstrated the presence of streptococci and bacillus coli. The discharge of bile-stained fluid from the wound, which was at first considerable, gradually lessened, the wound healed nicely, and on March 19 the patient left the hospital cured. (This patient subsequently developed a malignant growth of the viscera which, on examination, proved to be inoperable.)

Cholecystitis; cholelithiasis; cholecystectomy and drainage of cystic duct; cure.—Mrs. Clara F., 46 years old, was admitted on April 28, 1904. In this case there was a history of several attacks of pain in the right half of the abdomen, accompanied by constipation, once or twice by vomiting, and for six months previous to admission the patient had been troubled with belching and a sense of fullness in the epigastrium. When admitted to the hospital she stated that her illness had been of seven days' duration, and had begun with belching and epigastric pain, sharp and referred to the back. A few hours after the onset the pain became localized in the right hypochondrium and that area grew extremely tender. A little later she had chills, her temperature rose to 105°F., and the pain and tenderness in the right hypochondrium having become extreme she presented herself for treatment. Operation the same day.

Upon entering the peritoneum through the usual incision a large, distended gall-bladder presented; this was aspirated and four ounces of clear fluid and half an ounce of purulent fluid withdrawn. At the base of the cystic duct a very large stone, the size of a walnut, was felt and when it had been pushed back into the gall-bladder that organ was freed from its attachments and removed. The mucous membrane of the gall-bladder and cystic duct was gangrenous; pure carbolic was applied to the cystic duct, drains inserted and the usual toilet of the wound made. There was nothing to mar the uneventful recovery of the patient, and she was discharged cured on May 19.

Acute cholecystitis, cholelithiasis; cholecystectomy for chronic cholecystitis and cholelithiasis; death.—Annie S., 38 years old, married. Admitted July 19, 1904. With the exception of chronic constipation this patient had always been well until four years previous to admission, when she had occasional sudden attacks of pain in the right hypochondriac and epigastric region, radiating to the back and accompanied by nausea. She continued to suffer from these attacks for two years, and then for a year was entirely free from them. One year before admission the attacks returned and became more frequent, recurring every four to six weeks. Five days before coming to the hospital she had a typical attack of the pain and nausea with slight fever.

Physical examination demonstrated an elongated, tense, smooth, tender mass in the right hypochondrium just below the edge of the liver, extending downward and inward—the gall-bladder. This was tender to percussion and attached to its fundus was a softer, doughy mass, evidently omentum. The upper half of the right rectus was rigid and the liver extended 2 finger breadths below the free border.

On July 20 operation was performed, a vertical incision being made over the right rectus muscle, from just below the free border of the ribs to just above the level of the umbilicus; the peritoneum having been incised the gall-bladder presented and was aspirated, dark-brown grumous fluid being removed. Several large stones were felt in the cystic duct, some of which were pushed back into the gall-bladder but one could not be dislodged. Gall-bladder and duct were now removed, the cystic duct being clamped and not held by sutures. The clamp on the cystic duct and vessels slipped and profuse hemorrhage ensued. The hemorrhage was controlled but the loss of blood necessitated an intravenous infusion.

The gall-bladder was five inches long and contained four large stones and one stone embedded in the cystic duct. One of the stones at the fundus had become encysted and had caused ulceration until the viscus at this point was very thin. The remainder of the wall of the gall-bladder was ¾-inch thick and its mucous membrane congested and gangrenous in several places.

The patient's general condition was very poor, peritoneal sepsis ensued and she ceased to breathe two days subsequent to operation.

Acute cholecystitis; choledithiasis; cholecystectomy; cure.—E. M., 33 years old, married, in the second month of her eighth pregnancy, was admitted on August 7, 1904. The attack for which she sought treatment was the first of its kind from which this patient had suffered. It had begun five weeks previous to admission with epigastric and lumbar pain, general frontal headache, nausea, slight jaundice, chill, fever and constipation. A few days before admission she had had quite a severe attack, accompanied by cramp-like pain. On admission there was marked conjunctival icterus, rigidity over the right upper rectus, tenderness over the entire right hypochondrium, the gall-bladder being palpable as a smooth, very tender, tense, pear-shaped mass. She was operated upon on August 10, an incision being made between the fibres of the right rectus muscle. This exposed a bluish, tense gall-bladder projecting three and a half inches below a Riedel's lobe of the liver. There were dense adhesions around a dilated, thickened cystic duct and a few gall-stones were palpable; these were pushed into the gall-bladder and that organ removed. It was about six inches long, thick walled; its mucous membrane congested and in some places ulcerated; it contained three large mulberry stones about the size of a cherry.

An August 29 a rounded swelling was noted in the abdominal wall just below and to the right of the umbilicus in the line of the incision. This proved to be an abscess, and it was evacuated on September 10. With this exception there was nothing of note to record in the patient's convalescence and she was discharged cured on September 17.

This patient returned November 9, the small sinus which she had at the time of leaving the hospital in September having refused to heal in spite of curetting and the usual methods. On November 8 two tubular tents were inserted into the sinus; these were removed on November 9, and a piece of gauze then presented at the wound. This required considerable force for its extraction and was followed by the escape of one quart of thick, greenish, sanious pus. The sinus now healed nicely, and she was discharged on November 16.

INTESTINES AND GENERAL PERITONEAL INFECTIONS.

We have already referred, in previous reports, to the large number of patients with acute abdominal affections who are admitted to Mt. Sinai Hospital, and to the fact that whenever there is a hope of saving a life by an operation we have always given the patient the benefit of the doubt, no matter how poor his condition. As a result the mortality after operations in these affections is bound to be large.

Forty-six operations were done with sixteen deaths, or 34 per cent.; if we deduct from the fatal cases six that occurred within twelve hours from the time of admission, there were ten deaths, or 21 per cent. Of the patients that died within twelve hours of operation, two had general peritonitis from perforation of the intestine in typhoid fever, two had general purulent peritonitis, one had general peritonitis from volvulus of the sigmoid flexure, one had a gangrenous intussusception. Three patients died within forty-eight hours of admission, due to intestinal obstruction by gall-stones, to typhoid perforation, and to undiscovered causes. All had general peritonitis at the time of operation.

Among the forty-six cases there were nine of diffuse or general and six of local peritonitis in which the point of entry of the infection could not be determined. Of the nine cases of general or diffuse peritonitis the affection was chronic in five and all five recovered after laparotomy and evacuation of the fluid exudate; two of the tuberculous cases were apparently cured; one case of diffuse peritonitis due to the gonococcus recovered after laparotomy and drainage. The affection was acute in four, of which only two recovered. In one the staphylococcus aureus and bacterium coli were present, and in the other the gonococcus. In both patients who died there was a general purulent peritonitis with a pure culture of the pneumococcus in the fluid from the abdomen.

General purulent peritonitis (pneumococcus); laparotomy and drainage; death.—Dollie G., 16 years of age, admitted and died October 12, 1904. Three days' history of abdominal pain, vomiting, diarrhea; patient in very poor condition; physical signs of general peritonitis; immediate laparotomy; light green purulent fluid in peritoneal cavity; irrigation and drainage; death two hours after operation; no autopsy.

General purulent peritonitis (pneumococcus); laparotomy and drainage; death.—Annie B., 6½ years of age, admitted June 19, died June 21, 1903. Symptoms of peritonitis of five days standing. Laparotomy, irrigation and drainage for general purulent peritonitis; death twelve hours after operation. Culture from pus—diplococcus pneumoniae. No autopsy.

Special mention has been made of these two cases because we believe that diffuse pneumococcus peritonitis is a clinical entity and should be recognized as such, that the diagnosis can be made in many of the cases, and that operation should be performed only as a last resort if the diagnosis has been made. We have seen a considerable number of these cases, and have been impressed by the clinical picture they presented. The onset is very acute—the patients are suddenly "stricken down," vomiting and diarrhea are incessant, bulging of the umbilicus appears early, prostration is extreme, the abdominal signs point to diffuse affection. There may be a previous history of pneumonia or not, or there may be signs in the chest.

Of the six cases of localized peritonitis from undiscovered causes five recovered and one died.

Extraperitoneal abscess; incision and drainage; death.—Helen M., 59, admitted March 29, operated upon April 6, died April 7, 1904. Six weeks' history of pain in the abdomen, and fever; large abscess opened and drained; death, with symptoms of sepsis. No autopsy.

Six patients were operated upon for perforation of the bowel in the course of typhoid fever with two recoveries.

1. *Typhoid perforation; laparotomy; suture; drainage; death.*—Samuel H., 31, in third week of typhoid fever, had sudden pain and tenderness in right iliac region with obliteration of liver dullness and rise in pulse rate. Three hours later all symptoms more marked, leucocytes 5,800. Operation January 31, seven hours from first symptom; free fluid and gas in peritoneal cavity; perforation twelve inches from ileocecal valve one-eighth inch in diameter; Lembert sutures; irrigation with saline solution; drainage. Shock very marked; death twelve hours after operation.

2. *Typhoid perforation; laparotomy and suture; drainage; death from second perforation.*—Becky B., 9 years old, developed signs of perforation on 27th day of severe typhoid. She was transferred from the children's service and operated upon eight hours from the beginning of the symptoms; patient in very poor condition. October 1: Laparotomy and suture of perforation four inches from ileo-cecal junction, suture of three suspicious areas; feces and free gas in general cavity; saline irrigation; drainage. After eighteen hours condition of patient fair; no vomiting; abdomen softer and less tender; pulse 130, and of good quality. At the expiration of twenty-second hour sudden change in condition, collapse, death. Autopsy showed that there was a second perforation between two of the sutured areas; entire lower twelve inches of ileum filled with many large and deep ulcers; large amount of fecal matter in peritoneal cavity. Culture from fluid, bacterium coli.

3. *Typhoid perforation; laparotomy and suture; cure.*—Harry R., 9 years of age, admitted and operated on August 6, 1903, in the third week of typhoid fever, with symptoms of general peritonitis of about twenty hours standing. Laparotomy and suture of perforation in lower ileum; sero-purulent peritonitis. Duration of operation, fourteen minutes; recovery.

4. *Typhoid perforation; laparotomy and suture; recovery.*—Jacob F., 18, transferred from the medical service, and operated upon September 21, 1903. Perforation in lower ileum in fifth week of disease. Laparotomy and suture of perforation and of one area on the verge of perforation. Feces and free gas in peritoneal cavity. Duration of operation, eighteen minutes. After ten days of normal temperature, severe relapse with high temperatures and rapid pulse; recovery.

Another case of operation for probable typhoid perforation should here be mentioned. A young man in (probably) the fourth week of the disease came to the hospital on the medical side with a median abdominal abscess. The case was evidently one of typhoid. Incision and drainage was followed by recovery after some weeks, during which small intestine contents escaped through the wound. The actual point of perforation was neither sought nor found. The symptoms not having been very acute a delay of twenty-four hours was permitted before the operation.

5. *Typhoid perforation; laparotomy and suture; death.*—Jacob C., 16, operated on eight to ten hours after beginning of symptoms of perforation on 26th day of severe typhoid fever. October 30:

Laparotomy and suture of perforation twelve inches from cecum, saline irrigation; drainage, cultures from sero-purulent fluid in peritoneal cavity—staphylococcus aureus and bacterium coli. Death four days after operation, with symptoms of peritonitis. No autopsy. Duration of operation, twenty minutes.

6. *Typhoid perforation; laparotomy and suture; death.*—Rachel C., transferred from medical service, August 8, 1904, and operated upon about ten hours from first symptoms of perforation. Free fluid in peritoneal cavity; laparotomy and suture of perforation about ten inches from ileo-cecal junction; irrigation; drainage. Death about eight hours after operation. No autopsy. Cultures from blood and from fluid in abdomen—bacillus typhosus.

In our experience with perforation of the bowel in typhoid fever during the past five years we have been impressed by the following facts:

1. In most of the cases of perforation, the diagnosis may be made with probability within six to eight hours from the first suspicious symptom and often earlier.

2. Leukocytosis if present has but a limited value. It is but fair to say, however, that we have not in this class of cases made observation on the differential count.

3. Perforation is a surgical complication and operative interference should follow as soon as the diagnosis has been made, or if the diagnosis is probable—if the patient's condition is steadily becoming worse and the symptoms are of less than twelve hours' duration. If the symptoms are of more than twenty-four hours' duration when the patient first comes under observation, a few hours of delay while the patient is carefully watched is often justifiable.

4. If the operative manipulations are rapidly done, with as little exposure of the intestines as possible, the patients bear the interference remarkably well.

5. A sudden fall of temperature to the normal or near the normal within eight to twelve hours of the operation has considerable prognostic significance, and the absence of such a primary fall of temperature makes the recovery very doubtful.

6. In the patients that recover the abdominal signs disappear with considerable rapidity—usually within four to five days.

7. Healing is not essentially different from that after laparotomy for perforative peritonitis from other causes.

8. A light chloroform anesthesia is preferable to local anesthesia in most of the cases, as the necessary manipulations can be more rapidly performed and the shock is less.

INTESTINAL OBSTRUCTION.

Of eight cases of acute intestinal obstruction, four recovered, two of acute intussusception and two of intestinal obstruction by bands. Synopses of the fatal cases follow:

Acute intestinal obstruction by band; laparotomy and division of band; death.—Samuel R., 29, symptoms of acute obstruction of four days' duration. September 24, 1903; Laparotomy and division of band; death two days later with symptoms of peritonitis. Autopsy: healed ulcers of colon; peritonitis.

Acute intestinal obstruction due to gall-stones; communication between gall-bladder and duodenum; general peritonitis; cholecystotomy and drainage; death.—Abraham G., admitted November 17, died November 19, 1903. Eight days' history; signs of intestinal obstruction and peritonitis; patient in very poor condition; drainage of gall-bladder with evacuation of stones and pus; death on second day after operation. Autopsy: General peritonitis; perforation of gall-bladder into duodenum; two large stones obstructing bowel.

Gangrenous intussusception; resection and anastomosis with Murphy button; death.—Wm. K., 10 months old, admitted and died June 22, 1903. Resection of intussusception of twenty-four hours' standing; death two hours after operation from shock; no autopsy.

Volvulus of small intestine; peritonitis; reduction; death.—Pierry P., 21 years of age, admitted and operated on September 21, 1903, died September 22. Six days' history of acute intestinal obstruction; general condition very poor; signs of peritonitis; reduction of volvulus; death eight hours after operation; no autopsy.

Very many of the patients that are admitted to our hospital with acute intestinal obstruction are in such poor condition that any operative procedure which looks toward the permanent removal of the cause of the obstruction is inadvisable. We think that better results can be obtained in this class of cases by preliminary enterostomy. Unless the cause of the obstruction is easily found and can be easily removed (such as the untwisting of a volvulus, the reduction of an intussusception, etc.) it is better not to make a prolonged search perhaps with evisceration, but simply to take the most distended coil of intestine, anchor it in the wound, and open it.

Five patients with chronic intestinal obstruction were operated upon with one death. Twice exploratory laparotomy was done for inoperable tumors of the bowel; once for chronic peritonitis with adhesions; once resection of tumor of sigmoid flexure with fatal outcome; once resection of small intestine for stricture.

Circular ulcer of ileum; chronic intestinal obstruction; resection and anastomosis with Murphy button; cure.—Alois H., 23 years old, was struck in abdomen by dumb-waiter six months before. Four weeks before admission sudden abdominal pain and vomiting; for three weeks frequent pain, vomiting, constipation, visible peristalsis. June 29, 1904: Resection of loop of bowel with tight stricture, Murphy button anastomosis; convalescence uneventful; discharged July 28.

Carcinoma of sigmoid flexure; resection; anastomosis by suture; death.—Simon B., admitted December 3, died December 15, 1903. There was a ten months' history of chronic intestinal obstruction with loss of weight and presence of enlarging tumor in left iliac region. December 12: Resection of tumor, and end to end anastomosis by suture; drainage. Fecal fistula became established. Six days after operation patient suddenly collapsed after receiving an enema; immediate laparotomy and washing out of peritoneal cavity into which some of the enema fluid had escaped; death three days later. No autopsy.

Short histories of the other fatal cases follow:

Gangrenous infarct of spleen; general peritonitis; laparotomy; irrigation; drainage; death.—Joseph L., admitted December 16, died December 17. Symptoms of general peritonitis of three weeks' duration. Immediate laparotomy and drainage of necrotic infarct of spleen; irrigation of cavity. Death two hours later; autopsy showed large necrotic infarct of spleen and general peritonitis.

Pelvic abscess from perforation of intestine by pin; incision and drainage; death.—Zelmira B., 17 months of age, incision of abdominal wall and drainage of abscess on May 25. Condition poor before operation and did not improve; entire wound became gangrenous; fecal fistula; death on June 6. Post-mortem showed pin in abscess cavity and edges of opening in bowel gangrenous.

Fistula of jejunum; general peritonitis; entero-anastomosis; death.
—M. K., male, operated on in 1903 for echinococcus cysts of liver (q. v.). Four days before admission sudden pain in abdominal scar, redness, abscess, intestinal fistula. February 27: Resection of jejunum and entero-anastomosis by Connell suture; drainage. Death on third day, with symptoms of general peritonitis, ushered in by distension. No autopsy.

Pseudo-leukemia; cholelithiasis; multiple abscesses of spleen; laparotomy and drainage; death.—N. X., admitted July 26, died August 20, 1904. Typical history of cholelithiasis of two years' duration. Increasing pain and tenderness in left hypochondrium, with chills and fever for three weeks before admission. Liver and gall-bladder enlarged and tender; spleen much enlarged; not tender; blood count normal. July 29: Exploratory laparotomy for splenic tumor; gall-bladder distended, surrounded by adhesions, full of stones; spleen enormously enlarged, many fresh adhesions, large prominent fluctuating area on surface; numerous other smaller areas; large swelling in spleen contains pus; drainage of abscess cavity; removal of specimen for examination. Report of pathological department: Purulent inflammation. Condition became rapidly worse, preventing any further operation; high temperatures, rapid pulse. Blood culture negative; no leukocytosis; death August 20.

Finally, mention must be made of a patient with intra-abdominal omental torsion, who was admitted to the hospital with a history of eleven days abdominal pain with fever. He had had a hernia since childhood. The twisted omentum was excised and convalescence was uneventful.

Another case that is worthy of mention was that of a young woman who, in attempting to induce an abortion upon herself, pushed a silk bougie into the left retroperitoneal region as high as the left kidney. On account of pain and fever, she entered the hospital four months later, and by abdominal section the bougie was removed and the patient recovered.

APPENDICITIS.

The operative treatment of these cases has changed but little in the past two years. Fewer permanent packings, especially in the cases of diffuse peritonitis in which practically none are used, and immediate suture of the wound in the same class of cases have been followed by improvement in results. Then, too, the washing out of the free peritoneal cavity has been practically abandoned. Small incisions and no handling of the viscera are important points. As little delay as possible in acute cases has been our rule, and when for some exceptional reason this rule has been disregarded we have had cause for regret oftener than for gratification. Less haste to move the bowels when the patient is doing well and greater haste to perform enterostomy when acute obstructive symptoms appear seem to mark an improvement in practice.

In the two years there were 257 operations for appendicitis, with 14 deaths. This number includes the cases of peritonitis resulting from disease of the appendix.

Acute appendicitis; no operation; cure.—G. G., male, aged 79 years. This patient was admitted on October 31, 1903. The history given was that on October 23 he had been seized with indigestion, vomiting, localized pain in the right iliac region and fever. Constipation had also existed and the diagnosis of acute appendicitis was made.

Because of the patient's age and general feeble condition it was not deemed advisable to operate.

Under appropriate general medical treatment and poulticing, the mental confusion and hiccough, which were marked symptoms of the attack, disappeared, and on November 7 the patient was discharged cured.

This is an example of one of the rare forms of appendicitis in which operation is not indicated. The patient was senile and very feeble. The signs of peritoneal irritation were slight and the proper treatment seemed to be the poultice, for the purpose of hastening resolution or localizing and hastening the suppuration if this were inevitable. Had an abscess formed it was our intention to treat it by simple incision without general anesthesia.

Appendicitis; acute gangrenous peritonitis, purulent, general; appendicectomy; death.—O. L., male, 14 years old, was admitted on August 6, 1903, with a typical history of appendicitis of four days' duration, but no antecedent attacks. He was operated upon soon after admission. An incision one and a half inches long was made over the mass in the right iliac region, and on opening the peritoneum foul pus escaped. The appendix was found closely adherent to the pelvic wall and about one inch from the cecum was gangrenous, and was torn off in the manipulation. The remainder was then brought up and tied off close to the cecum and a cigarette drain inserted. The necrotic omentum which overlay the appendix was ablated and the abscess cavity thoroughly cleaned. Upon withdrawal of the packings which had been inserted up toward the liver they were found stained with foul serum, yet careful search did not reveal another abscess. On examination the appendix was found to be distended until it equaled the size of the small intestine, its cavity distended with pus, and at its proximal end was a gangrenous patch through which pus leaked from a large perforation.

Culture showed bacterium coli.

On August 7 the patient's general condition was fair, his temperature ranging between 102° and 103°. On the 9th it had become normal.

On August 10, however, a macular rash appeared on the chest, light yellowish-brown in color, which on the 11th changed to scarlet and became diffuse in character. German-measles being suspected he was sent to the isolation house.

The rash proved to be atypical, in some places vesicular, in others purpuric, and was probably due to sepsis. His general condition became gradually worse and he developed an acute nephritis. He took insufficient nourishment, complained bitterly of pain in the back. The febrile symptoms continued, temperature ranging between 102° and 103°. On August 14 desquamation was noted. Patient could not retain nourishment, even small quantities of liquid being vomited. Abdomen was distended, tense and tender. The wound was still discharging and the discharge had a fecal odor. Vomitus was now coffee-colored and projectile in character, and all the symptoms of peritonitis were present. The patient's condition grew rapidly worse, and on August 15 death took place. No autopsy was obtainable.

True necrosis (gangrene) of omentum such as existed in this case is a sign of grave prognostic import. In spite of free ablation the danger that sepsis has already invaded the circulation is great. The condition, though not so grave as a septic thrombosis of the mesenteriolum, belong in the same general class. It is unfortunate that no post-mortem examination was permitted.

Acute appendicitis with abscess and diffuse peritonitis; appendicectomy and drainage; death.—Louis M., 12 years old, was brought to the hospital on September 20, 1903. About a year before he had had an attack of pain in the left iliac region, which had lasted but one day. His present attack had an acute onset three days before admission, when he had severe cramp-like pain in the left iliac region, which later became lancinating. Twenty-four hours after the onset he began to vomit; had been feverish but had no chilly sensations.

On admission his general condition was fair; expression anxious. The abdomen showed general rigidity and distension, with moderate tenderness in the right iliac region and marked tenderness in left.

At the operation a few hours after admission several large abscesses were evacuated from between the coils of intestines and within the pelvis. The appendix was three inches in length and at least one inch in width, with a very large mesenteriolum. Its entire mucous membrane was gangrenous, and at the distal end there was a gangrenous ulcer through which purulent material was exuding. It contained considerable foul, necrotic material and two coproliths. The appendix was removed, the gangrenous stump carbolized, with a cigarette drain to stump and gauze drain in pelvis. No sutures. Wound strapped.

Culture showed bacillus pyocyaneus.

On September 22 the boy's temperature fell to 102°, but later rose to 104.4°; late in the afternoon he became very delirious and his pulse imperceptible. His pupils dilated and contracted at short intervals, his limbs became rigid, followed by periods of relaxation. Vigorous stimulation had no effect and he ceased to breathe at 5.30 P. M. No autopsy was obtainable.

The general practitioner has learned to suspect and fear appendicitis in every obscure acute abdominal infection. Yet, in this case, it is quite probable that the delay in seeking surgical aid was due to the history and presence of localized symptoms in the left iliac region, instead of in the right. We have noted maximum tenderness in regions other than that of the appendix in cases of peritonitis with multiple abscess. After visceral tension has been relieved by rupture of the appendix a walled off abscess in some other part of the abdomen may well be more painful and tender than the original focus.

The bacillus pyocyaneus should no longer be regarded as a harmless organism. It occasionally takes on virulent characteristics and may be the cause of general infection.

Acute gangrenous appendicitis; diffuse peritonitis; appendicectomy and drainage; death.—Jacob D., 20 years old, admitted September 4, 1903, having been suffering for two or three days with general abdominal pain, nausea, constipation, vomiting, chills and localized pain in right iliac region. At operation free purulent fluid was encountered and an adherent appendix was found. Upon breaking up the adhesions thick yellowish foul-smelling pus escaped. The thickened, gangrenous appendix was removed, the stump ligated and the wound drained.

Culture showed the bacterium coli.

He reacted well and on September 7, three days after operation, his general condition was good. On September 9, however, the temperature began to rise, and he vomited greenish material. There was considerable discharge from the wound, of a fetid odor. The wound was dressed twice daily but the discharge continued, the odor becoming more marked. He also continued to vomit occasionally and sank rapidly, dying on September 13.

Acute perforative appendicitis; general purulent peritonitis; appendicectomy; death.—Michael C., 5 years old, was admitted and operated upon July 29, 1903. There was no previous history bearing upon the case, except that two weeks ago after a fall he had had an attack of general abdominal cramps, lasting twenty-four hours. He had vomited once, greenish fluid, and had been feverish with chilly sensations. His present illness was of forty-eight hours' duration, and was ushered in suddenly with severe cramps in the abdomen, most marked on the right side. His abdomen had become distended and tender. He had vomited and had chilly and feverish sensations. Bowels had not moved since the onset of the attack.

His general condition was poor, and he was somewhat stuporous. The abdomen was rigid, distended, generally tender and tympanitic, except in the flanks, where there was movable dullness.

Operation.—A two-inch incision was made, and upon opening the peritoneum multiple abscesses were disclosed which contained foul-smelling yellow pus. These were evacuated and abscess cavities cleansed. The appendix was deeply congested, perforated, and its mucous membrane gangrenous. It contained a coprolith in the lumen near the tip. The appendix having been cut away the stump was carbolized, a cigarette drain inserted, the skin strapped and dry dressing applied. On July 30 the child's condition showed slight improvement, but the temperature continued to rise. In the evening he became quite noisy and very restless, pulse grew very rapid and temperature rose to 106.4°. Death took place at 5.20 P. M. on that day.

We have learned to dread multiple abscesses in peritonitis more than the diffuse peritonitis with few adhesions. When these cases do recover the convalescence is tedious, repeated operations are often necessary and the danger of relapse is great.

Acute gangrenous perforative appendicitis; general purulent peritonitis; appendicectomy and drainage; death.—Annie R., 11 years of age, admitted March 13, 1903, with a history of severe general abdominal pain which began one and a half days ago. The pain was not localized; there had been biliary vomiting with some fever but no chill. Bowels moved after enema; urination infrequent.

On admission her general condition was poor and she showed the peritonitic facies, also enlargement of all lymph nodes. The abdomen showed the usual signs of rigidity, distension, tenderness, dullness in right flank and iliac regions, tympany in left flank and some evidences of free fluid.

The child was operated upon on day of admission, a Kammerer incision, two inches long, being made low down. The abdominal wall was edematous, and on opening the abdomen there was an escape of foul, purulent fluid from all sides. The gangrenous appendix, which was thick and erect, showed no adhesions. There was a perforation near the base and the mucosa was so hemorrhagic and swollen as to completely obliterate the lumen. A coprolith was also found. The appendix was ligated and cut away and cigarette drain inserted. Next day the patient's general condition was poor, pulse rapid and of poor quality, repeated vomiting. The vomiting continued on the 15th and 16th, being of dark green fluid. Urination and defecation involuntary; temperature, 105°, and pulse, 180. She died on March 16, three days after admission. No autopsy.

Gangrenous perforative appendicitis; fibrino-purulent general septic peritonitis; appendicectomy; death.—Morris B., aged 16 years, was brought to the hospital on December 30, 1903, showing the anxious expression so characteristic of peritonitis and with physical signs that pointed to the urgency of operative measures.

He had had frequent attacks of diarrhea, but the history of the present illness dated back three days, when he had had a sudden attack of pain in the right iliac region, accompanied by vomiting. In spite of cathartics and enemata there had been no movement of the bowels since then, not even gas passing. There was considerable peristaltic unrest and he had a chill and some fever, but no jaundice. The lower half of the abdomen was symmetrically distended and tympanitic, also quite tense with general tenderness. Rectal examination showed the pelvis occupied by a soft tumor mass somewhat toward the left side.

Operation was deemed urgent and a median abdominal incision made. This was accompanied by the escape of considerable foul-smelling brownish fluid. On opening the peritoneal cavity, distended and markedly discolored intestines covered in scattered areas by large patches of easily detachable yellowish-green fibrin, presented in the wound. The pelvis and peritoneal recesses were filled with foul-smelling free fluid. The appendix was gangrenous and covered with fibrin and near its base was a large perforation.

The appendix was removed and the rent in the cecum repaired with silk sutures. Drainage of stump and pelvis; wound irrigated with salt solution; suture in layers.

The patient rallied well, but several hours later the pulse began to weaken, and in spite of vigorous and repeated efforts at stimulation he ceased to breathe the following morning.

The median incision was made because an accurate preoperative diagnosis was impossible and the septic peritonitis with intestinal obstruction was the prominent feature of the case.

Acute streptococcus appendicitis; pleurisy with effusion; appendicectomy and drainage; cure.—Flora L., 22 years old, single, was admitted and operated upon December 24, 1902. Her present illness was of two days' duration, although she had had a similar attack about a year before. She complained of general cramp-like abdominal pain, not localized but more severe on the right side. She had vomited once, but there was no chill, no cough and no dyspnea. Temperature, 104.4°F. There was neither jaundice nor glandular enlargement. She was fairly well nourished but had a septic appearance. The abdomen was rigid, slightly distended, tympanitic and generally tender. Rectal examination proved negative but pushing up the uterus caused great pain.

Operation.—A four-inch Kammerer incision was made and on opening the peritoneum a large quantity of whitish-yellow pus exuded. The appendix, four inches long, perforated, gangrenous and with a dense thick stricture, was found behind the cecum closely adherent and twisted upon itself. It was removed and the stump treated with pure carbolic. The pelvis was full of pus which was carefully sponged out. A cigarette drain was inserted with another leading down to the stump and the peritoneum sewed with catgut, the wound closed and dry dressing applied.

Culture from the peritoneal fluid showed streptococci.

From January 3 to January 7 the patient ran a temperature of from 101° to 104°. There was a profuse discharge and the dressings were changed twice daily and the wound irrigated. Physical examination was negative with the exception of a mass on the right side high up about the size of a lemon found on rectal examination. On January 8 an area of dullness in left lung from the angle of the scapula down, with increased fremitus and voice at base and bronchial voice and breathing over upper dull area, was noted and a little later the right lung was also found to be involved. January 12 the left chest was aspirated and about an ounce of clear straw-colored fluid rushed into the syringe; on the 15th the left chest was again aspirated and 22 ounces of slightly turbid straw-colored fluid obtained, the last 6 ounces withdrawn being sanguinolent. January 27 aspiration was again performed and 4 ounces of bloody serum withdrawn. On January 28 temperature was still 104.8°. From that time on the temperature fell gradually until February 6 when the patient was up and about. There was still a slight discharge from the wound and a sinus about two inches deep. On February 15 the patient was discharged cured.

Acute appendicitis; general septic peritonitis; death.—Harry H., aged 12½ years, was admitted July 25, 1903, in the fourth day of an attack of acute appendicitis. Constipation had been absolute since onset in spite of cathartics and enemata. The abdomen was distended, rigid and everywhere tender.

His general condition was so wretched that no operation was undertaken, and he died a few hours later in spite of active stimulation. No autopsy.

Chronic appendicitis, with abscess; chronic intestinal obstruction; chronic peritonitis; incision and drainage; entero-enterostomy; cured.—Israel S., aged 30 years, was admitted on June 23, 1903. Six years before he had had an attack of general abdominal pain and was ill two weeks during which his bowels did not move. Two years later he had a similar but milder attack.

His present illness had been of two weeks' duration and began with general abdominal pain and repeated vomiting. He had been very constipated but bowels moved a day and a half before admission. No gas passed since then. He had some fever but no chills or jaundice.

His general condition was good. Upon examination his abdomen was found to be slightly distended, both recti rigid and all regions of the abdomen, especially the right iliac fossa and left middle lumbar region, tender to pressure. A large mass was felt low down behind the right rectus muscle. Movable flatness in both flanks along the entire region of the colon. Under anesthesia a mass the size of a grape-fruit was readily felt in the right iliac fossa approaching closely to the median line.

On June 25 the patient was operated upon. A Kammerer incision three inches long was made and on entering the peritoneal cavity a mass was felt at the cecal site, which extended upward toward the liver. The incison was enlarged upward and the mass, which was firm, hard and covered by adherent omentum, was found to extend nearly to the hepatic flexure and seemed to be around the colon. Toward the left another mass was felt, which was made up of twisted adherent omentum, and one loop of small intestine was found partially collapsed. The omentum over the colonic mass was tied off and divided so as to get at the underlying gut. In the appendicular region between the coils of adherent intestine an abscess cavity was found, from which two ounces of foul-smelling pus were evacuated. The appendix was not sought. The partially collapsed coil of small intestine was anastomosed with a neighboring dilated coil by means of a McGraw ligature. Cigarette drains were inserted into the abscess cavity and the abdomen closed.

The man reacted well and his general condition continued excellent. The wound continued to discharge slightly until July 24. He was discharged cured on July 26, though a sinus two inches long still persisted.

Chronic appendicitis, with abscess; drainage and closure of intestinal openings; cure.—Seymour H., aged 3½ years, had a previous history of adenoids and hypertrophied tonsils for which he had been operated upon.

About four weeks prior to the time of his admission to the hospital (January 12, 1903) he had an attack characterized by fever, tumor, etc. Physical examination on day of admission revealed a hard mass a little above the umbilicus on the right side, neither tender nor movable. On January 13 laparotomy was performed. A 3½-inch incision having been made, the many adhesions in the right iliac fossa were broken up and the cecum was liberated it was found that the appendix was not attached to it, but corresponding to the stump of the appendix was a hole in the gut surrounded by a raw surface, and about one inch distant a smaller intestinal opening. A coprolith about ½ inch in diameter was found and removed.

The hole corresponding to the stump was cauterized and ligated and the raw surface and smaller hole sutured with catgut. Cigarette drain and layer suture of wound.

During the acute attack there had evidently been a rupture which freed the coprolith so that it rested in the pocket of adhesions. The appendix was not found.

The patient made an uneventful recovery and was discharged cured on February 3, 1903.

Sinus after appendicitis; appendicectomy; cured.—Minnie L., 9 years old, was admitted on February 5, 1903. The only previous history with any bearing on the case is that eight years before the child fell, sustaining a wound in the right lumbar region. The wound healed quickly and has never been the seat of trouble.

Her present illness began two weeks before admission, when she began to complain of pain in the right inguinal region; this pain increased steadily, was intermittent and was relieved by reclining. It never radiated and no tumefaction was ever noticed. There was no history of chill, vomiting or constipation. On admission the child's temperature was 103.6°, pulse 112; she was, however, free from pain.

Physical examination showed diffuse glandular enlargement, especially in right inguinal region. There was some dullness over the upper part of the sternum, considerable anemia, slight cyanosis and some clubbing of the fingers. There was also marked accentuation of second pulmonic sound.

Examination of the abdomen revealed an irregular scar about one and a half inches long in the right iliac region, just above McBurney's point, and in the direction of the fibres of the external oblique. It was adherent to the deeper tissue. In the right iliac region there was an area of dullness about the size of a silver dollar, and also tenderness but not very marked, except on deep pressure. Considerable tenderness on pressure in the groin but no pain on movement of the limb. Here there was also an indefinable mass.

Operation was performed on February 6. On opening the peritoneum, by a three-inch incision, thick, malodorous pus was found in the right iliac fossa. There was also a large mass of thickened omentum which was explored and several small abscesses opened. The appendix was not found. The right ovary was seen along the inner border of the mass. The pelvis contained adhesions. The omentum at the upper border of abscess was freely resected and the wound drained by cigarette drains.

On March 4 there was still a discharge of pus, although the sinus had decreased in size. It persisted, however, until June 4, when the sinus was widened and a tube inserted.

As there was no tendency to heal it was decided, on June 9, to operate again. The sinus was first thoroughly cleaned and sewn up; then an incision three inches long, about half an inch to the left of the old incision and parallel to it, was made, passing through the rectus. On opening the peritoneum the omentum was found adherent to the abdominal wall. A large portion was resected, exposing the intestines, which were covered by numerous small tubercles. The sinus was felt as a large mass leading backward to the base of the cecum, and it was dissected out. The excised mass consisted of the sinus and dense cicatricial tissue about the size of a peach. The appendix was sought in this mass but could not be found with any degree of certainty, having probably been entirely disorganized. A cigarette drain was inserted, the end coming out of the old incision. Closure of the recent incision by layer suture.

At the first dressing on June 12 there was suppuration and the sutures were removed and gauze and tube drainage inserted.

The discharge now gradually decreased, the patient's general condition improved and healthy granulations appeared in the wound, which healed steadily until the child was discharged well on July 11.

Adeno-carcinoma of appendix; acute appendicitis with abscess; appendicectomy and drainage; cure.—Nattie M., 17 years old, single, was admitted and operated upon on October 18, 1904. Six days before admission she had been seized with cramp-like pain in the abdomen, followed by chill and fever; later the pain became localized in the right iliac region.

The abdomen was slightly distended, generally tympanitic, with tenderness most marked in the right side. A moderately tense, movable mass was felt by rectum to the right of the uterus and extending up into the iliac fossa; vaginal examination demonstrated the same mass. On opening the abdomen the mass was found to consist of indurated tissue extending from the appendicular region into the pelvis, with a dense adhesion of ovary and tube. An abscess cavity behind the cecum was evacuated, the appendix found and removed. The appendix was three inches long and its distal end club-shaped; its peritoneal and muscular coats were much thickened and the mucous membrane showed a proliferation of lymphoid tissue; it also contained a coprolith. A culture showed the presence of bacterium coli, and microscopical examination of the appendix revealed the presence of adeno-carcinoma.

For some days there was considerable foul-smelling discharge, and on probing an abscess was evacuated containing an ounce of pus. The patient's general condition began to improve, however, the wounds healed nicely and she was discharged cured on November 16.

The new growth here was an accidental discovery. Carcinoma has been thus encountered eight or nine times at Mt. Sinai Hospital within the last four years. Yet clinical cancer of the appendix is extremely rare. What becomes of these cases when an accidental infection does not call for the removal of the appendix it would be interesting to know. The matter has been discussed by Moschcowitz in the *Annals of Surgery*.

Acute gangrenous perforative appendicitis; diffuse sero-purulent peritonitis; appendicectomy and drainage; enterostomy; intestinal secondary suture; cure.—Samuel D. G., 39 years old, was admitted on September 30, 1904. He acknowledged a specific history, two and a half years earlier, the medication having been continued up to the present. Two days before admission the patient was taken with nausea and vomiting, pain in the epigastrium and a feeling as of flatus in the abdomen. This was followed by a severe chill, some fever and headache. On physical examination the abdomen was found distended and tympanitic; there was movable dullness in the flanks and tenderness in both right and left inguinal regions. The diagnosis of acute diffuse peritonitis was made and operation was performed the same evening. Through a right iliac incision the appendix, completely gangrenous and with a perforation at its middle third, was removed. The opening of the peritoneum was accompanied by the escape of purulent fluid. Cultures from this fluid showed bacillus coli communis and streptococci.

The patient reacted well, but on October 4 his general condition became poorer owing to marked distension, and there was frequent vomiting of considerable quantities of greenish fluid. As these symptoms seemed to indicate intestinal obstruction a second operation was performed. The original wound was first inspected but no cause for the symptoms found. A median three-inch incision was then made above the umbilicus and on opening the peritoneum sero-purulent fluid escaped. A loop of greatly distended and congested gut was drawn up into the wound and incised. A small drainage tube was fixed in position by a purse-string suture and much gas and fluid escaped. This wound was packed without suture, the tube being led out so as not to cause soiling of the dressings. The distension was greatly relieved following this procedure and the patient improved. On October 6 this fistula was closed by the insertion of a layer of Lembert sutures. This was accomplished without pain and without the use of any anesthetic. The suture line held except for a very minute opening, which for some weeks permitted the escape of about fifteen minims of discharge in twenty-four hours. Otherwise healing was rapid and perfect. Patient was discharged well on the 18th of November.

Acute gangrenous appendicitis and abscess; diffuse peritonitis; appendicectomy and drainage; cure.—Max C., 6 years old, was admitted and operated upon on December 22, 1903. The history given was typical of appendicitis with an antecedent attack one year before. The present illness had been of four day's duration and examination of the abdomen revealed the usual signs. The gangrenous and adherent appendix was removed. An abscess was also drained. The patient had a glycosuria, but this gradually disappeared and he made a good recovery, being discharged cured on January 20. On January 9th bacillus pyocyaneus was demonstrated.

It is presumed that the glycosuria in this case was postoperative. There was more than a trace of glucose but no constitutional symptoms pointing to diabetes and with the general improvement the sugar disappeared. The case was an urgent one, and unfortunately the urine had not been carefully examined before operation.

Acute gangrenous perforative appendicitis with sero-purulent peritonitis; appendicectomy and drainage; death.—Frank G., 9½ years old, was admitted on the night of October 28, 1904, with a history of appendicitis of two days' duration. His general condition on admission was very poor, his pulse being irregular, very rapid and thready. There was marked distension and dilated superficial abdominal veins. There was movable dullness in both flanks with tympany and tenderness over the entire abdomen. Tenderness greatest in right iliac region.

The boy was operated upon on October 29, a short time after admission, and incision of the peritoneum was followed by a profuse discharge of purulent fluid. The appendix was found adherent but was ligated and removed. All its walls were gangrenous and there was a perforation at the apex. Culture showed bacterium coli.

In spite of all that could be done the boy sank rapidly and died on October 30.

Appendicitis; general peritonitis; death.—Morris S., 32 years old, was admitted on April 23, 1904, with a typical history of appendicitis of but 24 hours' duration. His general condition on admission was so poor that surgical interference was deemed inadvisable. He died a few hours after being admitted.

A fulminant case with profound sepsis. Another instance of the futility of rules for procedure according to the number of hours from the onset of the disease.

Appendicitis with abscess; incision and drainage; no appendicectomy; cure.—Isaac L., 22 years old, was admitted on July 26, 1904, with a history of three previous attacks of appendicitis. Seven days before admission he had had another attack with the usual symptoms and characteristic physical signs. A swollen edematous mass, covered with omentum, was found in the right iliac fossa and an abscess evacuated. Owing to the dense exudate the appendix could not be located. The wound was closed in the usual way and after an uneventful recovery the patient was discharged cured on August 13.

In most cases of this kind, when the breaking up of adhesions does not appear too formidable one would prefer to find and remove the appendix before considering the operation complete. In this case the adhesions were, however, so dense that the resulting traumatism would have been unjustifiable.

Appendicitis with abscess; incision and drainage; no appendicectomy; cure.—Chas. H., 9 years old, was admitted and operated upon August 7, 1904, with a typical history of appendicitis of one week's duration. A large abscess cavity behind the cecum was evacuated, but the appendix could not be found. Convalescence was uneventful and the boy was discharged cured on August 20.

Sinus after appendicectomy; excision and suture; cure.—Henry M. F., 27 years old, was admitted on June 4, 1904. This patient's father had died of pulmonary tuberculosis, otherwise his family history was negative. He had gonorrhea two years ago and at time of admission had a hacking cough but no expectoration. In March, 1903, he had been operated upon for acute appendicitis with abscess and was in bed three and a half weeks. He had left the hospital with the wound not entirely healed and, although it had been curetted, it had never since closed; the discharge from the sinus had a very disagreeable odor and contained vegetable fibres, demonstrating connection with the intestinal canal.

On June 7 it was decided to operate, and a four-inch incision was made along the inner margin of the former appendicular scar. The sinus was cut across and freed *en masse* from the cecum, leaving a small opening in this portion of the gut which was repaired by suture. The cord-like sinus was now dissected down to the right iliac fossa at the brim of the pelvis and cut across. The wound was closed as usual.

The patient's general condition was excellent, the wound healed nicely and he was discharged cured on June 20.

THE GENITO-URINARY ORGANS.

The cases here presented are all from the year beginning December 1, 1903. A number of interesting and instructive histories from the preceding year (beginning December, 1902), together with a discussion of operative technics, will be found in a paper in the *Medical Record* of June 18 and 25, 1904, entitled, "A Brief Report of Four Years of Genito-Urinary Work in the Second Surgical Division of Mt. Sinai Hospital," to which the reader is referred. Another year's work has changed very little our methods in this branch. We continue to practice the suprapubic prostatectomy with great satisfaction.

The cystoscope and ureter catheters* are used with increasing frequency, and we still avoid instrumentation of the ureter in the case of a presumably healthy kidney. When the "other" ureter cannot be properly observed with the cystoscope we make use of the intramuscular injections of indigo-carmine—4 c.c. of a 4% solution in sodium chloride 9-10%—which on cystoscopy 20 minutes after the injection gives an excellent indication of the renal activity.

Operations about the kidney, with the exception of nephropexy, present at best a high percentage of mortality, and should never be lightly undertaken. Pyelitis, even with considerable pain or fever, should usually be treated medically. Tuberculosis without mixed infection is not necessarily surgical, and in the absence of constitutional or very troublesome local symptoms the treatment should be general. If operation becomes necessary nephrectomy is the procedure which should be chosen, especially when the other kidney is sound.

In acute abscess of the kidney, so often pyemic (embolic) in character, early nephrotomy should be done with the hope of saving the affected organ.

When reflex anuria comes on with the obstruction of one ureter operation is not immediately indicated. Uremia is slow to appear,

---

*The excellent instrument devised by Dr. Follen Cabot, of New York, and manufactured by the Wappler Electric Controller Company, has given great satisfaction in this work.

and other means may be tried for two or three days in the hope of avoiding surgical interference, always assuming that the patient is not suffering from the results of nephritis. In simple mechanical obstruction or in cases in which by accident a solitary kidney has been removed, uremia may not appear for from 8 to 11 days or it may be absent altogether, the patient dying from other causes. If operation is undertaken at all in these cases both kidneys should be opened and each pelvis explored. Small stones in the renal pelvis, or even in the ureter, rarely call urgently for operation, although continued distress or frequent colic may finally demand relief through surgery. Many of these calculi will pass after persistent treatment for weeks, or even months, by water drinking.

Renal calculus; right nephrotomy; nephrectomy; death.—Samuel S., 46 years old, was admitted on February 18, 1904. He could give no previous history except that he had had gonorrhea and chancre 30 years before. Six months previous to admission he began to experience pain in the right lumbar region just at the edge of the last rib, the pain being increased after exertion. One month before admission he passed a few small stones and two weeks later the pain in the lumbar region became more marked. He never, however, had dysuria or hematuria, chills or fever. On admission his general condition was fair. In the right lumbar region, opposite the last rib, two inches from the middle line, was an area tender to deep pressure. The inguinal glands were enlarged and there were numerous scars on the abdomen, also old scar on penis.

On February 23 right nephrotomy was done and a stone removed one inch long and three-eighths inch in diameter. The kidney was very large and succulent. In three days secondary nephrectomy was done on account of severe sepsis, but the patient did not react well and died on February 27.

Nephrolithiasis; nephrolithotomy; cure.—Morris R., 53 years old, was admitted November 5, 1903. He had always been well with the exception of a slight cough which he had had for twenty-five years; also slight dyspnea on exertion and cardiac palpitation. Four months before admission he began to pass blood in the urine and about three months later he began to suffer with a dull aching pain in the right lumbar region, both of which symptoms persisted. He was admitted to the medical service on October 24. On October 27 he passed a small stone and was transferred to the surgical division on November 5. On November 7 he was operated upon for renal calculi through the usual transverse lumbar incision. The kidney was bound down by firm adhesions which were freed and the organ incised along its convex border; within the pelvis were numerous calculi varying in size from a pecan nut to a seed; these were removed, together with a quantity of calculus detritus. The kidney was sutured and replaced and the wound closed. The patient's general condition for some days was quite poor and he also developed a purulent otitis. This however, yielded to treatment and he made a gradual improvement, being discharged cured on December 5.

The prompt recovery in this case, after a simple nephrolithotomy, is worthy of note.

Tumor of ovary or kidney; exploratory laparotomy; unimproved.—Jette R., aged 10 months, had been healthy up to her fifth month when she had an attack of pneumonia and then a tumor in the left lower abdomen was noticed. The tumor increased in size, the child lost weight and for two months previous to admission vomited occasionally.

Examination of the abdomen showed the superficial veins dilated; there was a hard, rounded mass in the lower half, movable, with apparently another tumor attached above. The tumor seemed to spring from the pelvis.

The child was at first in the medical ward but was transferred to the surgical service, and on February 23 laparotomy was performed and a section removed from the tumor for examination. The pathologist's report was that there was no definite structure but that it resembled ovarian tissue slightly. The child was kept at the hospital until March 19, but her condition became worse, emaciation rapid and the tumor in the pelvis larger. She was discharged on March 20 unimproved.

Hypernephroma; nephrectomy; cure.—Jacob L., 51 years old, was admitted on April 6, 1904. For 8 years previous to admission he had had more or less pain of a dragging nature in the right loin and hypochondrium; five years before he had had a severe hematuria and had two or three subsequent attacks, the last one three days before admission. Physical examination was negative throughout except for a mass palpable in the right loin; the mass was about the size of an infant's head, freely movable and smooth, extending about four inches below the margin of the ribs.

On April 7 cystoscopy after an indigo-carmine injection showed an apparently well-functionating left kidney. Right nephrectomy was then performed through a lumbar oblique incision. The kidney and tumor mass, which apparently rose from the pelvis of the kidney and was lobulated, measured 15 cm. x 16 x 9 and was purplish-blue with tiny cysts on the surface and gray, depressed scar-like areas, the tumor mass proper being yellowish-red. Pathological report was hypernephroma. The patient made an uninterrupted convalescence and was discharged cured on May 26.

Cystic kidney; nephrectomy; pneumonia; death.—Theresa S., 59 years old, was admitted on April 6, 1904. This patient's illness began 14 months before admission, when she complained of a dull pain in the right side, increased on exertion. Some months later she felt a lump on that side which her physician told her was a tumor, and six weeks before admission the tumor was aspirated and purulent fluid obtained. Physical examination showed a large, hard, slightly movable and tender mass occupying the right hypochondrium and extending downward and outward.

On April 7, after an indigo-carmine test of the other kidney, a lumbar incision exposed the kidney, which was represented by a cystic mass the size of an infant's head. This was free, easily delivered, and the pedicle tied off. The ureter was markedly dilated at pelvis, filled with mucus and pus, and much thickened. Pathological examination demonstrated a cystic kidney and pyonephrosis.

The wound was healthy but the patient developed a pneumonia of the right lower lobe on April 9, and died the next day.

No autopsy was obtainable and this was unfortunate. It would have been interesting to learn whether the other kidney was also cystic though functionating. Without the pyonephrosis operation in this case would not have been indicated, the cystic condition being so frequently bilateral.

Left pyonephrosis; nephrotomy; secondary nephrectomy; death.—Henry C. M., 56 years old. This man gave a history of having had an external urethrotomy performed one and a half years before for stricture subsequent to an attack of gonorrhea. A slight urethral discharge had persisted since the operation and he had to urinate once or twice at night. For four years previous to admission his urine had been cloudy but he noticed that it was growing worse, and for five months before coming to the hospital he had had slight fever in the evening, lost weight and had become much paler; for two months he suffered with pain in the left lumbar region. The left kidney on physical examination was palpable, large, painful and tender; there was a slight mucoid discharge from the urethra. Cystoscopic examination showed an edematous area around the opening of the left ureter and pressure applied to the left kidney and ureter brought forth pus.

On October 21 left nephrotomy was performed and about a pint of pus evacuated, together with a flat stone about as large as a silver quarter. Culture from the pus showed bacterium coli and streptococci.

The man made fair progress until November 7, when his temperature rose to 102° and he complained of headache and pain in the stomach. Nephrectomy was deemed urgent and was performed on November 9. The kidney was so densely adherent to the surrounding tissue that much difficulty was experienced in the attempt to free it and there was considerable hemorrhage from the accidental rupture of an artery running to the upper pole of the kidney. The bleeding was finally completely checked, but in spite of vigorous stimulation the patient did not react and died on November 10.

Suspected stone in ureter; exploratory laparotomy; cure.—Edgar L., 21 years old, was admitted on August 9. A little more than a month previous to his present attack this patient had been in the hospital for a few days suffering with symptoms of renal colic, which, however, had subsided. On the morning of August 9 he was seized with severe cramp-like pains, beginning in the left lumbar region, radiating downward and inward toward the scrotum and down the thigh. He had been subject to attacks of this kind for about two and a half years, at intervals of four months, but recently the intervals had become much shorter. Although physical examination showed an area of tenderness midway between the left anterior superior spine of the ilium and the umbilicus there was nothing palpable.

On August 17 a three and a half inch incision was made over the left rectus muscle, and the peritoneum having been incised the entire length of the left ureter from the pelvis of the kidney to the bladder was palpated but no stone was found. The left kidney and right ureter were also palpated with a negative result. The wound was closed, primary union took place and the patient was discharged cured on September 1.

Prostatic hypertrophy; cystitis; pyelonephritis; right perinephric abscess; suprapubic cystotomy; death.—Mr. E., was admitted on August 9, 1904, and supra-pubic cystotomy performed for retention of urine. About a quart of foul-smelling turbid urine was evacuated. A large hypertrophied prostate was felt at the neck of the bladder. No attempt at removal was made. A drainage tube was inserted and the wound packed.

The man reacted well after operation but hiccough proved quite troublesome. On August 12 the temperature began to rise and the patient complained of marked tenderness in the right flank and loin. Three days after his general condition became worse, singultus continued, wound edges were necrotic, tenderness appeared in the right flank and his temperature rose to 102°. He sank rapidly and died six days after admission.

Extract from protocol of post-mortem examination made by Dr. E. Libman, six hours after death.—Prostate is much enlarged and contains a number of distinct fibrous nodules. Bladder is quite small, has a very thick wall and the mucosa is the seat of a diphtheritic hemorrhagic inflammation. There are a number of small recesses and to the left there is a large diverticulum about the size of a small orange, the wall of which is intensely inflamed. In each are several small phosphatic calculi. The orifice of the left ureter is markedly swollen and hemorrhagic. The left ureter contains several old calculi which do not completely block the ureter. The ureter is markedly dilated. The pelvis of the left kidney is somewhat dilated and the seat of a diphtheritic inflammation. The kidney itself is succulent and presents chronic interstitial changes. The right ureter is somewhat dilated and contains a few small calculi. There is no complete obstruction of the ureter. The right kidney is large and is the seat of an advanced pyonephrosis with distension of the pelvis and calyces; the latter show diphtheritic inflammation, and contain pus and small calculi. There is a perforation leading from one of the calyces into the paranephric tissues. There is a very marked paranephritis and a large abscess to the outer side of and below the kidney. This abscess has burrowed its way into the abdominal wall and the secondary abscess in the abdominal wall has caused a general peritonitis by rupture inwardly at a point a little to the right of and below the umbilicus. The paranephric abscess has also perforated the colon just above the cecum. The cecum is the seat of a marked diphtheritic inflammation and is much dilated. The lower 10 cm. of the ileum and flexure are acutely inflamed and contracted; the rectal end of the flexure is contracted.

Diagnosis: Hypertrophy of prostate, cystitis, pyonephrosis, paranephric abscess, rupture of the colon, abscess of abdominal wall, rupture into abdominal cavity, general peritonitis.

Sarcoma of bladder; excision of part of bladder; unimproved.—Sarah S., 3 years old, was admitted November 10, 1903. On October 21, 1903, this little girl had been discharged from the hospital after operation for papilloma of the bladder, undergoing sarcomatous degeneration, but less than a month later she returned with a recurrence. Examination on readmission showed a papillomatous excrescence on the right urethral wall. On November 14 suprapubic cystotomy was performed. The tumor, which was found on the left side of the bladder, was excised and the mucous membrane of the bladder sutured. A small papillomatous mass near the urethra was next cauterized with Paquelin and carbolic, and a tube inserted into the bladder emerging through the urethra; another small mass near the mouth of the urethra was tied off and cut away. The child reacted well and her general condition improved.

On December 23 she was again operated upon, the sutures being removed from the bladder and an abscess in the vagina evacuated. A papillomatous mass projecting from the urethra was excised and the stump cauterized. The neoplasm grew rapidly and on January 9 operative measures were again necessary. Two masses of hemorrhagic, papillomatous tissue which protruded through the suprapubic incision were excised. The bladder was filled with papillomatous tissue which extended into the urethra. Upon pathological examination of a portion of the excised tissue it was pronounced "sarcoma."

The growth remained unchecked and the child's general condition grew poorer. From January 21 to February 4 daily radium exposures were made but not with good result, the growth continuing to enlarge. She was discharged unimproved on February 9 and died at home eleven days later.

Perineal urethral fistula; hemorrhoids; plastic; clamp and cautery; cure.—Moses W., 70 years old, was admitted for the second time on January 5, 1904, having been a patient in this hospital from July 29 to August 23, 1903. Four months previous to his first admission he had fallen and sustained a laceration of the perineum from which urine and blood flowed. He was operated upon at another hospital, and was discharged with a granulating wound. Two months later he noticed that, although he urinated every two hours without straining, he passed but a small amount of fluid. Physical examination on admission, July 29, showed an oblique 5 cm. scar to the left of the perineal urethra and as the sound met with obstruction in the perineum, external urethrotomy for traumatic stricture was performed. He was discharged on August 23, the perineal fistula still open. He was readmitted January 5 with a sinus one-half inch in length back of the scroto-perineal junction. This was cauterized on January 8 with the Paquelin. On January 30 a plastic for the closure of the fistula was performed. No tissue was removed, but after making a sagittal incision about three-quarters of an inch beyond the anterior and posterior margins of the large fistula the skin was dissected away by the flap-splitting method. The deeper parts, including the urethral tissues, were inverted and sutured with fine chromic gut in several layers but the skin was left open, its edges simply lying in apposition. Permanent catheter for six days. Primary union took place and the patient was discharged cured on February 10.

Prostatic hypertrophy; suprapubic prostectomy; cure.—August N., 54 years old, was admitted on June 28, 1904. Four years previous to admission he had had urethritis and for fifteen years had been troubled with constipation and hemorrhoids. For about three years he had complained of pain in the back and sides, and burning pain on micturition, especially at the anterior portion of the urethra. He had to urinate 10 to 12 times a day and twice at night. There was but a small quantity at a time and the stream was small, forked and curling with dribbling afterward. The patient also complained of painful defecation and diminished sexual power, coition being painful and delayed.

On June 30 he was operated upon, suprapubic prostatectomy being performed. The bladder was opened and the prostate enucleated in the usual manner. On July 5 a small tube was placed in the bladder but it was removed on July 7, a soft rubber catheter being introduced through the urethra into the bladder and the suprapubic wound closed. The patient's condition improved steadily, although the catheter had to be used at intervals. On July 25 there was a rise of temperature; rectal examination showed a tense, tender mass in the pocket from which the prostate had been removed. This disappeared under massage, the temperature fell to normal and the man was discharged cured on July 25.

Following intercourse eight weeks after operation the patient presented himself to be treated for orchitis.

Hypertrophy of prostate; suprapubic prostatectomy; cured.—Louis M., 68 years old, was admitted on January 18, 1904. With the exception of hemorrhoids from which he had suffered for several years, the patient was in good health up to five years before admission when he had an attack similar to the one for which he sought relief. There was painful urination and retention of urine necessitating the use of the catheter. The urine was blood-tinged. For a week previous to admission the urine had contained small particles of blood and when it was retained for four or five hours he suffered great pain.

An enlarged tender prostate was demonstrated on rectal examination. Suprapubic prostatectomy was done January 19. Two days later the packings were removed, the bladder irrigated and a drainage tube inserted. The patient progressed nicely and the tube was removed on February 1. On February 8 the patient's temperature rose to 101.8° and the tube was re-introduced. Rectal examination showed marked induration over the prostate region but under manipulation this disappeared. The temperature also fell to normal in a few days, and on February 18 the drainage tube was permanently removed. The patient was discharged cured on February 26.

Prostatic hypertrophy; suprapubic prostatectomy; cure.—T. A., 65 years old, was admitted on May 11, 1904. Subsequent to an attack of gonorrhea in 1863 he was subject to bladder disturbance. In 1881 he had had an attack of cystitis with hematuria; urination frequent and very painful. Eleven years before admission he had a suprapubic cystotomy performed by a transverse incision, but it revealed only inflamed mucous membrane with sacculation. The somewhat enlarged prostate was cauterized with the Paquelin. Shortly thereafter he had a left orchitis which soon subsided. For a year the patient had to resort to catheterization and had a residual of 20 ounces, which had since decreased to 8 ounces. His bowels had been constipated and he had been subject to attacks of hematuria with frequent and painful micturition.

On May 13 suprapubic cystotomy was performed through a sagittal incision, and the prostate, the central lobe of which was much enlarged, removed. A drainage tube was inserted on May 14 and continuous irrigation instituted. On May 26 the tube was removed and the wound closed, the patient subsequently urinating naturally without pain. Catheterization after urination on June 10 revealed one ounce of residual urine. On June 27 there was a leakage of urine through the suprapubic incision following inability to pass urine through urethra. Sounds were used and the wound cauterized with the actual cautery. Following this procedure, the wound remained closed with no further leakage and the patient was discharged cured three months after admission. (Subsequently the wound reopened and remained open for some time. At the present writing, March 12, 1905, the patient is well.)

Senile prostatic hypertrophy; stones in bladder; suprapubic prostatectomy; cure.—A. M. R., 72 years old, was admitted on January 21, 1904. This old man for eight years before admission to the hospital had been troubled with frequency of urination, which increased in severity until he had to urinate every hour and a half to two hours during the day and five or six times at night. Five days before admission he was suddenly unable to pass any urine, and although an attempt was made at catheterization by his physician it was unsuccessful. Two days before he came to the hospital a Mercier catheter had been inserted, and about three quarts of bloody urine withdrawn. The introduction of the catheter was followed by some bleeding. He was still unable to urinate, and entered the hospital with a bladder distended up to the level of the umbilicus. On January 23 suprapubic cystotomy was done, and upon evacuating the contents of the bladder several small stones (phosphatic) were noted. The prostate was enucleated in the usual manner and a drainage tube introduced. The prostate was irregular, oval, its diameter two and a half inches, the lateral lobes greatly enlarged and the base very nodular. Small median lobes anteriorly.

In spite of his age the patient reacted well and made good progress, urinating per urethram on February 24. He continued to improve steadily, and on March 13 the wound was healed and he was discharged cured.

Adeno-carcinoma of prostate; suprapubic prostatectomy; death.—William A. H., 67 years old, was admitted on September 18, 1904. He gave a history of typhoid at 11, varioloid at 16 and had also had rheumatism. He had had swelling of the lower eyelids, headaches, had spots before his eyes and dyspnea on exertion. Urination had been normal up to a year and a half before admission when he began to experience increased frequency and difficulty in the act. At times he would have incontinence and then would be unable to void any, so that he had to resort to the catheter which he had to use more and more frequently. He also suffered from pain in the bladder and burning on micturition, and has lost weight and strength.

His general condition on admission was poor, and he looked yellowish and anemic. Examination of the genitals revealed a moderately large, tense cystic mass in the right scrotum, above the testicle and running up to the external abdominal ring. A large, hard, nodular mass the size of a plum could be made out on rectal examination.

On September 27 a suprapubic median incision was made, the bladder incised and an attempt made to shell out the prostate in the usual way; this was impossible, however, as it surrounded the urethra like a collar and was stony hard; the base of the bladder also seemed to be infiltrated and the prostate was removed in two sections. In removing the last portion of the prostate the bladder was torn through at the base into the peritoneal cavity. The incision was extended upward, the peritoneum opened in the median line and packing placed in the peritoneal and vesical rent.

In spite of vigorous stimulation the patient did not react and died in shock a few hours after the operation, though the loss of blood had been small.

Pathological report on excised portions of prostate was adeno-carcinoma. No autopsy was permitted.

This case being a malignant one does not come under the heading of operations for the relief of senile hypertrophy.

Adenoma of bladder, rectum and prostate; extirpation of bladder; death.—Philip W., 34 years old, was admitted on April 27, 1904. With the exception of the usual diseases of childhood and hemorrhoids, with which he had been troubled for seven years before admission, this patient said that his health had been good until about ten weeks before he came to the hospital. He had complained then of constipation and pain on defecation and of a protuberance like a bunch of grapes when straining at stool. Seven weeks before admission he began to experience pain on micturition and had twice passed a little clotted blood before urinating. For three weeks before coming to the hospital he had diarrhea, the stools being tinged with blood, and he also at times had a whitish discharge from the rectum. Since the beginning of his illness he had lost fourteen pounds, and felt very weak with frequent nausea and vomiting, chills and night sweats.

On physical examination, a tumor mass, hard, nodular and slightly tender, was made out in the left iliac fossa, following the course of the sigmoid flexure; on the anterior rectal wall, just within the anus, was a hard, nodular and slightly tender mass which extended higher than the finger could palpate, probably adherent and involving the prostate and bladder.

On May 4 he was operated upon by a perineal section for the removal of a specimen of the tumor for examination. The pathologist's report was *acute inflammation*.

The patient being unable to urinate voluntarily a silver catheter was used. Catheterization became more and more difficult, and on May 9 suprapubic cystotomy for retention of urine had to be done. About a quart of urine was evacuated and a small papilloma on the bladder was excised. A tube was inserted and the wound packed as usual. Pathological report on the papilloma was negative.

Although drainage was good the capacity of the bladder decreased, the mass in the rectum still remaining as before.

It was decided to operate again on May 31 for the removal of new growth of the prostate by suprapubic incision. The bladder was entered along the old scar, the incision enlarged above and below and a large fungating papillomatous mass, soft and friable, was felt in the position of the prostate. An attempt was then made at enucleation, but owing to its friability only small portions could be removed at a time by the finger, hence as much as possible was taken away by curette. Pathological report on the specimen submitted showed cystic adenoma.

On June 1 it was decided to make an attempt to extirpate bladder and rectum. The suprapubic wound was enlarged upwards and downwards, the bladder was freed from its connections on all sides, the ureters were cut across close to their entrance into the bladder and attached to the skin on either side, the bladder was divided at its neck and removed, together with the adjoining rectum. Clamps were applied to control the bleeding and the wound packed with sterile gauze.

The patient lived a month after this operation, but his general condition became very poor, and on July 1 he suddenly went into collapse and died.

This man was in very miserable condition. In a more favorable subject a recovery might have been expected in spite of the severity of the operation. Having survived a month, the case may almost be considered one of operative recovery.

FEMALE GENITALS.

Of the thirty-seven operations on the female genitals the following four are of interest:

Twisted ovarian dermoid cyst; purulent peritonitis; salpingoöphorectomy; death.—Mildred B., 4 years old, admitted February 7, 1904. The child had been suddenly seized with severe abdominal pain and vomiting three days before the operation. At the operation a large cyst of the left ovary was found, with two twists of the pedicle. There was considerable chocolate-colored fluid in the abdomen. The cyst, together with the left tube, was removed. Death took place in forty-eight hours. The cyst was the size of a large orange. It contained bloody fluid, rolls of hair, irregularly formed teeth and particles of bone. At the autopsy, pus was found between the layers of the abdominal wall, and in the general peritoneal cavity. The pus was found to contain streptococci in pure culture.

Traumatic perforation of uterus; laceration of intestines; resection of intestines; death.—Hattie A., 30 years old, admitted November 13, 1904. Two hours before admission, the patient had been curetted outside of the hospital for an abortion. The uterus had been perforated by the curette, and a loop of small intestine, which had been mistaken for the umbilical cord, had been cut across. The patient was brought to the hospital in the ambulance in a condition of shock. The abdomen was immediately opened by a median incision. On opening the abdomen, there was a gush of free blood. The patient was put in Trendelenburg's position, packings introduced, and the uterus delivered into the wound. A laceration was found at the fundus extending down the posterior surface of the uterus. Through this hole a loop of small intestine passed into the vagina. The uterus was so tightly contracted around it that the opening in the uterus had to be enlarged before the loop of gut could be pulled back into the abdomen. The other end of the cut loop of gut was found in the pelvis, and the bleeding was found to have come from the torn mesentery. About seven inches of gut were resected from each end of the lacerated intestine, and the ends united with a Murphy button, reinforced by Lembert sutures. On examining the gut on either side of the anastomosis several perforations were found and were closed with silk sutures. Owing to the poor condition of the patient it was deemed inadvisable to remove the uterus, or to attempt to repair the laceration. A gauze packing was introduced into the pelvis, walling off the uterus from the general abdominal cavity. The abdomen was closed with through and through sutures. At the close of the operation an intravenous saline infusion was given. Death took place eight hours later. No autopsy.

Pelvic abscess; peritonitis; incision and drainage; death.—Meta S., 42 years old, admitted August 31, 1904. In the right iliac fossa there was a tender mass of the size of a cocoanut. An incision was made through the right rectus and a large amount of pus was evacuated. Death occurred six hours later.

Ruptured ectopic gestation; sepsis; salpingo-oöphorectomy; death.

—Therese K., 42 years old, admitted May 1, 1904. On opening the abdomen a large number of old clots were found. Rupture had probably taken place ten days previously, and there was evidently some infection as evidenced by the continuous rise in temperature before operation. The right tube was found perforated and it was removed, together with the sac. The pulse and temperature remained high after the operation, and the patient died of sepsis four days later.

RECTUM AND ANUS.

Of the 148 operations on the rectum and anus, the following is the only one that ended fatally:

Hemorrhoids; Whitehead operation; death by suicide.—Morris L., 38 years old, admitted May 18, 1903. The man had been suffering from hemorrhoids and slight prolapse of the rectum for three years. Under gas and ether the Whitehead operation was performed with chromic gut sutures. The patient reacted well from the operation, and his pulse and temperature remained normal. There was no wound infection. The man seemed perfectly rational, when, seven days after operation, he committed suicide by jumping out of the window.

Adeno-carcinoma of rectum; excision of rectum; cure.—Abraham K., 63 years old, admitted March 31, 1904. Two and a half months before admission the patient had begun to complain of pain in the rectum and blood in the stools. Five weeks before admission he had been operated on for hemorrhoids. After the parts had healed the man still complained of pain, and on examination a hard mass was found within the rectum, about two inches from the anus. It presented an ulcerated appearance, and there was a grumous discharge. The man had lost 17 pounds in six months. Operation April 2, 1904. An incision was made from the anal margin along the left side of coccyx to the first sacral vertebra. Subperiosteal excision of the coccyx. Anteriorly the rectum was freed bluntly from prostate and urethra. The posterior hemorrhoidal vessels were ligated, and the dissections gradually carried to the upper level of the sacrum, the vessels as far as possible being ligated before division. The rectum was then drawn down and clamped. The man was now placed in the lithotomy position, the rectum cut across above the clamp, and again just above the anal orifice. The upper part of the rectum was now drawn down through the anal orifice and sutured to the mucous membrane around the anus with several silk sutures. These sutures were passed with the rectum outside of the anus. The rectum was now replaced and a small tear in its lateral wall repaired. A few sutures were placed at the upper angle of the wound, and the rest of the wound packed with gauze. A tampon canula was allowed to remain in the rectum. On examining the specimen it was found that the excision had been done two inches above the growth and one inch below it. The tumor was as large as a silver dollar and occupied the posterior and the right rectal wall; it was ulcerated and there was induration around it. The microscopic diagnosis was adeno-carcinoma. The lower two inches of the rectum became necrotic, although there had been no tension on the sutures, and sloughed away, leaving the lower end of the rectum in the upper part of the wound. Convalescence was delayed by a troublesome diarrhea. On May 19, 1904, the patient left the hospital with a superficial wound. A few months later he was in good condition and had gained seventeen pounds. He had fair control of formed stools.

HERNIA.

During the two years the following herniotomies were performed:

Inguinal, non-strangulated	72	(35 double)
" strangulated	16	
Femoral	3	(2 double)
" strangulated	3	
Umbilical	6	
" strangulated	3	
Ventral	10	
Epigastric	1	

The usual procedure in cases of inguinal hernia has been the Bassini operation. In six cases the Halsted modification was carried out. Chromic catgut was regularly used for the deep sutures, plain catgut for the superficial fascia, and silk for the skin. In some cases the skin was approximated with strips of zinc oxide plaster. Of the seventy-two cases of non-strangulated inguinal hernia, sixty-two healed by primary union. In ten cases there was a slight infection which in no case interfered with the healing of the deeper parts. It is interesting to note that the majority of these infections took place during the year 1903, and only a few during 1904, although there were more herniotomies performed during the latter year. In most of the cases no drain was used; occasionally a little strip of rubber tissue was left at the lower angle of the wound.

In the femoral hernias, the regular procedure has been the suturing of Poupart's ligament to the pectineal fascia. Here also chromic catgut has been used, and the superficial fascia has been sutured with plain catgut.

The only two deaths among the herniotomies were the following:

Large inguinal hernia; secondary operation with silver wire filigree; nephritis; death.—I. M., a man 53 years old, had been operated on at Mt. Sinai Hospital in November, 1902, for a large indirect inguinal hernia. At that time the sac contained many coils of small intestine, together with the cecum and ascending colon, the latter firmly adherent to the sac. The appendix, the testis and the spermatic cord were removed. The adherent cecum with the attached part of the sac were reduced into the abdominal cavity, and the sac closed with chromic gut. The wound was packed and no radical cure was attempted. The man was readmitted to the hospital on August 16, 1904. He then stated that for several months the hernia had been increasing in size so that he could no longer work and could hardly walk. Under anesthesia in Trendelenburg's position, the many loops of small intestine were with difficulty returned into the abdominal cavity, and the sac tied off with a purse string suture. On account of the distance between the conjoined tendon and Poupart's ligament, it was not possible to make use of the Bassini sutures. Accordingly, a running suture of silver wire was introduced between these two structures without approximating them. A silver filigree was then sutured with chromic gut to the superficia fascia, and a small gauze drain left at the lower angle of the wound. Silk was used for the skin sutures. For three days the lower end of the bed was kept elevated, and the patient's condition was good, although the temperature remained around 102°F., and the pulse around 120. On the fourth day the man became restless and uncomfortable, respiration labored and rapid, 32 to 36. The bowels had been moved freely and gas had also been passed. However, about 72 hours after operation vomiting set in, and the abdomen became somewhat distended, but it was not tender. The wound was dressed and was found clean. The urine contained albumin and many granular casts. The general condition gradually became worse, vomiting continued, although the bowels moved freely. Death took place five days after operation. There was no autopsy.

Incarcerated inguinal hernia; fecal fistula; herniotomy; death.—Pearl F., female, 80 years, admitted July 20, 1904. The patient had had a double inguinal hernia for twenty years. There had never previously been any difficulty in reducing the hernias. Four days before operation the hernia on the left side had become irreducible. Vomiting, which promptly set in, had persisted. Owing to the advanced age of the patient (80 years) it was not deemed advisable to give a general anesthetic. Under local anesthesia, the sac was opened and a badly strangulated loop of small intestine found with a small perforation. The strangulation was relieved, and the opening in the gut was sutured with three layers of silk sutures. The wound was packed after reducing the loop of gut just within the abdomen. No attempt was made at a radical cure. Five days after operation fluid fecal matter was found in the wound, and thereafter the fecal fistula persisted. She lived for twenty-eight days, finally dying of exhaustion.

OPERATIONS ON THE EXTREMITIES.

Two hundred and eight operations were performed upon the extremities with fourteen deaths.

Thirty-three amputations were performed with four deaths, namely:

Amputation of arm.................. 2 times, 1 death.
" " fingers .... 3 " 0 "
" " thigh .... 10 " 3 "
" " leg .... 11 " 0 "
" " foot .... 3 " 0 "
" " toes .... 4 " 0 "

Synopses of the histories of the fatal cases follow:

Wounds of arm and leg; septic osteomyelitis of ulna and radius; amputation of arm; death.—Jacob B., 6 years old, admitted March 19, died March 27, 1903. Infected wounds of arm and leg with osteomyelitis of bones of forearm from injury by street car. After primary incisions and drainage, osteotomy of bones of forearm but without improvement in symptoms of sepsis. Later, amputation through lower third of left forearm. Death eight days later.

Diabetic gangrene of foot; amputation of thigh; death.—Ida B., 62 years of age, admitted October 10, died November 1, 1903. Three months' history of gangrene of toes; after two weeks' treatment, gangrene began to spread rapidly up the foot and leg. October 24: Amputation of thigh through lower third; wound strapped; after operation acid intoxication, then coma, and death on November 1. No autopsy.

Arterio-sclerotic gangrene of left leg; amputation of leg; reamputation through thigh; gangrene of right leg; amputation of right leg; cerebral embolism; death.—Nathan S., 50 years of age, admitted

December 19, died February 14, 1904. Spreading arterio-sclerotic gangrene of six weeks' duration. December 26: Amputation of left leg, wound strapped. January 9: Amputation of left thigh at lower third on account of gangrene of stump; wound strapped and widely drained; union by second intention. January 19: Amputation of right leg through upper third for gangrene of that leg; union good, by granulation; sudden death from cerebral apoplexy on February 14. No autopsy.

Sarcoma of femur; exarticulation at hip; death.—Joseph K., 36 years of age, admitted February 10, died February 14, 1904. History of traumatism of knee four months before; large tumor of lower end of femur; section removed and proved to be osteo-sarcoma. Exarticulation at hip on February 13, after primary ligation of femoral vessels. Death twenty-two hours after the operation. No autopsy.

A considerable number of patients are admitted to our service every year with gangrene of the lower extremities due to diabetes or Raynaud's disease. The mortality following amputations for diabetic gangrene has been considerably reduced from the time that we had methodical examinations of the urine made for acetone and diacetic acid, and delayed the operative interference until these substances had disappeared from the urine or had become much diminished. The only death during the last two years was that of the patient Ida B., whose history has been abstracted above. This patient had only a trace of acetone and diacetic acid when she was admitted to the ward, and for four days before the amputation of the thigh was performed the acetone and diacetic acid were absent from the urine, although the quantity of sugar remained undiminished. After the operation the acetone and diacetic acid increased very much and remained present in large quantities until the patient's death in coma eight days after the operation.

After amputations for diabetic gangrene or for Raynaud's disease we seldom close the wound by sutures, but drain widely and approximate the edges with sterile adhesive plaster strips.

During the past year we have given the method of Mosetig-Moorhof for the treatment of chronic osteomyelitis and of chronic bone cavities a considerable trial. The method consists of filling the bone cavity with a mixture of iodoform, sesame oil and spermaceti after the walls of the cavity have been thoroughly prepared and all diseased tissue removed. Twelve operations were done by this method and the results, although still far from ideal in most of the cases, have been very satisfactory. A complete account of our experience with the iodoform wax filling will be found in another part of this volume, to which the reader is referred for details.

In the following are given abstracts of the histories of other fatal cases after operations on the extremities, and in almost all it will be seen that the patients succumbed to their disease and not to the operative interference.

Cellulitis of forearm and ankle; pyemia; incision and drainage; death.—Sarah L., 2 weeks of age, was admitted April 13, 1903, with pyemic abscesses over the lower end of the left ulna and ankle. The little patient's condition was very poor. The abscesses were incised and drained. High temperatures and rapid pulse persisted and death occurred four days later.

Tuberculosis of elbow and of os calcis; septicemia; arthrotomy and osteotomy; death.—Sarah F., 7 years of age, admitted June 8, 1903, with discharging sinuses of the left elbow and ankle, and signs of sepsis. Both regions were thoroughly drained, but the patient's symptoms grew worse until death occurred two days after operation. Autopsy showed, besides the local disease in the elbow and ankle, parenchymatous degeneration of the kidneys, infarcts in both lungs, and petechiæ in the heart muscle.

Carcinoma of rectum; metastatic carcinoma of femur; exploratory osteotomy; death from exhaustion three months later.—Rosie G., 37 years old, admitted December 13, 1902, died March 29, 1903. The patient had had pain in her left leg for nine months and had been unable to walk for four months before admission. She had become emaciated, a fusiform swelling had appeared on her left thigh, which gradually increased in size. The entire limb became edematous, swollen and tender, and sinuses formed over the tumor from which much pus was discharged. December 13: Osteotomy of femur and aspiration of hip joint; specimen of tumor removed and proved to be carcinoma. A small nodular mass was later discovered in the rectum which gradually increased in size under observation. The patient slowly emaciated and died from exhaustion about three months later.

Osteomyelitis of femur; staphylococcemia; meningitis; drainage of femur by osteotomy; death five days later.—Hyman D., admitted May 16, died May 23, 1902. Injury to thigh one week before. Red and fluctuating swelling over anterior aspect of left thigh, with high temperature. Abscess of thigh drained on the day of admission;

culture showed staphylococcus aureus in blood; two days later osteotomy of femur; medulla full of pus. In forty-eight hours symptoms of meningitis; lumbar puncture fluid contains staphylococcus aureus and streptococcus; death in three days. No autopsy.

Tuberculosis of knee: arthrotomy (Mayo) and drainage; general miliary tuberculosis: death.—Aaron I., 30 years old, admitted January 11, died February 11, 1903. Eight months' history of pain, swelling and tenderness in left knee; for past few weeks high temperatures and symptoms of acute infection of knee joint. January 13: Mayo's operation; joint found distended, with pus which contained many tubercle bacilli. High temperatures and profuse sweats persisted. After intravenous injection of formaline solution no improvement. Condition became gradually worse; signs in lungs of a diffuse inflammatory process. Death on February 11.

Cellulitis of leg: sepsis; incision and drainage; death.—Etta R., 19 months old, admitted September 26, died September 29; splinter of wood removed from foot six days before; on admission, cellulitis of foot and leg. Incision and drainage; high temperatures and rapid pulse persisted and death occurred on September 29.

Pelvic abscess due to suppurating hip disease; incision and drainage; death from exhaustion.—Millie G., admitted November 24, 1903, died April 4, 1904. Numerous sinuses around hip of several months' duration, which secreted much pus. December 15: incision and drainage of pelvic abscess; sinuses and profuse discharge persisted for several months until patient left the hospital on April 4, much improved in her general condition. She was readmitted on October 1 in poor condition with numerous suppurating sinuses. On October 21 the sinuses were thoroughly curetted and drained. Four days after the operation there occurred a profuse hemorrhage from one of the sinuses which could only be controlled by very tight packing and which must have been due to rupture of a large blood vessel. The patient's condition thereafter became steadily worse, she died on October 27. No autopsy.

Chronic suppurative osteoarthritis of hip; osteotomy; resection of hip; death.—Walter B., 12 years of age, was admitted on August 24, 1904, with sinuses of the hip of four years' duration. August 26: Osteotomy of femur. September 7: Resection of hip joint; upper end of femur and acetabulum much diseased. Death from shock about 20 hours later. No autopsy.

Osteomyelitis of femur and pelvis: osteotomy and drainage; resection of hip; death from exhaustion six weeks later.—Abe S., 1½ years of age, admitted June 22, died November 9, 1904. Six months' history of abscesses and sinuses around hip; marked emaciation. June 24: Incision and drainage; no improvement; suppuration and sinuses, with high temperature persisted. In spite of arthrotomy and drainage on August 17 and resection of hip on September 21, condition did not improve. The patient emaciated rapidly, death occurred from exhaustion, on November 9. No autopsy.

ON THE TREATMENT OF CHRONIC OSTEOMYELITIS AND OF CHRONIC BONE CAVITIES BY THE IODOFORM WAX FILLING.*

By Charles A. Elsberg, M.D.,
ADJUNCT ATTENDING SURGEON.

It is a basic principle in surgical technic never to leave cavities or dead spaces in a wound if it can be avoided. In most cases where we leave behind cavities, these have collapsible walls, so that, after a short time, the walls come into contact with each other and the space becomes obliterated. As examples of cavities of this kind may be mentioned the bed from which a tumor has been removed or the dead space left after the evacuation of the contents of an abscess. Sometimes a part of the wall of the cavity is rigid, as in the chest after an empyema operation; we then seek to make the cavity smaller by causing the maximum of expansion of the lung, and if this does not suffice, we resect a number of ribs so as to collapse the soft parts of the chest wall and thus obliterate the space that has remained.

It is far different, however, with cavities left in the bones, and more especially in the long bones after operations for disease in those structures. Bone cavities have rigid, unyielding walls, in which blood and secretions are only too apt to collect and stagnate and to serve as a nidus for bacterial growth. In deficiencies in the bony skull, osteoplastic methods are often successful, but in the case of the long bones they are seldom feasible. In the majority of the cases these cavities in the long bones have to heal by the slow and tedious process of granulation; repeated operations and months of treatment are often necessary to obtain healing. The best way to keep these cavities relatively aseptic and thus favor the growth of healthy granulations is to change the dressings as infrequently as possible.

From the very earliest times, attempts have been made to obliterate

---

*Read at the February meeting of the Surgical Section of the New York Academy of Medicine.

these cavities by filling them with tissues from some other part of the patient's body, or by the introduction into them of foreign substances. Large pieces of bone or bone chips, muscle or fat were taken from one part of the patient's body and introduced into the cavity, but successes were few and failures many. Later the moist blood clot method of Schede was highly recommended. The good results with the method were, however, rare and the procedure has been almost entirely abandoned. The skin flap method recommended by Neuber has occasionally yielded good results, but in many cases there is not sufficient skin for the formation of satisfactory flaps. Bone derived from animals and prepared in a number of ways was next tried but without success. Attempts were made to fill the cavities with a variety of foreign substances, such as glass, ivory, rubber, cork, lead, sponge, celluloid, plaster-of-Paris, gold-foil, copper, amalgum, gelatin, etc., but satisfactory results were obtained in only exceptional cases. The materials introduced almost always acted as foreign bodies, caused increased secretion and suppuration, and were either extruded or had to be removed.

During the last three years, Mosetig-Moorhof, of Vienna, and his assistant have published the results that they have obtained with an iodoform wax filling for bone cavities. Impressed by the claims of these authors, the writer determined to give the method a trial.

The steps of the procedure as described by Mosetig-Moorhof, are the following: The limb is prepared in the usual manner and rendered bloodless by the Esmarch constrictor. The bone is exposed, the periosteum turned back, and all diseased bone removed with the chisel, spoon, etc., until the walls of the cavity are formed by healthy bone. The cavity is then thoroughly washed out with sterile salt solution, and its walls rubbed with sponges wet with two per cent. formalin solution. The bleeding from the bone is next stopped by hot irrigation, the insufflation of sterilized hot air, and tight packing with gauze. The soft parts are now carefully examined, all diseased skin, sinuses, etc., excised, until the wound in the soft parts is formed by healthy tissue. As soon as the bleeding from the bone has entirely ceased the filling is introduced. This filling consists of a mixture of 60 parts of iodoform, 40 parts of spermaceti and 40 parts of sesame oil. The mixture is prepared by heating the spermaceti and the oil of sesame over a water bath for one-half hour, then adding the iodoform to it, and preserving the mixture in a sterilized bottle or special retainer. When the filling is to be introduced, the mixture is melted by immersing the bottle in hot water, and while still fluid is poured into the cavity, until the latter is entirely filled. Within a few minutes the mixture solidifies. The periosteum, or, if this is impossible, the soft parts are closed over it, the skin wound closed with or without drainage, and a dry compression bandage applied. The Esmarch constrictor is then removed. The wound is dressed after seven to ten days and in the majority of the cases will be found to have healed by primary union. If the wound has been drained, which is advisable in most cases, the sinus left will heal in the course of a few weeks. In a certain number of cases the wax mixture is slowly extruded in the course of several weeks by the active growth of new tissue around it, and the mixture seems to act as a powerful stimulus to this growth. Iodoform poisoning was never seen, in spite of the large percentage of that substance in the mixture, as the iodoform is very slowly absorbed out of the filling, but traces of iodine were sometimes to be found in the urine for the first two or three days after the operation. Healing usually occurred without much elevation of temperature or pulse, although occasionally there was observed a marked rise of both temperature and pulse for one or two days.

As a result of his investigations and experiments on animals, Mosetig-Moorhof was able to determine that the wax mixture slowly disappears as new tissue grows into it from the bone, and the gradual disappearance of the mixture could be nicely followed in X-ray pictures.

Mosetig-Moorhof declares that his method is applicable to all forms of chronic bone disease, inclusive of the tuberculous variety, and also to chronic tuberculous affections of the joints, but the method is not applicable to acute bone disease in which the cavity cannot be rendered aseptic. In order to insure successful results, great care must be observed that the walls of the cavity shall consist of healthy bone, and that the soft parts of the wound shall be thoroughly freshened; the oozing from the bone must be very carefully stopped before the wax mixture is inserted, so that no blood shall collect between the wax mixture and the walls of the bone cavity.

During the past year, the writer has used this method on the surgical service of Dr. Lilienthal at the Mount Sinai Hospital in three cases of chronic osteomyelitis of the hip; four of chronic osteomyelitis of the femur, one of tuberculous disease of the tibia, one of chronic disease of the ulna, and one of chronic tuberculosis of the bones of the elbow-joint. All of the patients had been repeatedly operated upon in various hospitals, including our own, without permanent cure.

The results that I have obtained with the method of Mosetig-Moorhof, although not as good as those of this author, have shown much improvement over former methods of treatment, so that I feel warranted in recommending the method for further trial. I think it probable that with increasing experience the various steps of the method may be much improved upon.

It is better to remove the Esmarch constrictor from the limb before the wax mixture is introduced so that the hemostasis in the bone cavity may be more perfect and the oozing from the bone be perfectly controlled when the normal circulation is established. In the second place, I have not made use of dry hot sterilized air in controlling the oozing from the bone cavity because this required more complicated apparatus than I had at hand. The bleeding has been entirely controlled in our cases by irrigation with hot saline solution, irrigation with peroxide of hydrogen, and packing of adrenalin and dry sterile gauze. In our cases the wax mixture often did not harden as quickly as claimed by Mosetig-Moorhof, and considerable time was often lost in waiting for the mixture to become firm. During this time slight oozing was apt to occur from the bone and to leak through the mixture while it was still semi-fluid. Even if the filling seemed fairly hard, the central portions were still soft, so that considerable of the softer portions of the filling were squeezed out when the soft parts of the wound were being closed, and the solidity of the filling was thus rendered imperfect. I now pour the melted mixture into a basin of sterilized cold water and mold it with the hands until it has about the consistency of putty. I then press bits of the mass into the walls of the cavity and thus stop the very slightest oozing from the bone and fill up all small spaces (in the same way that we use Horsley's bone wax in cranial surgery). When this has been done, the cavity is lined by a thin layer of wax and is absolutely dry. Then the cavity is tightly packed with the filling in the same way that the dentist fills a cavity in a tooth.

I have never used more than 20 per cent. of iodoform in the wax mixture because in my earliest cases I had one of well-marked iodoform poisoning. I have tried also to use a mixture of iodoform and spermaceti without the oil, and a mixture of iodoform and paraffin without the oil, but the results have not been as good as those obtained with the mixture of equal parts of spermaceti and oil containing 20 per cent. of iodoform.

In three of the cases here reported there was a considerable rise in the temperature and pulse, after the operation, which lasted for from two to four days. All but two of the patients had small quantities of iodine in their urine for one or two days after the insertion of the filling; in one case there were marked symptoms of iodoform poisoning for twenty-four hours. The patients almost uniformly complained of a burning sensation in their wounds for a few days but thereafter declared that they felt better than after any one of their previous operations.

In six patients the wounds healed by primary union except for the drainage opening. In four of these cases the filling remained *in situ*; in one, a small part of the wax was extruded and the wound then healed up; in the sixth case, all of the filling was extruded in the course of two weeks and the wound then rapidly closed.

In a patient who had a large cavity occupying almost the entire tibia, the result of a tuberculous osteomyelitis and numerous operations, I introduced the filling, but was able to close only about two-thirds of the wound in the soft parts. The wax filling remained in place for about two weeks and was then gradually pushed out of its bed by the active growth of granulations around it. The shell of bone that was left was very thin and during the manipulations incident upon the last operation a fracture had occurred. At the end of four weeks the fracture was firmly healed, and six weeks later the large wound was entirely healed and the cavity was filled with new tissue so that the scar was hardly depressed. During the healing, the discharge was serous or sero-purulent in character and small in amount. This case demonstrated the powerful stimulating effect of the mixture, and the rapidity of growth of new granulation tissue. I have observed this same effect in other cases. In three of the cases that I operated upon the method resulted in failure. One patient had a large cavity in the lower end of the femur after several operations for osteomyelitis two years before. In spite of three operations, I never succeeded in rendering the cavity aseptic; after each operation the wound reopened and the wax was extruded. At the present time, the filling inserted at the third operation is being gradually extruded with considerable purulent discharge. In a case of chronic disease of the ulna, the filling remained in place for a number of weeks, but on reopening the wound, at a second operation, it was found that a sequestrum had been left behind. After the last operation a sinus has persisted for four weeks and, although no bare bone is to be felt and there is very little discharge, the operative procedure must be considered a failure.* In a third case, one of sinuses of the hip-joint of many years' duration, the wax filling gradually escaped and a sinus still persists.

In the case of a child of six years, who had several sinuses left after resection of the hip-joint for suppurating tuberculous arthritis (the sinuses had persisted for two years in spite of repeated operations, so that the patient was considered incurable), the wound was entirely healed three weeks after the filling had been introduced. Owing to a misunderstanding, the little patient was allowed to walk around without a hip-splint, so that direct pressure was made upon the wax filling. Some months later a sinus reformed from which the wax is being extruded at the present time, but there is little discharge. The general condition of the child, which was very poor when she was operated upon, is now excellent, and I have little doubt that the sinus will soon close. This case must, however, be included among those in which the operation was not or was only a partial success.

With the exception of the cases just mentioned, all of the other patients have remained well up to the present time, the most recent case was operated upon two months ago and the first case more than three years ago.

A careful consideration of the results that I have obtained in the cases I have operated upon, has convinced me that the method of Mosetig-Moorhof is worthy of a more extended trial than it has received up to the present time. It must be remembered that the cases in which this operation was tried were cases in which all other methods of treatment had failed. The general condition of the patients is very much improved because the long-standing and continual suppuration is stopped. If the operation is successful, the patient's stay in the hospital is much shortened. Even if the filling is extruded, the healing process will be much hastened.

Success will depend to a great extent upon the thoroughness with

*After the above was written the wound closed rapidly. It was healed in three weeks, and has remained healed up to the present time.

which the operation is done. The procedure is a slow and painstaking one, and it is not unusual for the operation to take one to two hours. If the patient's condition does not allow of so prolonged an anesthesia, the operation may have to be done in two stages. The greater the care that is taken in the preparation of the bone cavity for the filling, the better will be the results that will be obtained. I believe that, with increasing experience, the cures obtained by this method of operation will become more and more frequent. A more detailed account of my experiences is reserved for a future publication.

GYNECOLOGICAL SERVICE.

December 1, 1902, to December 1, 1903.

JOSEPH BRETTAUER, M.D.,
GYNECOLOGIST.

HIRAM N. VINEBERG, M.D.,
ADJUNCT GYNECOLOGIST.

```
Patients admitted ............................................ 522
Diseases treated ............................................. 567
    Cured ................................................ 475
    Improved ............................................. 36
    Unimproved ........................................... 39
        1. Treated ............................... 23
        2. Not treated (refused, 12; inoperable, 4).. 16
    Died ................................................. 17
Number of operations......................................... 494
```

DISEASES.

	Not operated.	Cured.	Improved.	Unimproved.	Died.	Total.
Vulva (2 cases).						
Carcinoma of vulva, carcinomatous inguinal glands	..	..	..	..	1	1
Vulvitis	1	..	1	..	..	1
Urethra and Bladder (2 cases).						
Urethral caruncle	..	1	..	..	..	1
Cystitis	1	..	1	..	..	1
Vagina (86 cases).						
Rectocele	1	38	..	*1	..	39
Cystocele	1	41	1	*1	..	43
Vaginitis	1	..	1	..	..	1
Carcinoma of vagina	1	..	..	†1	..	1
Uretero-vaginal fistula	..	1	..	..	..	1
Vesico-vaginal "	..	..	..	1	..	1

*Refused treatment.   †Inoperable.

	Not operated.	Cured.	Improved.	Unimproved.	Died.	Total.
Perineum (8 cases).						
Complete laceration	..	2	..	..	..	2
Incomplete "	2	4	..	*2	..	6
Rectum (8 cases).						
Hemorrhoids	..	6	..	..	..	6
Carcinoma rectum, intestinal obstruction	..	..	..	..	1	1
Fistula in ano	..	1	..	..	..	1
Uterus (308 cases).						
Cervix (47 cases).						
Injuries: 1. Lacerations	1	28	..	*1	..	29
Inflammations: 1. Eroded	2	1	..	1	..	2
2. Hypertrophied	..	8	..	..	..	8
New Growths:						
Benign: Polyp	..	1	..	..	..	1
Malignant: Carcinoma	..	2	5	..	..	7
Body (263 cases).						
A. *Abortions:* 1. Incomplete	..	27	..	..	..	27
2. Inevitable	..	3	..	..	..	3
3. Threatened	1	1	..	..	..	1
4. Incomplete, bipartate uterus	..	1	..	..	..	1
B. *Inflammations:* 1. Post-abortive endometritis	2	10	1	*1	..	12
2. Chronic endometritis	8	60	4	*4	..	68
3. Post-partum sepsis	3	2	..	..	4	6
4. Metritis	..	1	..	..	..	1
5. Post-partum sepsis, nephritic abscess	..	1	..	..	..	1
6. Post-abortive endometritis, perforation, general peritonitis	..	..	..	..	2	2
7. Para- and perimetritis	4	4	..	..	..	4
C. *New Growths:*						
I. Benign: 1. Polyp	..	3	..	..	..	3
2. Fibroid uterus	4	40	1	*3	..	44
3. Sloughing fibroid, sepsis	..	..	..	..	1	1
4. Fibroid, ovarian cyst, general peritonitis	..	..	..	..	1	1
II. Malignant: 1. Carcinoma	..	1	..	..	..	1
2. Sarcomatous degeneration of fibroid	1	1	..	1	..	2
D. *Displacements:*						
1. Anteflexion and stenosis	2	27	..	*2	..	29
2. Retroflexion and retroversion	6	37	2	*4	..	43
3. Prolapsus	2	10	1	*2	..	13
Ovaries (38 cases).						
Cyst: Simple	1	18	..	*1	..	19
Dermoid	..	2	..	..	..	2

*Refused treatment.

	Not operated.	Cured.	Improved.	Unimproved.	Died.	Total.
Ovaries—*Continued*.						
Twisted pedicle	..	2	..	..	..	2
Tubo-ovarian	..	3	..	..	..	3
Dermoid with pregnancy	..	1	..	..	..	1
Intraligamentous	..	3	..	..	..	3
Inflammations: 1. Tuberculosis	..	1	..	..	..	1
2. Abscess	..	3	..	..	1	4
New Growths:						
Malignant: Sarcoma	1	1	..	1	..	2
Carcinoma	..	..	..	1	..	1
Tubes (51 cases).						
Pyosalpinx	1	4	..	*1	..	5
Hydrosalpinx	1	1	..	1	..	2
Diseased appendages	10	14	6	4	1	25
Tubercular "	..	1	..	..	1	2
Ectopic pregnancy	..	14	..	..	2	16
Diseased appendages, retroversion	..	..	..	..	1	1
Pelvic Peritoneum and Cellular Tissue (40 cases)						
Abscess	..	17	1	..	..	18
Exudate	5	3	2	2	..	7
Hematocele	..	6	..	..	..	6
Pelvic peritonitis	9	3	6	..	..	9
Miscellaneous (22 cases).						
Chronic appendicitis	..	8	..	..	..	8
Inguinal hernia	..	1	..	..	..	1
Carcinoma of stomach	1	..	..	†1	..	1
" " colon	1	..	..	†1	..	1
Auto intoxication	1	1	..	..	..	1
Multilocular cyst of gastro-colic omentum	..	..	..	..	1	1
Incarcerated pessary	..	1	..	..	..	1
Intestinal obstruction, volvulus	..	1	..	..	..	1
Abdominal sinus	2	..	2	..	..	2
" abscess	..	1	..	..	..	1
Ventral hernia	1	1	..	†1	..	2
Tubercular peritonitis	..	..	1	..	..	1
Parotid cyst	..	1	..	..	..	1

*Refused treatment.   †Inoperable.

Operations.

Urethra and Bladder (1 operation).

Cauterization of urethral caruncle... 1

Vagina (81 operations).

Anterior colporrhaphy 42
Posterior   "   38
Plastic for vesico-vaginal fistula..................................... 1

Rectum (7 operations).

Clamp and cautery for hemorrhoids................................... 6
Incision and drainage for fistula in ano.............................. 1

Perineum (6 operations).

Tait for complete laceration... 2
Emmet for incomplete laceration..................................... 4

Uterus (284 operations).

Cervix (51 operations).

Trachelorrhaphy 28
Amputation 8
Curettage and paquelinization for carcinoma......................... 5
Excision of polyp... 1
Discision and dilatation for stenosis............................... 9

Body (233 operations).

Curettage for incomplete abortion, inevitable abortion, post-abortive endo-
    metritis, chronic endometritis................................103
Curettage for diagnosis... 2
Excision of polyp... 3
Abdominal hysterectomy: 1. Fibroid uterus......................... 32
                            2. Carcinoma cervix 3
                            3. Metritis 1
                            4. Perforation of uterus................ 2
                            5. Diseased appendages 8
Vaginal hysterectomy: 1. Fibroid uterus........................... 10
                            2. Diseased appendages 1
Myomectomy 2
Alexander's operation for retroversion and retroflexion............. 17
Vaginal fixation of round ligaments................................. 9
Ventral suspension of round ligaments............................... 6
    "   fixation 16
Dudley's operation for anteflexion and stenosis..................... 18

Ovaries and Tubes, Pelvic Peritoneum and Cellular Tissue (92 operations).

Abdominal section for:
    Simple ovarian cyst... 17
    Dermoid cyst 3
    Twisted pedicle 2

Ovaries and Tubes, Pelvic Peritoneum and Cellular Tissue—*Continued.*

Abdominal section for:
    Tubo-ovarian cyst 3
    Intraligamentous cyst 3
    Tuberculosis of ovary... 1
    Abscess of ovary.. 4
    Sarcoma of ovary... 1
    Pyosalpinx 4
    Hydrosalpinx 1
    Diseased appendages 7
    Tubercular " 2
    Diseased " hysterectomy 8
    Ectopic pregnancy 16
Vaginal section for:
    Ovarian cyst 1
    Pelvic abscess 18
    " exudate 2
    Hematocele 6
    Exploratory, carcinoma of ovary...................................... 1

Miscellaneous (23 operations).

Appendectomy for chronic appendicitis..................................... 8
Bassini's operation for inguinal hernia................................... 1
Incision and drainage of cyst of gastro-colic omentum..................... 1
Removal of incarcerated pessary... 1
Colostomy for intestinal obstruction, volvulus............................ 1
Incision and drainage of abdominal abscess................................ 1
Radical operation for ventral hernia...................................... 1
Laparotomy for tubercular peritonitis..................................... 1
Nephrectomy for uretero-vaginal fistula................................... 1
Colostomy, intestinal obstruction, carcinoma of rectum.................... 1
Resection of colon and intestinal anastomosis for fecal fistula........... 1
Excision of abdominal sinus... 1
Incision and drainage for nephritic abscess............................... 1
    "   "   "   " suppurating carcinomatous glands.............. 1
Laparotomy for post-operative hemorrhage.................................. 1
Excision of parotid cyst.. 1

GYNECOLOGICAL SERVICE.

December 1, 1903, to December 1, 1904.

Joseph Brettauer, M.D.,
GYNECOLOGIST.

S. M. Brickner, M.D.,
ADJUNCT GYNECOLOGIST.

```
Patients admitted ............................................. 362
Diseases treated .............................................. 473
    Cured .............................................. 409
    Improved ........................................... 27
    Unimproved ......................................... 24
        1. Treated ................................. 7
        2. Not treated (refused, 4; inoperable, 13).. 17
    Died ............................................... 13
Number of operations.......................................... 420
```

Diseases.

Vulva (5 cases).	Not operated.	Cured.	Improved.	Unimproved.	Died.	Total.
Epithelioma	..	1	..	..	..	1
" and kraurosis	..	1	..	..	..	1
Atresia of hymen	..	1	..	..	..	1
Bartholinian abscess	..	1	..	..	..	1
" cyst	..	1	..	..	..	1
Urethra and Bladder (3 cases).						
Urethral caruncle	1	..	..	*1	..	1
Tubercular cystitis	1	..	1	..	..	1
Incontinence of urine after prolonged labor	..	..	..	1	..	1
Vagina (92 cases).						
Cystocele	..	40	..	..	..	40
Rectocele	..	41	..	..	1	42
Congenital atresia of vagina	..	1	..	..	..	1
" absence of vagina and uterus	1	..	1	*1	..	2

*Refused treatment.

	Not operated.	Cured.	Improved.	Unimproved.	Died.	Total.
Vagina—*Continued.*						
Sarcoma of vagina	..	..	1	..	..	1
Abdomino-vaginal fistula	1	1	1	..	..	2
Recto-vaginal fistula	..	..	..	2	..	2
Utero-vaginal fistula	..	2	..	..	..	2
Perineum (8 cases).						
Laceration, complete	..	3	..	..	..	3
" incomplete	..	4	..	..	..	4
" " infected	1	..	1	..	..	1
Rectum (4 cases).						
Hemorrhoids	..	3	..	..	..	3
Fistula in ano	..	1	..	..	..	1
Uterus (233 cases).						
Cervix (37 cases).						
Injuries: lacerated cervix	1	21	..	§1	..	22
Inflammations: hypertrophied cervix	..	7	..	..	..	7
Senile cervicitis	..	1	..	..	..	1
New Growths:						
1. Benign: polyp	..	2	..	..	..	2
2. Malignant: carcinoma	1	2	1	*1	1	5
Body (196 cases).						
A. *Abortions:* 1. Incomplete	2	18	..	..	..	18
2. Inevitable	..	2	..	..	..	2
3. Threatened	2	2	..	..	..	2
B. *Inflammations:* 1. Post-abortive endometritis	..	11	..	..	..	11
2. Chronic endometritis	2	41	2	..	..	43
3. Post-partum sepsis	4	..	..	..	4	4
4. Metritis	..	2	1	..	..	1
5. Pyometra	..	1	..	..	..	1
C. *New Growths:*						
I. Benign: 1. Polyp	..	2	..	..	..	2
2. Fibroid uterus	3	33	..	*3	..	36
3. Subserous fibroid	..	4	..	..	..	4
4. Submucous fibroid	..	4	..	..	..	4
5. Sloughing fibroid	..	1	..	..	1	2
6. Fibroid, pregnancy	1	..	..	†1	..	1
II. Malignant: 1. Carcinoma	..	1	..	1	1	3
2. Sarcomatous degeneration of fibroid	..	1	1	..	..	2

*Refused operation.
†Pregnant
§Inoperable (nephritis).

Body—Continued.		Not operated.	Cured.	Improved.	Unimproved.	Died.	Total.
D. Displacements:	1. Anteflexion and stenosis	..	15	..	..	..	15
	2. Retroversion and retroflexion	3	29	..	‡3	..	32
	3. Prolapsus uteri	1	8	..	*1	1	10
E. Malformations:	Infantile uterus	1	..	..	1	..	1

Ovaries (32 cases).

		Not operated.	Cured.	Improved.	Unimproved.	Died.	Total.
Cyst:	1. Simple	..	11	..	..	..	11
	2. " bilateral	..	3	..	..	..	3
	3. Dermoid	..	3	..	..	..	3
	4. Twisted pedicle	..	3	..	..	..	3
	5. Tubo-ovarian	..	1	..	..	..	1
	6. Parovarian	..	3	..	..	..	3
	7. Corpus luteum	..	1	..	..	..	1
Inflammations:	1. Abscess	..	1	..	*1	..	2
	2. Tubo-ovarian abscess	..	1	..	..	..	1
New Growths:							
Malignant:	1. Carcinoma	1	..	..	†1	..	1
	2. " and intestinal obstruction	..	..	1	..	..	1
	3. Sarcoma	..	..	1	..	..	1
	3. Myxosarcomatous degeneration of cyst	..	1	..	..	..	1

Tubes (44 cases).

	Not operated.	Cured.	Improved.	Unimproved.	Died.	Total.
1. Pyosalpinx, unilateral	1	4	1	..	..	5
2. " bilateral	..	1	..	..	..	1
3. Hydrosalpinx	..	3	..	..	..	3
4. Diseased appendages	4	14	4	..	..	18
5. Acute salpingitis	2	..	2	..	..	2
6. Ectopic pregnancy	..	15	..	..	..	15

Pelvic Peritoneum and Cellular Tissue (26 cases).

	Not operated.	Cured.	Improved.	Unimproved.	Died.	Total.
Pelvic abscess	2	8	1	..	1	10
" " sepsis, lung abscess	..	..	..	..	1	1
Exudate	4	3	..	*1	..	4
Hematocele	..	2	..	..	..	2
Infected hematocele	..	2	..	..	1	3
Parametritis	2	1	1	..	..	2
Pelvic peritonitis	4	2	2	..	..	4

Miscellaneous (26 cases).

	Not operated.	Cured.	Improved.	Unimproved.	Died.	Total.
Chronic appendicitis	..	5	..	..	..	5
Cyst of breast	..	1	..	..	..	1
Nihil	1	..	..	*1	..	1
Persistent abdominal sinus	..	1	1	..	..	2
Fibromyxoma of abdominal wall	..	1	..	..	..	1
Carcinoma transverse colon, perforation, general peritonitis	..	..	..	..	1	1
Acute catarrhal appendicitis	..	1	..	..	..	1

*Refused operation.
‡2 cases refused operation; 1 case diabetes.
†General condition of patient did not warrant operation.

Miscellaneous—*Continued*.	Not operated.	Cured.	Improved.	Unimproved.	Died.	Total.
Constipation	1	1				1
Pyelitis in pregnancy	1		1			1
Neurasthenia	2			2		2
Floating kidney		1				1
Hemophilia	1		1			1
Acute gangrenous perforative appendicitis with abscess, diffuse peritonitis and two large twisted pedunculated fibroids		1				1
Ventral hernia		2				2
Nephroptosis	1			*1		1
Eclampsia in a mother		1				1
" " " baby		1				1
Carcinoma of breast		1				1
Papilloma of bladder			1			1

OPERATIONS.

Vulva (5 operations).

Excision of epithelioma of vulva	2
" " imperforate hymen for hematocolpos and hematometra	1
" " Bartholinian cyst	1
" " " gland	1

Urethra and Bladder (1 operation).

Gersuny's operation for incontinence after prolonged labor	1

Vagina (88 operations).

Anterior colporrhaphy	39
Posterior "	42
Vaginal fixation of uterus for cystocele	1
Excision of diaphragm in upper third of vagina causing atresia vaginæ	1
Plastic for congenital absence of vagina	1
Curettage and paquelinization for sarcoma of vagina	1
Plastic for recto-vaginal fistula	2
Excision abdomino-vaginal sinus	1

Perineum (7 operations).

Tait for complete laceration	3
Emmet for incomplete laceration	4

Rectum (4 operations).

Clamp and cautery for hemorrhoids	3
Incision and drainage for fistula in ano	1

*Refused operation.

Uterus (217 operations).

Cervix (36 operations).

Trachelorrhaphy for laceration.. 21
Amputation for hypertrophy... 7
Excision of cervical polyp.. 2
Curettage and paquelinization for carcinoma............................ 4
"   for senile cervicitis.. 1

Body (181 operations).

Curettage for incomplete abortion, inevitable abortion, post-abortive endometritis, chronic endometritis and metritis.......................... 70
Induction of abortion for tuberculosis of lungs........................... 1
Curettage for diagnosis... 3
Atmokausis for metrorrhagia after double salpingo-oöphorectomy........ 1
Dilatation of cervix and drainage for pyometra........................... 1
Excision of uterine polyp... 2
Abdominal hysterectomy: 1. Fibroid uterus............................ 25
                       2. Metritis................................... 1
                       3. Carcinoma uterus 2
                       4. "   cervix (Wertheim) 2
                       5. Sarcomatous degeneration of fibroid....... 2
Vaginal hysterectomy: 1. Fibroid uterus............................. 10
                     2. Metritis................................... 1
                     3. Complete prolapse of uterus................ 1
                     4. Carcinoma uterus 1
Abdominal myomectomy 2
Vaginal myomectomy: 1. Subserous 4
                    2. Submucous 2
Alexander's operation for retroversion and retroflexion................. 15
Fixation of round ligaments to abdominal wall.......................... 2
Ventral fixation 19
Dudley's operation for anteflexion and stenosis......................... 15

Ovaries and Tubes, Pelvic Peritoneum and Cellular Tissue (80 operations).

Abdominal section for:
    Simple ovarian cyst.. 11
    Double   "   " 3
    Dermoid cyst 1
    "   "   hysterectomy 1
    Twisted pedicle 3
    Tubo-ovarian cyst 1
    Parovarian   " 3
    Corpus luteum cyst.. 1
    Tubo-ovarian abscess, hysterectomy............................... 1
    Myxosarcomatous degeneration of cyst............................ 1
    Sarcoma of ovary... 1
    Ectopic pregnancy 13
    "   "   with double ovarian cyst, hysterectomy........... 1
    Hydrosalpinx 2
    Pyosalpinx 5
    Diseased appendages 10
    "   "   hysterectomy 3
    Hematocele, hysterectomy 1

Ovaries and Tubes, Pelvic Peritoneum and Cellular Tissue—*Continued.*

Vaginal section for:
- Dermoid cyst 1
- Ovarian abscess 1
- Ectopic pregnancy 1
- Hydrosalpinx 1
- Diseased appendages, hysterectomy............................. 1
- Pelvic abscess 9
- Infected hematocele 3
- Hematocele 1

Miscellaneous (21 operations).

- Appendectomy for chronic catarrhal appendicitis...................... 5
- Excision of mammary cyst.. 1
- Curettage of abdomino-vaginal sinus..................................... 2
- Excision of myxofibroma of abdominal wall............................ 1
- Colostomy for intestinal obstruction caused by carcinoma transverse colon 1
- Appendectomy for acute catarrhal appendicitis......................... 1
- Nephropexy 1
- Nephrectomy for uretero-vaginal fistula................................. 2
- Myomectomy and appendectomy for gangrenous perforative appendicitis and two twisted pedunculated fibroids............................ 1
- Laparotomy, radical cure for ventral hernia............................ 2
- Amputation of breast for carcinoma...................................... 1
- High forceps for eclampsia, after induction of labor.................. 1
- Suprapubic cystotomy and paquelinization for papilloma of bladder. 1
- Colostomy for intestinal obstruction caused by carcinoma of ovaries and intestines 1

A STUDY OF THE RESULTS OF ABDOMINAL HYSTERECTOMY FOR FIBROID OF THE UTERUS WITH AND WITHOUT DRAINAGE.

By Joseph Brettauer, M.D.,
GYNECOLOGIST MT. SINAI HOSPITAL.

This study was undertaken with a view toward ascertaining the difference in the immediate results of abdominal hysterectomy, or rather in supra-vaginal amputation for fibroids of the uterus, upon the comfort, rapidity of convalescence, and general condition of the patient, in those cases in which drainage through the vagina was instituted, and in those in which it was omitted. The cases included are those which have been operated upon in my service at the Mt. Sinai Hospital, covering a period of two years, from December 1, 1902, to December 1, 1904. There are in all 54 cases. There was no mortality, complications of an inflammatory or other character were very few, and generally speaking the total results could hardly be improved upon. It may be well to state that no differentiation has been made between the cases operated upon in the old hospital, where the facilities were far inferior to those in use in the present hospital, which came into clinical use on March 26, 1904. Of the 54 operations, 32 were performed with gauze drainage through the cervix, and 22 without.

For the thorough appreciation of any set of statistics referring to operations, the technics of the operator are an essential; I shall, therefore, briefly describe my own mode of procedure in a typical case of abdominal hysterectomy. This does not differ materially from that of other operators, except in a few unimportant details; the length of the abdominal incision is regulated by the size of the tumor; very little time is taken up for preliminary hemostasis; the ovarian artery and round ligament on both sides are ligated with silk, and the bladder peeled off from the anterior surface of the uterus. A small posterior flap of peritoneum is then dissected from the cervix at about the height of the insertion of the sacro-uterine ligament, the uterine arteries are ligated with silk, and the uterus amputated in such a way as to leave a crater-like cervical stump. When drainage was practiced a piece of iodoform gauze was now put through the cervix, the upper end left long enough to cover the cervical stump, with the idea that it should act more as a compression for the slight oozing, than as actual drainage; the anterior and posterior peritoneal flaps are then united by a running catgut suture, starting at the ligature over the ovarian artery so as to invert both this ligature and the round ligament, leaving no raw surface or free pedicle within the abdominal cavity. When drainage is not resorted to, the cervical stump is closed with a running catgut suture, and the peritoneal flaps united as in the other cases. After removing the appendix a running catgut suture closes the parietal peritoneum, interrupted silk sutures unite the fascia, and the skin is either sewed by a running suture, strapped, or united with Michel's clamps, dependent upon the amount of adipose tissue in the abdominal wall.

It is well to say at the outset that the immediate results of abdominal hysterectomy by all operators are satisfactory in the main; the mortality is not high in uncomplicated cases, and the convalescence undisturbed; to substantiate this, I will refer only to the comprehensive statistics of Winter,* who has collected 689 cases of supravaginal amputation with a total mortality of 32, or 4.6 per cent. His table includes 105 operations by Henricius, with 2 deaths; 118 by Hofmeier, with 5 deaths; 122 by v. Rosthorn, with a mortality of 4; 77 by Wyder, with 6 deaths; 100 by Olshausen, with 6 deaths, and 167 by himself, with a mortality of 9.

Pulse.—The study of the pulse rate for the first five days after operation, furnishes us with the interesting fact that the heart's action is practically the same in both sets of cases. In drained cases the average low pulse is 85, the average high pulse is 97, and the average for five days after operation, 91; in undrained cases the average low pulse is 88, the average high pulse 99, while the general average for the first five days is 93. In neither series of cases could any particular course be made out, the morning pulse often being higher than the evening. The highest pulse rate was observed during the first 48 hours after operation. Comparing the two figures, we

*Zeit. f. Geb. und Gynek., vol. 51.

are justified in concluding that drainage as employed by us, or its absence, does not perceptibly affect the heart's action; as the pulse affords the most reliable index to the course of convalescence, this is undoubtedly a most important consideration.

Temperature.—The temperature charts show an average high temperature of 100.8°, an average low temperature of 99.8°, and an average temperature for five days after operation of 100.3°; the temperatures being identical for both sets of cases. The highest temperatures in all cases were registered within 48 hours after operation, this being due to absorption, or possibly to imperfect hemostasis. A fact worthy of mention is that we have invariably noted a rise in temperature of from two to three degrees within 48 hours after operation.

As far then as pulse and temperature, the two great criteria for judging the patient's condition, are concerned, we find that the results are practically the same, whether drainage is employed or not.

Gastric Disturbances.—In all cases the combined anesthesia of nitrous oxide and ether was employed. A certain amount of nausea and vomiting,* due entirely to the anesthesia, is the rule for the first 24 hours after operation, and will not be considered further. If nausea and vomiting persist for days they are certainly due to the operative procedure; to the manipulation of the pelvic organs and intestines, and to the breaking up of adhesions, etc. We find that of the drained cases 72.4 per cent. were not nauseated at all, while 14.5 per cent. were noticeably affected; 61 per cent. did not vomit at all, while 29 per cent. vomited very severely; one patient vomited so excessively for six days that a serious complication resulted, which will be described later. Of the undrained cases, 41 per cent. were not nauseated at all, while 18 per cent. were nauseated to such an extent that great distress was experienced; one was nauseated for eight days. Three patients did not vomit at all, and six vomited excessively. The drained cases certainly appear to advantage in these important factors to the comfort of the patient. There were 20 free from nausea, and 19 free from vomiting, while we find among the undrained cases only 9 free from nausea, and three free from vomiting; prolonged nausea and vomiting were also more frequent in the undrained cases. While it is true that individual idiosyncrasies exist among patients as regards their actions after operations, it would appear, nevertheless, that

*The records as to nausea and vomiting are somewhat imperfect.

cases in which the supra-vaginal stump was drained with gauze, enjoy more gastric comfort than those in whom this method was not resorted to.

Intestinal reaction.—A very important factor in the comfort of patients after abdominal section, is the abdominal distention due to the accumulation of gas in the intestines. In the majority of uncomplicated cases of fibroid, Trendelenburg's position is employed immediately after opening the abdominal cavity; this causes the intestines to recede into the upper half of the peritoneal cavity, where they are covered with moist pads, and do not receive any insult further than exposure to the air; on this account severe symptoms due to extreme distention are naturally very rare. Reviewing the history charts, we find that among the drained cases there were 7 with no distention whatever, 13 moderately, and 12 considerably distended; however, only two patients were greatly distressed by this symptom. Of the undrained cases, three had no meteorism, 8 were slightly distended, and 11 distended to a considerable degree. It is evident that as far as post-operative distention is concerned, it makes little difference whether drainage is employed or not.

For relief of the distention we resorted to the use of the rectal tube, low and high enemata, and in a few cases to calomel and salines. Forty and seven-tenths per cent. of the drained cases, and 40.8 per cent. of the undrained cases, had their bowels moved by low enema on the third day; in only 9 cases of the drained and 8 of the undrained was it found necessary to resort to this procedure before the third day, for the relief of abdominal distention. In general, the principles* which I have repeatedly expressed in regard to moving the bowels were strictly adhered to, and no difference in any respect was found between the two classes of case.

Pain.—In all cases of both series there was a moderate amount of pain present, due to the operative procedure. Small doses of Magendie's solution, given at frequent intervals, relieved the pain in all instances; this medication was invariably discarded after the second day.

Catheterization.—One might expect that the period during which catheterization was necessary, would be of longer duration in those

---

*"The Question of Early Catharsis After Celiotomy," by the author (New York Jour. Gyn. and Obst., 1894).

cases in which gauze was employed for drainage; this, however, is not borne out by the facts; if there is any difference, we find it in favor of the drained cases. It is shown that the average length of time in which catheterization was necessary, was 1.3 days in the undrained and 1.5 days in the drained cases, a difference hardly worthy of consideration. Only one patient urinated voluntarily of the drained cases, and two of the undrained; no cystitis developed in either series.

It is evident that in respect to catheterization, both series are almost equal.

Convalescence.—Primary union resulted in the great majority of cases in both series. In all drained cases, after the removal of the pelvic gauze, there was a vaginal discharge with more or less odor, necessitating the employment of irrigations, which were never necessary in the undrained cases. This discharge was profuse, lasting sometimes for weeks.

Of the undrained cases the average length of time in bed was 20 days for 19 patients (the records of the exact time are not complete), the longest time was 38 days for one patient, in whom the fascial sutures tore through on account of excessive vomiting, and the shortest stay was 14 days. Among the drained cases the average time in bed was 17½ days, the longest period was 30 days, and the shortest 11 days; these figures, however, are of no import, as, firstly, the records are incomplete, and, secondly, one patient's complications necessitated such a prolonged stay in bed that the figures were materially influenced.

Complications.—Although in the main the convalescence from the operations was smooth, a number of patients developed complications which in some instances gave rise to pain and distress, and in others ran a prolonged course, which kept them in bed longer than was the usual rule. Among the drained cases there were two cases of wound infection, one in which silk and one in which silkworm gut had been used to close the skin wound. Both cases showed the staphylococcus aureus on culture. In a third case a hematoma developed under the skin, which had been closed by clamps. The hematoma did not become infected, and the wound healed promptly after evacuating the blood. In only one instance was the whole wound infected, the others being sharply localized. All of these cases ran a low temperature for from 6 to 9 days.

In the undrained set of cases there were 5 instances of wound disturbance. Two of the wounds became infected with the staphylococcus aureus, one of the patients running a temperature between 100.5°F. and 101.5°F. for 19 days. In one case the entire wound, though not infected, tore open to the fascia (this had been sutured with silk). In another the upper angle of the fascia separated, giving rise to a prolapse of omentum. This was repaired immediately on its discovery, and the skin wound, which was small, healed by granulation. In still another case the fascial sutures were torn through on account of vomiting, with a prolapse of the intestine.

Among the drained cases, one patient with a chronic myocarditis developed an embolic process in the left pleura, the exact nature of which was not determined. She had a temperature varying from 99° to 102° for ten days, during five of which she vomited constantly. She was discharged cured. One patient, on the twelfth and thirteenth days, vomited without assignable cause. Another patient had frequent urination for two weeks, but there was no cystitis. One patient developed a broncho-pneumonia of ether origin, which lasted for ten days, and another had a severe bronchitis for a week, also probably due to the anesthetic.

Among the undrained cases there was one patient who had frequent urination for two weeks without the development of a cystitis. Another had a curious edema of the labia majora which lasted for three days and disappeared as rapidly as it had come. Another had a severe erythema toxicum for four days, and still another had a superficial burn of the abdomen of unascertainable origin.

The pelvis gave rise to few disturbances. In the drained set of cases, one patient developed an exudate on the left side, with a temperature of 102.2°, which gradually reached normal in seven days. At the time of discharge the exudate could scarcely be felt and gave no pain or discomfort. Another patient had a retroperitoneal hematoma which became infected and gave rise to a temperature of 104.8°, with a correspondingly rapid pulse. This was relieved by posterior section, and the patient left the hospital well.

Among the undrained cases one patient had a small stump exudate, which disappeared before she left the hospital. Another developed an exudate on the right side, with a temperature of 101°, lasting for five days; this exudate too had almost disappeared when the patient was discharged.

Deaths.—There were no deaths among the 54 cases.

In conclusion I wish to say, from the observations made in these two series of cases, that generally speaking there is not the slightest difference in the immediate post-operative course, whether drainage is practiced or not.

Before starting these two series, I always employed drainage, more for the purpose of controlling the small amount of oozing than for actual drainage; during this time a few instances occurred where a retro-peritoneal hematoma formed and became infected after the removal of the gauze from the cervix. This complication, though not of any serious consequence, was always unpleasant; to-day, therefore, it appears preferable to me to sew up the stump in all cases, so as to assure a more perfect hemostasis.

SYNOPSIS OF DEATHS.

Service of Joseph Brettauer, M.D.,
ATTENDING GYNECOLOGIST.

DECEMBER 1, 1902, TO DECEMBER 1, 1903.

CASE I.—*Post-partum pelvic inflammation; septicemia.*—R. W., age 24, admitted February 28, died March 7. She was normally delivered on February 22, and on February 25 was taken ill with a severe chill and high fever. On admission there was a foul, profuse, yellowish discharge from the very large soft uterus, and a dense exudate filled the left broad ligament. Exploration of the uterus resulted in the expulsion of some small pieces of necrotic tissue; the general condition, which on admission was already very precarious, gradually became worse. Chills twice daily, with remittent temperature, continued; no further surgical intervention. The blood culture was negative. No autopsy.

CASE II.—*Puerperal streptococcemia.*—P. D., age 25, admitted March 28, died April 11. Four weeks previous to admission she was normally delivered of a full term child, and on account of foul discharge from the cervix was curetted one week later; this was immediately followed by severe chills, high fever and constant vomiting. On admission these symptoms were still marked; the general condition was miserable, pulse 140 and thready, temperature 105°; behind and to the left of the uterus there was a large, hard exudate; blood culture showed streptococci in large numbers. All treatment was without result, the patient dying two weeks after admission. No autopsy.

CASE III.—*Puerperal septicemia.*—S. W., age 21, admitted April 18, died April 20. Very soon after the delivery of a full term child, the patient became very ill with abdominal pain and nausea, followed by a severe chill. On admission, her general condition was extremely wretched, pulse and temperature high, and the vulva, vagina and lacerated cervix were covered with necrotic areas. There was a small exudate in the left fornix, the uterus was soft, large and extremely tender. The patient failed rapidly, and died 28 hours after admission.

Post-mortem examination revealed a septic condition of the vagina, uterus and tubes, and a general peritonitis.

CASE IV.—*Puerperal septic endometritis; perforation of uterus; peritonitis* (Vineberg).—B. H., age 21, admitted July 7, died July 9. Three weeks before admission, normal confinement; five days later chills and high fever recurring twice daily. On admission there was a free yellowish discharge from the uterus, and a slight bulging in Douglas' cul-de-sac. The uterus was curetted and accidentally perforated by the instrument; four hours later the patient's general condition was very much worse, and an abdominal hysterectomy was done; cloudy fluid was found in the abdominal cavity. She grew rapidly worse, and died 48 hours after the second operation.

CASE V.—*Puerperal septicemia.*—R. S., age 31, admitted November 9, died November 9. Two weeks prior to admission was normally delivered of a full term child; she was curetted for hemorrhage one week later, which was immediately followed by severe sepsis. On admission she was pulseless and cyanotic, practically moribund, and died two hours later. Post-mortem showed perforation of the uterus, hemorrhagic peritonitis, and a pyelonephritis.

CASE VI.—*Ruptured ectopic gestation.*—M. E., age 29, admitted March 19, with the history that eighteen hours before she had had a sudden sharp pain in the left iliac region, and had fainted frequently since. The history obtained from her husband made the diagnosis positive. She was taken at once to the operating room, and the pregnant ruptured left tube removed in a few minutes; intravenous and subcutaneous infusion was resorted to, but in spite of this the patient died four hours after leaving the operating room. Post-mortem examination revealed a most acute anemia as the cause of death.

CASE VII.—*Cyst of gastro-colic omentum; post-operative shock* (Brettauer).—I. L., age 68, admitted May 7, died May 8. On May 6 an incision was made through the abdominal wall, which revealed a broadly adherent omentum, under which was found a multilocular cyst originating in the gastro-colic omentum; part of the cyst had ruptured previously, the omentum acting as a protecting agent and preventing fluid from entering the general peritoneal cavity; distinct signs of a localized peritonitis were present. As the general condition of the patient was very poor, it was deemed inadvisable to remove the remaining part of the cyst, therefore it was simply incised, the walls sewed to the skin, and the cavity drained. The patient did not react after operation, gradually grew weaker, and died in collapse twenty-four hours after.

CASE VIII.—*Tubal pregnancy; general peritonitis* (Stark).—R. N., age 30, admitted April 15, died June 7. The patient was operated upon on April 22, when the left appendages were removed; one week after operation the abdominal wound broke down and was drained; from this time until May 10 there were constant temperature and increased rapidity of the pulse, at times accompanied by chills; at the bottom of the suppurating wound a gauze pad was found, which was gradually removed. Rapid improvement followed. During a dressing on June 3 the peritoneal cavity, which had heretofore not been affected by the suppurating process, was in some way entered by the physician in charge; this accident was followed by a most acute general peritonitis, and death three days later.

CASE IX.—*Fibroid uterus; ovarian cyst; hysterectomy; general peritonitis* (Vineberg).—P. D., age 48, admitted July 18, operated upon July 20, died July 25. The history states that during the operation part of a multilocular ovarian csyt burst during removal; signs of intestinal obstruction appeared soon after operation. On July 24 the abdomen was reopened and drained. Autopsy revealed general peritonitis.

CASE X.—*Tubercular salpingitis; ovarian abscess; sepsis* (Frank).—L. L., age 30, admitted August 30, died September 6. Patient had been suffering severely for eight years previous to admission with pelvic pain; both appendages were diseased; general condition good. On September 2 a large right tubo-ovarian abscess and a left pyosalpinx were removed. The operation was a very difficult one, owing to the presence of extensive adhesions; a slight tear in the rectum was made and immediately repaired. The patient showed signs of septic infection immediately after operation, and died after four days. The pathological report proved the condition of the left appendages to be tubercular.

CASE XI.—*Perforation of uterus; general peritonitis* (Frank).—E. L., age 36, admitted September 6 in a moribund condition, with a history of curettement for incomplete abortion one week prior to admission. As a last resort a hurried abdominal section was made, and two perforations in the wall of the uterus with gangrenous edges were discovered, together with a general purulent peritonitis. The patient died soon after being put back to bed.

CASE XII.—*Tubo-ovarian abscess; general peritonitis* (Vineberg).—S. S., age 24, admitted September 1, died September 7. Four weeks previous to admission the patient apparently had a miscarriage, which was followed by pains in the left iliac region. On examination an enlarged uterus was found to the right, behind which, filling both fornices, was a large fluctuating mass. A posterior vaginal section was done, a large amount of foul-smelling pus was evacuated, and the cavity irrigated and packed; this procedure was followed within twenty-four hours by symptoms of general peritonitis. An abdominal section was then done, but was of no avail, the patient dying of septic infection on September 7. Auptosy showed a general purulent peritonitis, and a large abscess cavity in Douglas' cul-de-sac.

CASE XIII.—*Retroversion; diseased appendages; pelvic peritonitis; shock* (Vineberg).—L. C., age 38, admitted September 7, died September 11. The patient was admitted for retroversion of the uterus. Her general condition was poor; she had an enlarged liver and a chronic endocarditis. The left appendages were found diseased and were removed, and the uterus fixed to the abdominal wall; on account of the presence of some fetid fluid in the cul-de-sac, the pelvis was drained. The patient died two days after operation. Post-mortem revealed a fatty heart, a cirrhotic liver and a chronic nephritis.

CASE XIV.—*Sloughing fibroid; septicemia* (Vineberg).—T. B., age 36, admitted September 5. Hysterectomy for sloughing fibroid was done on September 6, and a posterior vaginal section two days later, during which the bladder was injured. The patient died on September 19.

CASE XV.—*Carcinoma of rectum; intestinal obstruction* (Brettauer).—R. S., age 50, admitted October 21, died October 24. On admission the patient was suffering from acute intestinal obstruction of three days' standing; she was extremely cachectic, had a large mass in the region of the liver, and a stricture high up in the rectum, probably malignant. Under local anesthesia the obstruction was relieved by a right iliac colostomy; patient died three days later. Autopsy showed carcinoma of the rectum, a stricture which practically closed the entire lumen, and metastatic growths in the liver.

CASE XVI.—*Right tubo-ovarian cyst; left hydro-salpinx; secondary hemorrhage* (Brettauer).—S. P., age 22, admitted November 20, died November 29. Double salpingo-oöphorectomy was performed; five hours after, a secondary hemorrhage was discovered. The abdomen was immediately reopened, and the right ovarian artery, from which the ligature had slipped, retied. In spite of vigorous stimulation the patient succumbed three days later to extreme acute anemia.

CASE XVII.—*Recurrent carcinoma of inguinal glands* (Brettauer). A. L., age 50, admitted September 15, died January 11, 1903. Primary operation for carcinoma of vulva on June 3, 1899. Present examination showed a large growth in the inguinal region, firmly adherent to the underlying tissue; this was practically inoperable, particularly as the patient's general condition was extremely poor. During the six weeks of her stay at the hospital, several profuse hemorrhages from the ulcerating tumor took place. Patient died from exhaustion.

SYNOPSIS OF DEATHS.

DECEMBER 1, 1903, TO DECEMBER 1, 1904.

CASE I.—*Puerperal streptococcemia.*—R. F., age 22, admitted January 24, died February 13. Two weeks previous to admission patient was delivered of a full term child, and was taken sick five days after delivery. On admission there was found a double Bartholinian abscess, a left cervical tear extending into the fornix, and a large, soft, tender uterus. Temperature 104°, pulse 140; general condition poor. A blood culture taken immediately after admission showed the presence of streptococci in large numbers. After a few days a systolic murmur at the apex developed, and petechiæ in the conjunctivæ and skin were noted. At no time since admission to hospital was operative interference deemed advisable. Autopsy revealed ulcerative endocarditis; no microscopical changes in the peritoneal cavity, uterus or appendages.

CASE II.—*Puerperal septicemia; pneumonia.*—L. K., age 32, admitted February 10, died February 17. Patient was delivered of a full term child on February 1, and taken sick with chills on February 5. On admission, examination showed a double-sided pneumonia; blood culture negative; locally, a bilateral tear of the cervix into the fornix was found, which, however, did not appear infected. Patient's temperature continued high, and she died one week after admission.

CASE III.—*Puerperal streptococcemia.*—S. B., age 36, admitted February 18, died February 21. Patient was normally delivered on February 7, chills and high fever developed seven days later. On admission, examination showed an irido-cyclitis, and hypopion; a systolic murmur at the apex, and petechiæ in the conjunctivæ; blood culture showed a large number of streptococci; temperature 103°, pulse 130; a large uterus, with a deeply lacerated cervix, was found locally. Autopsy showed septic changes in all organs.

CASE IV.—*Puerperal septicemia; pneumonia.*—B. B., age 38, normally delivered one week previous to admission on April 7. Patient was moribund on admission, and died eleven hours later. Post-mortem showed suppuration in both broad ligaments, and a double-sided pneumonia.

CASE V.—*Pelvic abscess; abscess of lung; septicemia* (Brettauer).—K. M., age 33, admitted February 5. Patient was curetted some time before admission for a profuse yellow discharge, which dated back to a period of amenorrhea of four months' duration; the curettement was followed by intense cramp-like pains and high fever, alternating with chills. On admission the patient was in very poor general condition, emaciated, temperature 102°. The uterus was small, soft, with a wide open cervix; to the right and somewhat anterior was a soft tender mass the size of an orange. Pressure over the abdomen, over the uterus, and over the mass, caused a profuse purulent discharge from the cervix. During an intra-uterine irrigation, small pieces of bone, evidently pieces of parietal bones, were discharged. The poor condition of the patient prohibited any radical interference. The cervix was split on February 17, and a broad communication between the abscess cavity in the broad ligament and the cervix was established. Within the next few days the patient developed a double parotitis, and signs of consolidation in both lungs; purulent expectoration was noticed soon after, and the patient died of exhaustion on March 1. Autopsy showed an abscess in the lower lobe of the right lung, bilateral broncho-pneumonia, a purulent parietal thrombus in the upper part of the vena cava, and a large abscess cavity in the right broad ligament, with normal appendages. Etiologically we assume that pregnancy had occurred, that the fetus died *in utero* and was retained; the sac became necrotic, and the broad ligament was secondarily infected.

CASE VI.—*Prolapse of uterus; pulmonary embolism* (Brickner).—F. L., age 54, admitted April 28 in good general condition. An anterior and posterior colporrhaphy and Alexander's operation were performed on May 3 for prolapse of the uterus. The convalescence was uneventful until the evening of May 12, when she was suddenly seized with a clonic convulsion, became cyanotic, respiration shallow and irregular, pulse imperceptible. She died a few minutes after the onset of the attack. No autopsy.

CASE VII.—*Submucous necrotic fibroid* (Brettauer).—H. S., age 46, admitted June 25. For the past five years has suffered from severe menorrhagia, the abdomen gradually increasing in size; suffering from dyspnea for the past six months; general condition poor, extremely anemic. A mitral insufficiency was found. The abdomen was symmetrically enlarged, due to a large fibroid uterus, which reached above the umbilicus; the cervical canal was extremely dilated, and from the opening a gangrenous polypus protruded which filled the entire vagina. On June 27 an attempt was made to remove this gangrenous mass without anesthesia; this, however, could not be accomplished, as it was found more difficult than was anticipated. Ether was administered and the submucous fibroid removed piecemeal, until the patient's condition forbade any further procedure; the uterus was packed and the radical operation postponed. Though the patient had lost comparatively little blood during this operation, she died of shock six hours after. Autopsy showed chronic endocarditis and nephritis.

CASE VIII.—*Carcinoma of cervix; hysterectomy; secondary hemorrhage* (Brickner).—D. K., age 45, admitted June 25, died July 14. On July 13 abdominal hysterectomy was performed; three hours later, patient's pulse became imperceptible, and there were signs of hemorrhage from the vagina; the abdomen was reopened; no ligature had slipped, but there was an aberrent vessel in the broad ligament outside the ligature, which was then tied. The patient died two hours later.

CASE IX.—*Carcinoma of uterus; hysterectomy; myocarditis* (Brickner). E. C., age 54, admitted July 11. On July 19 abdominal hysterectomy was done for carcinoma of the cervix; the shock of the operation was apparently not overcome, the patient dying twenty-four hours after. Autopsy revealed a marked fatty degeneration of the heart and liver, and parenchymatous and interstitial degeneration of the kidneys.

CASE X.—*Rectocele; cystocele; suicide* (Brickner).—G. F., age 31. Plastic operation was performed on July 19, from which patient recovered and was up and about, apparently well. On August 1 she jumped out of the window of the ward (fifth floor), dying two hours later.

CASE XI.—*Carcinoma of transverse colon; general peritonitis* (Brickner).—F. R., age 34, admitted September 11. On September 12 an exploratory laparotomy on account of intestinal obstruction revealed a general peritonitis, carcinoma of the transverse colon with metastases high up in the rectum. A right colostomy was performed, but the patient collapsed immediately afterward, and died in five hours. Post-mortem showed, besides the already mentioned conditions, a pulmonary tuberculosis.

CASE XII.—*Infected hematocele; septicemia* (Brettauer).—B. U., age 35, admitted November 25. Salpingo-hysterectomy was performed on November 29, for a ruptured left tubal pregnancy. Death in twenty-four hours from acute sepsis.

CASE XIII.—*Pelvic abscess; tuberculosis of lungs* (Brettauer).—L. S., age 21, admitted December 1. Four weeks previous to admission a pelvic abscess was opened by posterior vaginal section, and the patient left the hospital after three weeks at her own request; she then showed signs of tuberculosis at the right apex. She was readmitted in a week, the process having gone further, and her general condition grown much worse. Although both appendages were diseased, no further operative interference was possible. She had several attacks of hemoptysis and died on January 29.

SPECIAL CASES.

Volvulus of the large intestine complicating pregnancy; recovery.—A. S., 37 years old, was admitted to the hospital February 13, 1903. Her family history is negative. She had typhoid fever during childhood. She has had seven children. At the time of her admission to the hospital she was seven months pregnant. She had always been more or less constipated. During the last two weeks before admission to the hospital she had had great difficulty in moving the bowels, and for two days prior to admission no gas passed. The abdomen began to distend, and she had quite intense colicky abdominal pains. She was admitted at 8 P. M., six hours after she had a severe collapse, which necessitated the free use of stimulants. On admission temperature was normal, and the pulse 110 to 120; she had an anxious expression, cyanosis, rapid and short respiration, abdomen distended, but not tender, and with slight rigidity. There was a tympanitic sound over the entire abdomen, even over the pregnant uterus, which could barely be made out by palpation. Bimanual examination showed the uterus crowded down in the pelvis, the cervix patent for about two fingers. A high enema in the knee chest position gave no result. At 10 P. M. I decided to deliver the patient, hoping this might possibly relieve the obstruction; though there were no uterine contractions, I found, to my astonishment, the membranes protruding through the vulva; I opened them and easily delivered the child which lived a few hours only. With the hand in the rectum as far up as the sigmoid, I could distinctly feel the obstruction about 14 inches above the anus. On opening the abdomen in the median line I found the sigmoid flexure and the descending colon with its mesocolon twisted 360 degrees; it was black for from 26 to 28 inches. There was some fluid in the peritoneal cavity. The patient's condition not being favorable,

I untwisted the gut, laid it upon the abdominal wall and covered it with gauze, sewed the upper part of the wound, and united the gut at the nearest normal-looking surface with the parietal peritoneum in the lower angle of the wound, and packed the rest with gauze. When the distended gut was being untwisted an assistant introduced a rectal tube through which gas and bloody fluid escaped. As soon as I had walled off the lower angle of the wound and covered the upper, I made a small opening in the gangrenous gut, and by a purse-string suture fastened a tube into the transverse colon. After forty-eight stormy hours the patient began to revive. Day by day I cut off pieces of the sloughing transverse colon, and after the tenth day the central slough came off entirely. Strange as it may seem the upper part of the incision healed by primary union, though it had simply been impossible to prevent the fecal contents from coming into contact with the parts. After a few weeks the patient, with the exception of the artificial anus in the median line, was in good condition. The finger could easily be introduced into the colon, but the rectal opening had contracted so as to allow only a small probe to enter. My intention was to open the abdomen again, and if the conditions found were favorable, to unite both intestinal ends by suture. To be able to work clean and so insure a more satisfactory result I made a colostomy in the region of the cecum, fastening the cecum to the parietal peritoneum on April 8, and opening it by cautery on April 9. As soon as the intestinal functions were fully established and free defecation had taken place through the new anus, I began to prepare the patient for the final operation, by daily washing out the ascending and transverse colon as well as the rectum.

On April 29 I incised the scars in the median line, carefully dissected several adherent coils of small intestine, and removed a piece about one inch in length from the colon and about one quarter of an inch from the rectum, and united the freshened edges of suture with heavy silk, according to Cornell's method, re-enforcing the line by two rows of Lembert's sutures. For protection against a possible leakage a small Morris drain was put in the lower angle of the wound which was then closed in layer suture. No untoward symptoms followed this rather serious interference, which had lasted two hours. After the patient had passed flatus by rectum for several days she had a copious formed movement per *vias naturales* on May 19, and daily after that. The temporary anus in the region of the appendix was allowed to close, and the patient was discharged cured on June 7.[*]

This case, unique in my experience, presents a number of very interesting features. While at first it seemed more than probable that the enlarged pregnant uterus was responsible for the occurrence of the volvulus, nothing was found on opening the abdomen to substantiate this presumption; as we found out through close inquiry later, the usual chronic constipation from which the patient suffered for

[*] When seen on December 1, 1904, the patient was quite well.

years, was the foremost etiological factor; secondly, the avoidance of infection of the puerperal genital canal in the presence of an abundance of septic material in close proximity; thirdly, the absolute freedom from any operative complications in four consecutive abdominal sections within three months.

Twisted pedunculated fibroids; acute perforative, gangrenous appendicitis; sero-purulent peritonitis, limited to the pelvis (Brickner). N. O., admitted July 16, 1904, with the history of an ovarian cyst with a twisted pedicle, and operated upon with this diagnosis. The condition found was that of two huge pedunculated fibroids of the uterus super-imposed upon each other, the pedicle of the upper one being twisted once. The tumors weighed 1920 grammes. They blocked the entire pelvis, completely shutting it off from the general abdominal cavity. After their removal the pelvis was seen filled with sero-purulent fluid of a dirty color and foul odor; the right appendages were violently inflamed, the fimbriæ of the tube lying in an abscess cavity. These were removed and the vermiform appendix was seen adherent to the pelvic wall, perforated at its center, and gangrenous to its base. Several small subserous fibroids were removed and the wound drained through the abdomen. Recovery was uneventful and the patient discharged on August 13.

The interesting features of the case were the incorrect diagnosis, and the fact that a pathological condition, the two large pedunculated fibroids, was life-saving, preventing a general peritonitis by shutting off the general abdominal cavity from the pelvis.

Eclampsia in new-born children, with eclampsia in the mother.—Baby R., one of twins born September 29, 1904, of a mother who was admitted with an intra-partum eclampsia. The birth was accomplished by accouchement force, this child being delivered by high forceps. It was deeply asphyxiated at birth; six hours post-partum there was a general convulsion lasting two minutes, with marked divergent strabismus and nystagmus; four hours later another convulsion took place; one more convulsion was noted eight hours later. The nystagmus and strabismus lasted for three days, and were followed by pronounced icterus and digestive disturbances. Within five days these conditions had disappeared and the infant left the hospital on the tenth day, nursing satisfactorily. A report received from the mother two months later stated that the child was normal in every way and was gaining steadily in weight.

The second child was born within a few minutes of the first by breech presentation; there was asphyxia pallida at birth. The child breathed satisfactorily after one-half hour's effort at resuscitation, it lived about fifteen hours, requiring frequent attention to its respiration. It had many convulsions of a typical eclamptic character, including adductor spasm, the thumbs being folded within the palms, and the legs being crossed.

Unfortunately, no autopsy was obtained.

Rupture of abdominal wound, due to excessive vomiting after hysterectomy.—Mrs. K., 43 years of age, admitted June 6, 1904, suffering from a very large uterine fibroid which caused considerable metrorrhagia and pain. A typical abdominal hysterectomy was done on June 7; the narcosis (gas and ether) was rather difficult, and very often disturbed by attacks of vomiting. Retching and vomiting were practically incessant for three days after. A high enema and the rectal tube were partly effectual, some fecal matter and a large amount of gas being expelled, without relieving a marked abdominal distention. On June 10 lavage of the stomach was resorted to successfully, several previous attempts having proved ineffectual. On the afternoon of the same day the abdominal dressing was found to be saturated with blood; investigation revealed a gaping of the entire four-inch incision in all its layers, with coils of intestine protruding

In view of the fact that of the four such cases comprising my experience with this complication, the only one which terminated fatally was one which was resutured, I concluded to refrain from immediate suture, especially as it would have necessitated a second narcosis, followed most probably by the same nausea and vomiting. The intestine was replaced in the abdominal cavity, and held there by a flat piece of iodoform gauze, and the wound tightly strapped. Vomiting and nausea ceased from that day; the bowels were moved forty-eight hours later by enema, and the patient's condition was very satisfactory. After the sixth day the intra-abdominal gauze was gradually removed, the edges of the wound being approximated by plaster straps. An uneventful convalescence followed, the patient being discharged on July 18, and on July 30 the wound had entirely closed.*

*December 1, 1904: As yet no ventral hernia has appeared, the linear scar being apparently very firm.

AN ANALYTICAL AND CLINICAL STUDY OF THIRTY CASES OF ECTOPIC PREGNANCY

By Samuel M. Brickner, A.M., M.D.,
ADJUNCT GYNECOLOGIST.

In the two years ending December 1, 1904, thirty cases of ectopic gestation were admitted to the first gynecological service of the Mt. Sinai Hospital. It has seemed worth while to review these cases critically in their clinical and diagnostic lights for the purpose of determining the relative value of the varying symptoms presented in this interesting condition.

Sterility.—All authors, except the most recent, agree that a certain period of sterility is coincident with or favorable to the development of an ectopic pregnancy. In more recent light, however, it seems more correct to ascribe the sterility often preceding an extra-uterine pregnancy to some uterine or tubal lesion which is itself, possibly, responsible for the abnormal pregnancy, i.e., a severe endometritis, a retroversion, inflammatory disease of the appendages, etc. Another reason for the alleged sterility lies unquestionably in the methods used to prevent conception, which, some patients have frankly avowed, failed in the present instance. It is impossible in the present paper to go into the question of the etiology of ectopic pregnancy. Miholitsch (*Zeit. fur Geb. und Gynekol.*, vol. 49, p. 42) has made out a good case for an accessory lumen or lumina in the tube. Ballantyne ("Antenatal Pathology and Hygiene," "The Embryo," p. 618) suggests that if the ovum be detained in the tube till the trophoblast—by which the ovum attaches itself to the uterine wall—be fully formed, or if this be formed prematurely, the ovum may effect a lodgment upon the tubal mucosa. It may be that we shall never know positively the source or sources of tubal pregnancy; but whether Webster ("Ectopic Pregnancy," 1905) is right in his atavistic theory, or whether congenital or inflammatory conditions are at fault, the fact remains that in some cases we find absolutely no deviation from the normal, while in others we see, accompanying the abnormal pregnancy, the grossest pathological conditions which, in themselves, should make for sterility.

In the present series of cases the longest period of sterility was eleven years, the shortest period since the preceding pregnancy eight months. The average sterile period for the thirty cases was 3.49 years. Seven of the patients, or 23 per cent., had never before been pregnant, so that it is impossible in their cases to speak of any period of sterility. Four others had had spontaneous abortions only, the periods of sterility being respectively eight months, three and a half years, two years and six years. One of these had had two attacks of gonorrhea, and another had suffered from fever in the recovery from her first abortion, presumably from some inflammatory process.

From these figures it is evident that previous sterility in cases of tubal pregnancy is certainly not dependent upon any one factor and that it is not necessarily a premise to extra-uterine gestation. But I would like to emphasize this point in this class of case, that the inaptitude to conception when it does occur, is probably the underlying cause of the ectopic pregnancy, and that the tubal pregnancy, on the other hand, does not depend upon the sterility. In other words, the anamnesis of the patient should not mislead the physician because a period of relative sterility has been noted.

Para.—Of the thirty patients, seven had never been previously pregnant, and four others had aborted but had never gone to term. Twelve had had one child, six had given birth to two children, and one had had four, one five, and one eleven full term births. One of the patients had been previously operated for tubal pregnancy on the other side and had never otherwise been pregnant. Two patients had had abortions before a final gravidity which went to term.

Age.—The oldest patient of the series was 41, the youngest 21 years of age, the average age of the thirty cases being 27.9 years. I have appended as the briefest form of expression, the following table:

Age	21	22	23	24	25	27	28	30	31	32	33	34	35	37	41
Cases	1	2	5	2	1	4	1	4	1	1	1	4	1	1	1

Tube involved.—Among the thirty cases there was one hematocele, the character of the operation for which (posterior vaginal section) did not permit a determination of which tube had been involved. Another case was an intramural pregnancy with the typical history of an ectopic pregnancy. Of the remaining twenty-eight, fourteen pregnancies were found on the right side and the same number on the left, a distribution so even that it is impossible to speak of a predilection for the condition to attack either side.

Dysmenorrhea.—In but twenty-three of the cases is any note made of the character of the usual menstruation. Of these, fourteen are said to have no pain with the menstrual flow and nine are given as having had painful menses. These figures have no especial significance except, possibly, to indicate that the fourteen patients, at least, were not suffering from any gross pathological changes in the pelvic organs.

The bleeding.—The subject of metrorrhagia has naturally been carefully studied. In three of the cases the data are missing. In twenty-seven cases the average length of time preceding admission at which the patient last menstruated was 7.24 weeks. The shortest time at which the regular period had taken place was two weeks prior to admission. This was a case of tubal abortion in which there had been no external bleeding whatever. Two patients had menstruated last as long as three months before applying for admission, in one of them a hematocele was found, in the other a hematosalpinx of the left side. Between these extremes every variety of irregularity in menstruation is noted.

In every case but one there is a history of irregularity in the menstrual flow, and this point is of great importance in the consideration of the history of patients suspected of being the bearers of a tubal pregnancy. The usual statement, crudely put, involves a skipping of the period at the regular time with some bleeding before the time for the arrival of the next regular period. The variations show the most widely different phases. Thus, in one case (No. 184, a tubal rupture*), the last menses before admission had taken place seven weeks previously, and there had been no bleeding or spotting of any kind up to the hour of operation. The other extreme is seen in No. 186, a tubal abortion, in which there had been constant bleeding for eleven weeks prior to admission after an amenorrhea of two

*The numbers refer to the gynecological cases for the year.

weeks. Between these two forms every variety of hemorrhage can be found.

It must be noted, however, that *profuse bleeding in ectopic pregnancy is a rarity*, and that its presence may usually be regarded as a sign that the condition is rather one of interrupted uterine pregnancy. In our series but four patients reported their bleeding as profuse, and in none of these did it last more than two weeks out of five or six weeks of unusual hemorrhage. A further study of the cases reveals the fact that *profuse bleeding is recorded only in cases of rupture of the tube or of hematocele*, and it also appears that the bleeding became more profuse at the presumptive time of rupture or abortion.

Scant bleeding or spotting is the rule in the majority of cases of ectopic pregnancy, while a moderate metrorrhagia is also not infrequently noted. In our thirty cases, eight patients reported slight spotting, four profuse bleeding, eleven moderate hemorrhage and two no bleeding whatever. One patient (No. 183, ruptured tube one day before admission), had bled profusely only the day before her operation.

The question of intermittent or of constant bleeding has been carefully investigated. Of the thirty cases, there are notes of 26 on this point. Sixteen of the patients bled constantly for a certain length of time and the flow subsequently became intermittent. In ten cases the bleeding was of an intermittent nature only. In the former series of sixteen we find many varieties in the character of the flow, some bleeding a little every day, some bleeding constantly for a time the flow later becoming intermittent, and others bleeding for a time with subsequent entire cessation of the flow. There is evidently, then, no type of vaginal bleeding in cases of ectopic pregnancy, the main element which marks it being its great irregularity.

The appended table shows clearly the type of bleeding in the twenty-six cases.

In the table the period of amenorrhea is likewise given. This naturally varies with the length of the pregnancy, but there are evidently other factors which come into play. The varyingly intense congestion of the uterine mucosa in different cases (Cazeaux, *Revue prat. d'obstetrique et de pediatrie*, Nov., 1903) accounts for the hemorrhage from this organ and for its appearance at different times in different cases. It is probable, too, that the casting off of the

Case No.	Probable Duration of Pregnancy.	Period of Amenorrhea.	Type of Bleeding.
284	1 month	None	Constant.
285	2 months	1 month	Constant for 1 month.
276	1 month	1 month	Constant.
275	5 weeks	1 week	Constant for 1½ weeks.
274	5 weeks		Intermittent.
273	11 weeks	2 weeks	Constant for 6 weeks.
272	2 months	6 weeks	Constant for 2 weeks.
278	6 weeks	2 weeks	Constant.
279	3 weeks	6 days	Constant for 6 days.
280	2½ months	9 weeks	Constant for 2 days before admission.
281	5 weeks	17 days	Intermittent.
282	7 weeks	2 weeks	Constant for 2 weeks; amenorrhea for 19 days; constant since.
178	9½ weeks	2 weeks	Constant for 5 weeks.
179	8 weeks	6 weeks	Intermittent.
181	2 months	5 weeks	Constant for 3 weeks.
182	2 months	1 week	Intermittent
184	1 month	2 weeks	Constant for 2 weeks.
185	3 months	2 weeks	Intermittent.
186	3 months	7 weeks	Intermittent.
271	2½ months	3 weeks	Intermittent
269	8 weeks	5 weeks	Constant for 3 weeks.
270	6 weeks	4 weeks	Intermittent.
187	1 month	11 days	Constant for 5 days, then intermittent.
189	7 weeks	4 weeks	Constant for 3 weeks.
192	7 weeks	4 weeks	Constant.
277	7 weeks	4 weeks	Constant for 2 weeks.

uterine decidua has some bearing on the metrorrhagia. In the present series of cases the longest period of amenorrhea was nine weeks, the average for the thirty cases being 3.4 weeks. In one instance there was no amenorrhea at all, the flow starting at once upon the cessation of the menses.

Pain.—Next to irregular bleeding, the most characteristic symptom of ectopic pregnancy is pain of one character or another. The character of the pain varies considerably. Three of the patients described their pains as *like those of labor*, differentiating them sharply from the cramplike pain sometimes seen in tubal pregnancy. It is likely that these labor pains are only the accompaniment of the expulsion of shreds of uterine decidua or of blood from the uterus, for all these patients added that their pains were followed or accompanied by the appearance of blood. In two of these cases there was found a ruptured tube, in one a tubal abortion.

Eight patients described their pains as *sudden and sharp*, localized, as it appeared, over the affected tube, and varying from two weeks to two days before admission in its appearance. Of these, four presented ruptured tubes, two, tubal abortions, and one each a hematosalpinx and an unruptured tube.

Eleven patients complained of *cramp-like pains in the abdomen*. In some of the cases this was not sharply localized but extended over the entire abdomen or its lower part. In the greater number of instances, however, the cramps were referred to the region of the affected tube. Their intensity, too, varied, some patients complaining of intense pain, others averring that it was only uncomfortable. Of these eleven cases five were found at operation to be hematosalpingitides, three were tubal ruptures, two were tubal abortions and one was an unruptured tube. The cramp-like pain is now generally and quite properly accredited to the effort of the tube to rid itself of its contained ovum, or if this has already escaped, of the clot remaining in its lumen.

Bearing down pains were noted by four patients, two of them in cases of ruptured tubes, two in cases of tubal abortion. Of these one was an intraligamentous rupture with the development of a large mass, one was an hematocele, and the other two showed moderate amounts of blood in the general peritoneal cavity.

One patient complained of pain only when sitting, which was relieved by lying down, and two patients had greater pain on walking than at other times, one of these (a patient with a ruptured tube) having noted a sense of fullness in the pelvis on standing and walking. But a single patient said she had no pain whatever, her tube being the seat of a hematoma.

There are, as will be seen, no typical or classical pains by which we can distinguish the various forms of ectopic gestation. In cases of hematoma and tubal abortion cramp-like pains appear to be more common, but they are seen also in other forms of extra-uterine pregnancy. It is unfortunate that we can find no differential points to distinguish the various types of clinical signs; the examining finger must after all remain the principal guide to accurate diagnosis.

Twelve patients stated the character of their pains as *constant or intermittent*, four saying they were continuous and six intermittent, two having pain which varied in its intermittency, at times being constant. There seems to be no relation, however, between the lesion and the constancy or intermittent character of the pain.

There were frequent complaints of *vomiting after onset of pain*, twelve patients emphasizing this fact. Of these, six were the subjects of ruptured tubes, one of an unruptured tube, two each of a hematosalpinx and a tubal abortion, and one of an intramural pregnancy. Unquestionably this vomiting was of so-called reflex character, provoked often by the presence of blood in the general peritoneal cavity, all the patients but one having this condition present. It is likely, too, that the pelvic peritonitis which often accompanies ectopic pregnancy may account for the vomiting.

Symptoms of pregnancy.—Six of our patients considered themselves pregnant at the time of their admission. They had reached this conclusion on account of their symptoms—the amenorrhea, nausea, and vomiting, frequent urination and painful breasts.

It does not always follow that an ectopic pregnancy is necessarily accompanied by the usual recognized symptoms of intra-uterine pregnancy. Indeed, these symptoms are often strikingly absent. I have carefully gone over the histories of these thirty patients, however, and find that while in seven no record at all is given the remaining twenty-three showed some interesting facts. Thus, eleven of them suffered from *nausea and vomiting* while five had no such phenomena. Three had noticed *enlargement of the breasts* but seven had not observed this, nor had any of the patients noted the darting signs so common in early pregnancy. Four complained of *frequent urination* while nine did not suffer from this annoyance.

The following table shows clearly the relation of type of pain to the lesion found at operation:

	Labor Pains.	Sharp and Sudden Pain.	Cramp-like Pain.	Bearing-down Pain.
Tubal rupture	2	4	3	2
Tubal abortion	1	2	2	2
Hematosalpinx	..	1	5	..
Unruptured tube	..	1	1	..

A resumé of these figures shows quite plainly that while the phenomena of early pregnancy are not by any means incompatible with the presence of an ectopic pregnancy, they are absent more frequently than they are found; a history of pregnancy, on the other hand, does not militate against the diagnosis of a pregnancy located in the tube.

OTHER SYMPTOMS.

Pulse and temperature.—In the cases of freshly ruptured tubal pregnancies the pulse was naturally much accelerated. In three of the cases it was imperceptible at the wrist at the time of operation, but these patients all recovered, a demonstration of the oft repeated observation that women stand the loss of blood well. In other cases, usually those of rupture, the pulse was often 120 or higher at the time of admission. Unless there has been considerable bleeding, however, there seems to be no especial tendency toward rapidity of the pulse in tubal pregnancy.

The temperature, on the other hand, is usually somewhat elevated. Eighteen of our thirty cases had temperatures above the normal before operation. Eight of the thirty patients were operated upon immediately after admission and their temperatures were, therefore, not taken. Fifteen of the eighteen who had elevated temperatures had blood in the general peritoneal cavity either from rupture of the tube or from tubal abortion. Their temperatures were as follows:

99–100°	100–101°	101–102°	104°	
9	8	1	1	(infected hematocele.)

It is plain, therefore, that omitting consideration of inflammatory conditions, the preoperative temperature in cases of tubal pregnancy is due to the presence of blood in the free peritoneal cavity. While it is needless to consider the elements which cause a rise of temperature in the presence of a foreign body of any kind in the peritoneum, we know that blood and even salt solution will bring this about. It must not be forgotten, however, that, as mentioned above, a pelvic peritonitis of more or less severity is a usual complication of tubal pregnancy and this may serve too as a causative factor of the temperature.

The practical bearing of moderately elevated temperature, when infection of any kind can be excluded, in the differential diagnosis of tubal pregnancy, is evident. A normal or ordinary uterine abortion, with which this condition is most frequently confused, gives rise to no deviation of temperature. Given a history, then, suggestive of tubal pregnancy, with a moderate rise of temperature, the suspicion will be strengthened if the other essentials for the diagnosis are present.

Tenderness.—One point which has been brought out with great clearness in this study is that the mass which is felt next to the uterus in cases of tubal pregnancy is almost invariably tender. The text-books but barely mention this fact; indeed, few of them speak of it at all.

We have found that *tenderness on palpation* is a very constant finding in all our cases of ectopic gestation. Among the thirty cases a note is made in twenty-three of the result of the pelvic examination in this particular. In twenty-two of these the record distinctly states that tenderness or sensitiveness was present over the mass adjacent to the uterus, in the great majority of cases exquisite tenderness being complained of. This was entirely independent of the character of the lesion present; it was found equally in cases of tubal abortion, of ruptured and unruptured tubes, and of hematoceles. The cause of this sensitiveness lies, undoubtedly, either in the compression of the distended tube or in the peritoneal adhesions so often present.

Whatever its origin, it offers a practical diagnostic point taken in connection with a history suggestive of ectopic gestation.

Abdominal rigidity.—Ectopic pregnancy seems to offer an exception to many intra-abdominal lesions in that the abdominal wall is not often rigid. Rigidity is noted in six of our cases, while in five the abdominal wall was especially lax. In other words, the abdominal wall may or may not be rigid but its absence or presence has no diagnostic significance.

Previous Pelvic Disease.—In view of the widespread belief or, at least, frequent assertion, that inflammatory pelvic disease is a prominent factor in the causation of extra-uterine pregnancy, I have carefully investigated the histories and operative findings in the thirty cases to ascertain the extent to which this held true. Two of the patients gave a history of fever following a former puerperium; in one of these a hydrosalpinx was found opposite the affected tube, in the other the pelvic organs were normal. One patient only had had previous gonorrhea and another had been operated for pyosalpinx on the other side a year previously.

But one patient in the whole series presented a typical history of pelvic inflammation. She had had repeated abortions, and after her third labor had suffered from a purulent endometritis. At the operation for her tubal pregnancy, there was found an intense pelvic peritonitis on the left side with an unruptured tubal pregnancy in the tube which ran over a large ovarian cyst. On the right side there was a smaller, adherent ovarian cyst. No other patients presented pelvic inflammations of any kind.

We have, then, but five patients, or 16 per cent., who gave any evidence of previous pelvic inflammatory processes.

Whatever may ultimately prove to be the etiological factor or factors of ectopic pregnancy, it is certainly evident that a previous gonorrhea or pelvic inflammation alone are not responsible for it. It seems rational to believe that not one, but many elements enter into the causation of the condition. In one case it may be endometrial, or pelvic inflammation, or a congenital or acquired tubal anomaly, while in another it may be atavistic or improper or premature nidation of the ovum, or the fault may even lie with the spermatozoa. We do not know, and it is unwise and unscientific to allege that any one of the elements named or other factors are responsible for the many cases of ectopic pregnancy constantly coming under observation.

CONCLUSIONS.

1. Sterility does not necessarily precede the development of ectopic pregnancy. If it does exist its cause is often the same as the cause of the abnormal pregnancy.

2. The main element of the bleeding in ectopic gestation is its great irregularity, there being no type. As a general rule it is not profuse. It may be constant or intermittent, and its character or profuseness has no relation to the type of the lesion. A chilly feeling often accompanies the bleeding, and vomiting and nausea may accompany the first flow. The uterine flow has apparently no connection with the death of the fetus.

3. The pain in tubal pregnancy is usually localized over the site of the lesion. It has no definite character; it may be cramp-like over the affected tube, it may simulate labor pains, it may be sharp and sudden, or it may be of a bearing down nature. The pain during a tubal abortion and that concomitant with the presence of a hematosalpinx is usually cramp-like.

4. The usual symptoms of pregnancy may be present. They are frequently absent but their absence does not militate against the possibility or probability of an ectopic pregnancy.

5. Tenderness on palpation of the mass adjacent to the uterus is of great diagnostic value when taken in connection with the history and the other pelvic findings.

6. A rise of temperature between 99° and 100°, in the absence of signs of infection, is worthy of consideration in the diagnosis.

7. The causative factors of tubal pregnancy are probably numerous. Not one element but many may bring about the condition in different instances. It is likely that atavistic tendencies, congenital or acquired anomalies, pelvic inflammations, ovarian and tubal disease, all play a role in individual cases; but none of these factors alone is sufficient to explain all cases.

8. We have as yet no definite data by which we can differentiate diagnostically between all the varieties of ectopic gestation. Occasionally this may be done, but it is impossible always to distinguish between an unruptured tube and a tubal mole. An hematocele and a freshly ruptured tube can almost always be differentiated from the other usual lesions.

The value of Werth's dictum, to regard every unruptured tube in the light of a malignant neoplasm, has not diminished with the years.

SPECIAL CASE.

H. N. VINEBERG, M.D.,
ADJUNCT GYNECOLOGIST.

Extra-uterine pregnancy; full term; total extirpation of placenta and uterus; recovery.—Mrs. R. S., aged 28, married 6 years. Menses set in in the twelfth year, regular four weekly, amount scanty, attended with pain in both hips; had never missed a period until September 1, and has not menstruated since then. She had never had either nausea or vomiting; had never felt any fetal movements. Was supposed to have had labor pains of some kind in April; was an inmate of a prominent city hospital during May; had been examined by several of the attending staff but no conclusions were reached.

The patient was brought to me on July 27, 1904. Her physician said that on June 19 she had pain resembling labor pains lasting the entire day, but there was no discharge of blood from the vagina then or at any other time. The patient had lost a great deal of flesh, her usual weight being 140 pounds but she now weighs only 112 pounds. The patient said that her abdomen began to enlarge two months after cessation of menses and the enlargement continued to increase until about a month ago; since then the abdomen has diminished somewhat in size. At the time of her visit to me she was very anemic, cheeks sunken and she presented a somewhat cachectic appearance.

On examining the abdomen it was found to be distended to a size corresponding to pregnancy at about full term. On palpation two distinct masses could be made out, the larger one on the right side reaching to near the liver, the smaller one on the left side reaching about half way between the umbilicus and the ensiform cartilage. No fetal movements could be felt and no fetal heart sounds heard. In the right lower quadrant a distinct bruit could be heard.

On vaginal examination the whole of Douglas' cul-de-sac was filled with a slightly nodular mass, somewhat hard and continuous with the pelvic wall; it was not movable. In front of this and projecting above the symphysis the uterus could be outlined. It was enlarged to the size of a gravid organ at about the eighth week. It was patulous and as far as the finger could reach it was found empty, but the finger could not reach much beyond the internal os. The breasts were enlarged and on pressure milk flowed from the nipples.

The question of diagnosis was not as easy as it would seem from subsequent events. The cachectic appearance of the patient, the loss of flesh and the hard nodular mass felt filling the pelvis could readily lead to a diagnosis of a malignant growth with a condition of "missed abortion." However, I was inclined to look upon the case as one of extra-uterine pregnancy going beyond term and advised immediate operation. The patient entered Mt. Sinai Hospital two days later, and was operated upon by me on the 31st.

On opening the abdomen a dark, bluish membrane was found extensively and closely adherent to the abdominal parietes, so that it was difficult to tell when the peritoneal cavity was entered. Finally, when the peritoneal cavity was entered the condition was not so easily made out. This bluish membrane covered the two masses above described and the enlarged uterus lay in front of them. On palpating the abdominal contents I decided that the head of the fetus lay toward the left side, and accordingly incised the bluish membrane at that point, and seized the child's head, which lay deep in the left pelvic fossa, hidden in part by the uterus, and rapidly extracted the child. At this time the placenta, which was extensively adherent to the right side of the abdominal wall, was torn in a measure and bled very profusely, so that it had to be clamped. Making a rapid survey of the condition, I concluded that my only chance of getting the patient off the table alive would be to do a rapid hysterectomy and enucleation of the placenta which occupied the right broad ligament, the entire pelvic cavity, and extended up on the right side to a line with the umbilicus. I, therefore, began by ligating the left ovarian vessels, the left uterine artery, then cut the uterus across, ligated the right uterine artery and rapidly enucleated the placenta from below upward as one would a large intra-ligamentous cyst. There were extensive adhesions of the membrane with the intestines; these were in part cut with the scissors and in part torn through, but some of the membrane could not be removed and it was sutured into the edges of the abdominal wound. The portion of the cervix that was left was quite patulous and readily admitted a strip of iodoform gauze. The abdomen was closed with through-and-through sutures excepting at its central part, to which the membranes were sutured.

In spite of rapid work, the whole operation not taking more than thirty-five minutes, the patient had to be given two intra-venous saline infusions.

The patient made a satisfactory recovery and was up out of bed at the end of three weeks. The abdominal fistula took about two weeks longer to close entirely.

A. Sittner* collected all cases of abdominal pregnancy from 1813 to 1900. He divided the cases into various periods. For purposes of comparison we may take the period from 1891 to 1900. There were

*Archiv. f. Gyn., Bd. lxiv., p. 527.

26 patients in whom the placenta was left *in situ*, with a mortality of 34.5 per cent. During the same period there were 37 patients in whom the placenta was removed at the time of the operation, with a mortality of only 10.8 per cent. Taking another period, 1896 to 1900, there were 12 patients with placenta left *in situ*, with a mortality of 33.3 per cent., and 16 patients with removal of the placenta, with a mortality of only 5.5 per cent. In several of the patients in which the placenta was removed, the uterus was also removed when it was extensively adherent to the gestation sac, or in other instances when it had to be done to arrest hemorrhage.

It will be thus seen that the mortality is increased sixfold when the placenta is left *in situ*, and on analyzing the individual cases, the best results were obtained when the neighboring organs were also removed. In many cases, however, such a radical procedure is not called for. It is only called for when the placenta develops within the folds of the broad ligament and is extensively attached to the pelvic organs. Cases are sometimes seen in which the placenta and gestation sac form a well-defined tumor with a pedicle. These are the simplest cases, from a surgical standpoint, and are as easily handled as a simple ovarian cyst.

THE GENITO-URINARY SERVICE.

H. GOLDENBERG, M.D.,
VISITING SURGEON.

MARTIN W. WARE, M.D.,
ADJUNCT SURGEON.

Thanks to the munificence of the gift of the late Mr. Joel Goldberg, patients afflicted with genito-urinary ailments are cared for in a ward by themselves with twelve beds, capable of eventually accommodating fifteen patients. The equipment specially provided for by this bequest has made it possible to attain such excellent asepsis that the most we can say for this service, of such recent date, is that urethral fever has been reduced to a minimum, thereby materially shortening the stay of patients in the hospital and lowering the mortality from such cause.

The efficiency of the service, furthermore, has been maintained at its height by the co-operation of the X-ray department and the laboratory, to the heads of both of which the best thanks are tendered.

	Total.	Cured.	Improved.	Unimproved.	Died.
1. Diseases of the Penis.—3 CASES; 0 DEATHS.					
1. Phimosis	1	1	..	..	..
2. Hypospadias	2	..	1	1*	..
2. Diseases of the Urethra.—22 CASES; 1 DEATH.					
1. Urethritis, acute (gonorrhea)	1	..	1*	..	..
2. Urinary fistula (secondary)	4	2	1	1*	..
3. Rupture of (traumatic)	1	..	1	..	..
4. Stricture of	7	7‡	..	..	..
5. Rupture of (secondary to stricture)	3	2	1	..	..
6. Polyp of	2	1	1	..	..
7. Periurethral abscess	3	2	..	..	1
8. Spasmodic stricture	1	..	1*	..	..

*Not operated.   ‡2 cases not operated.

	Total.	Cured.	Improved.	Unimproved.	Died.
3. Diseases of the Prostate.—13 CASES; 2 DEATHS.					
1. Hypertrophy	8	1	2†	3‡	2
2. Inflammation of (acute)	1	1*	..	..	..
3. Abscess of	2	2	..	..	..
4. Tuberculosis of	1	..	..	1*	..
5. Prostatism	1	..	1*	..	..
4. Diseases of the Bladder.—13 CASES; 4 DEATHS.					
1. Inflammation of	4	1*	2*	1*	..
2. Tuberculosis of	2	..	2*	..	..
3. Calculus of	5	3	..	..	2
4. Carcinoma of	2	..	..	..	2
5. Diseases of the Kidney.—5 CASES; 1 DEATH.					
1. Pyelonephritis	1	..	..	..	1*
2. Tuberculosis	3	2	1*	..	..
3. Calculus of	1	1	..	..	..
6. Diseases of the Testicle.—35 CASES; 0 DEATHS.					
1. Epididymo-orchitis, acute	13	8*	4*	1*	..
2. Tuberculosis of	4	2	1*	1*	..
3. Sinus following orchidectomy for tuberculosis	2	..	2†	..	..
4. Hydrocele	3	3	..	..	..
5. Varicocele	11	10	..	1*	..
6. Hydrocele and varicocele	1	1	..	..	..
7. Hematocele of tunica vaginalis	1	1	..	..	..
7. Diseases of the Rectum.—4 CASES; 1 DEATH.					
1. Hemorrhoids	2	2	..	..	..
2. Periproctitic abscess	2	1	..	..	1
8. Diseases of the Inguinal Lymph Nodes.—3 CASES; 0 DEATHS.					
1. Suppuration of	3	3	..	..	..
9. Unclassified Diseases.—9 CASES; 0 DEATHS.					
1. Inguinal hernia	1	1	..	..	..
2. Syphilis (not treated)	2	..	..	2*	..
3. Neurasthenia sexualis	2	1*	1*	..	..
4. Abdominal tumor	1	..	..	1*	..
5. Subacute appendicitis	1	1	..	..	..
6. Arthritis (gonorrheal)	1	..	1*	..	..
7. No diagnosis (refused examination)	1	..	..	1*	..
Total	107	60	24	12	9

*Not operated.   †1 case not operated.   ‡2 cases not operated.

1. Operations on Penis.

	Total.	Cured.	Improved.	Unimproved.	Died.
1. Circumcision for phimosis............................	1	1	..	..	..
2. Urethroplasty for hypospadias........................	1	..	1	..	..

2. Operations on Urethra.

	Total.	Cured.	Improved.	Unimproved.	Died.
1. External urethrotomy for stricture of.................	4	3	1	..	..
2. Internal urethrotomy for stricture of.................	5	4	1	..	..
3. External urethrotomy for rupture of....	1	1	..	..	..
4. Secondary suture of perineum.........................	6	4	2	..	..
5. Excision of urinary fistula...........................	1	1	..	..	..
6. Incision and drainage for periurethral abscess........	3	2	..	..	1
7. Multiple incision and drainage for extravasation of urine...	2	2	..	..	..
8. Ecrassement for polyp of.............................	1	1	..	..	..

3. Operations on Prostate.

	Total.	Cured.	Improved.	Unimproved.	Died.
1. Suprapubic prostatectomy for hypertrophy of...........	2	..	1	..	1
2. Perineal prostatectomy for hypertrophy of.............	3	1	1	..	1
3. Bottini operation for hypertrophy of..................	1	..	1	..	..
4. Incision and drainage for prostatic abscess...........	2	2	..	..	..

4. Operations on Bladder.

	Total.	Cured.	Improved.	Unimproved.	Died.
1. Suprapubic cystotomy and drainage for calculus of.....	4	3	..	..	1
2. " " for tuberculosis of................	1	..	..	..	1
3. " " and drainage with partial resection of bladder and implantation of ureter...................	1	..	..	..	1
4. Litholopaxy for calculus of...........................	1	..	..	..	1

5. Operations on Kidney.

	Total.	Cured.	Improved.	Unimproved.	Died.
1. Nephrectomy for tuberculosis of.......................	2	2	..	..	..
2. Nephrotomy for calculus...............................	1	1	..	..	..

6. Operations on Testicle.

	Total.	Cured.	Improved.	Unimproved.	Died.
1. Orchidectomy for tuberculosis of......................	2	2	..	..	..
2. Excision of secondary sinus (tuberculosis) of.........	1	..	1	..	..
3. Winkelman operation for hydrocele.....................	4	4	..	..	..
4. Injection of carbolic acid for hydrocele..............	1	1	..	..	..
5. Excision of veins for varicocele......................	11	11	..	..	..
6. Incision and drainage for hematocele of tunica vaginalis....	1	1	..	..	..

7. Operations on Rectum.

	Total.	Cured.	Improved.	Unimproved.	Died.
1. Clamp and cautery for hemorrhoids.....................	2	2	..	..	..
2. Incision and drainage for periproctitic abscess.......	2	1	..	..	1

	Total	Cured	Improved	Unimproved	Died
8. Operations on Inguinal Lymph Nodes.					
1. Incision and drainage for suppuration of	2	2	..	..	..
2. Curettage for necrosis of	1	1	..	..	..
9. Operations on Inguinal Hernia.					
1. Bassini operation	1	1	..	..	..
10. Operations on Appendix.					
1. Appendectomy	1	1	..	..	..
Total	72	55	9	0	8

POISONING BY WOOD ALCOHOL.

A CASE OF COMPLETE BLINDNESS (TRANSITORY) WITH RECOVERY OF VISION

By CARL KOLLER, M.D.,
ADJUNCT ATTENDING SURGEON (EYE AND EAR DEPARTMENT).

The knowledge of the poisonous properties of wood alcohol, and especially of its deleterious effects on the vision, is of very recent date; in fact, it is within only about five years that it has become generally recognized by the medical profession. Of the fifty-four cases collected from literature and tabulated by Buller in his and Casey A. Wood's valuable monograph on "Poisoning by Wood Alcohol" (read at the fifty-fifth annual session of the American Medical Association, in 1904), only four cases antedate the year 1899. These four were published respectively in 1879, 1888, 1897 and 1898. The other fifty cases were published between 1899 and 1904. Upon inquiry instituted among the profession in the United States and Canada, Wood has been able to add one hundred and eighty-one cases of partial or complete blindness, blindness followed by death, or death without history of previous blindness—all of recent years. It is very likely that sporadic cases occurred in former years (and were perhaps attributed to other causes). The present alarming increase in blindness and death caused by poisoning with wood alcohol is due directly to refinement in its manufacture by which it is rendered odorless. The nauseous odor adhering to the product by the old process limited its use to purposes of the arts and trades, for instance, as a solvent of shellac, etc.; and, although poisoning by the fumes occasionally did occur, poisoning by drinking was quite out of the question.

Since an odorless product under the name of "Columbian Spirits," colonial spirits, or eagle spirits has been put on the market, its uses have been largely increased, and not only its legitimate use but it has to a very large extent entered into the adulteration of alcoholic beverages, into the manufacture of flavoring substances meant for consumption, and into the preparation of proprietary remedies in which only ethyl alcohol should have been used. Many cases of blindness and death have followed the ingestion of Jamaica ginger, lemon extract, essence of lemon, essence of peppermint, bay rum, cologne water, witch hazel, etc.

The sensation produced in this city quite recently, through the sudden death of a considerable number of men (variously stated at 17 to 25), in a certain district, who had fallen victims to the consumption of whiskey adulterated with wood alcohol, is still fresh in everybody's memory. Under these circumstances, the publication of the following case, which presents some interesting features, appears sufficiently justified.

S. G., a Russian Hebrew, forty-two years of age, presented himself on October 28, 1904, at Dr. I. Abrahamson's clinic for nervous diseases in the Mt. Sinai dispensary. He was totally blind but perfectly rational. He had no idea what had caused his condition, and the history which he gave lacked, therefore, the most important element. He stated that he used tobacco and alcoholics very moderately, drank tea excessively, and enjoyed, in general, very good health, occasionally suffering from rheumatic pains. There was no history of syphilis.

He was referred to the eye department for an examination of his eyes, and, the true state of affairs being here suspected, the following history was elicited from him:

On Saturday, October 2, after the morning service, he took, at the house of some friends, a small quantity (about two ounces) of whiskey, but did not feel anything unusual until after eleven o'clock. P. M., when returning home from a meeting which he attended the same evening he felt chilly and nauseated, and vomited. He drank some tea and went to bed. The next day (Sunday) he went, according to his every-day custom, to morning and also to evening service, but neither ate nor drank. During the night he woke and noticed that the gaslight seemed dim. On Monday morning he rose at seven o'clock and as it appeared rather dark to him he asked if it was raining. Then he noticed that his vision was at fault, but ascribed it to his abstaining from food the previous days, and drank some tea. He could not read the ordinary print of the newspaper, although he was able to distinguish the large letters. He felt chilly and extremely weak and his hands were cold. As the day wore on, vision became worse, but toward evening of the same day he could indistinctly see, although not recognize, human figures. On the next morning (Tuesday) he was completely blind, all perception of light being gone. Various physicians were consulted but the condition remained unchanged. Total blindness persisted for the following four days. On Friday, October 28, he came to the dispensary. The *status præsens* was as follows:

"The pupils are widely dilated and absolutely without reaction. The optic nerves of both eyes present the picture of a neuroretinitis of moderate intensity. The outlines of the discs are indistinct; the radiating nerve fibres are opaque and somewhat edematous; the blood-vessels (arteries and especially the veins) congested. In the macular region of both eyes are dispersed numerous yellowish, bright-shining little spots, similar to the picture described as chorioiditis guttata."

On his way home from the clinic he saw with his right eye the first ray of light. This caused him to change his attitude toward our request for a sample of that whiskey of which he had partaken two days before the visual disturbances began, and at a subsequent visit he brought a quantity of it sufficient for chemical analysis. Dr. Carl Goldmark, chief of the dispensary pathological laboratory, made a qualitative test which showed the presence of methyl alcohol in the whiskey. As the test is very decisive and easy of execution, it might be useful to describe it in a few words. Dr. Goldmark says about it:

"The test depends upon the synthetic production of methyl salicylate (artificial oil of wintergreen). Beringer devised the method of producing methyl salicylate by taking half an ounce of salicylic acid, dissolving it in two ounces of absolute methylic alcohol, and then gradually adding one ounce of sulphuric acid.

"On this basis the suspected fluid was tested. To about two drachms of it, half a drachm of salicylic acid solution and one drachm of sulphuric acid were added in a test-tube. The odor of the oil of wintergreen was at once apparent, and became more pronounced the longer it stood."

Later, Dr. S. B. Bookman, of the Mt. Sinai pathological laboratory, made a quantitative analysis of the sample by fractional distillation, and found that it contained 34 per cent. of pure methyl alcohol. Our patient had, therefore, taken about 20 c.c. of pure methyl alcohol.

Potassium iodide was prescribed, and the patient was directed to take hot baths to induce free perspiration, and to nourish himself well. As a result of this course of treatment there was a gradual improvement in vision for the following two months. He did not present himself for an eye examination until December 21, when sent for; but, on November 18, we heard of him, that the right eye had steadily and quickly improved since the day of his first visit, and that the left eye had begun improving about two weeks later. When he was examined on December 21, vision of the right eye was 15-20, and that of the left 15-30. The outlines of the fields of vision were normal. The ophthalmoscopic examination showed a decided change. The discs were well outlined, and in their temporal halves very pale. The big vessels showed no abnormal calibre, perhaps the arteries were somewhat narrower than they should have been. The bright yellowish spots in the macular region of both eyes were decidedly increased in number.

The patient was lost sight of until sent for by the end of April, that is six months after the onset of the affection. His examination on April 23, 1905, gave the following result: The pupils were more than average size, about 6 mm. in diameter, in an ordinarily bright room. When his face was turned toward the strong light of the window, they became slowly narrower, 3 mm. in diameter. The reaction to strong changes of light was very sluggish. The vision of the right eye was 4-12 and with $+1$ sph. $\supset$ cyl. $+0.5$ ax. hor. it was 4-8, this improvement of the vision with a convex correcting glass in a man of forty-two years, who had not used glasses before, evidencing a weakness of the accommodation which is in keeping with the weakness of the pupillary reaction. The vision of the left eye was 6-36, the refraction the same as in the right eye, but the glass made no improvement. The field of vision of the right eye was normal in its outlines, no relative central scotoma. The field of the left eye showed moderate concentric contraction (about 15 degrees); no perception of green color; red recognized, and no relative central scotoma could be ascertained with this color. The ophthalmoscopic examination showed the optic discs opaque and very pale, bluish, edges fuzzy; lamina cribrosa visible; arteries narrow, especially those of second order; those of the third order hardly visible. A connective-tissue sheath accompanied the arteries a short distance from the nerve head. The veins were larger than usual, especially in the left eye. The retina was very thin, appeared atrophic. In the macular region of either eye were very numerous yellowish-white dots.

That methyl alcohol is a poison dangerous to eyesight and to life is now generally conceded, although not long ago it was disputed, sincerely by some and from interest by others, the chief contention being that not the methyl alcohol itself but admixed "impurities" produced the poisonous results. Of such, acetone was chiefly accused. The uncertainty was largely due to the fact that taken in small quantities methyl alcohol is innocuous to a great many persons, although taken in large quantities or habitually in moderate quantities it must be acknowledged as poisonous without exception. On the other hand, there are a great many people for whom a very small quantity (half a teaspoonful) would constitute a dose sure to bring on the gravest consequences. This difference, or "idiosyncrasy," well known in regard to every other poison, in the case of methyl alcohol is most likely due to the difference of secondary chemical compounds formed in the alimentary canal and in the blood of the different persons into whom it is ingested. One of these is formaldehyde, but whether it is or is not the chief factor of methyl alcohol poisoning is not decided.

In reviewing all the cases on record, Casey A. Wood comes to the conclusion that there are three degrees of wood alcohol poisoning: "(1) An ordinary, mild intoxication, with perhaps some dizziness, nausea, and mild gastro-intestinal disturbance, terminating in perfect recovery within a few days, but occasionally followed by more or less serious damage to vision. (2) A toxic effect more pronounced in every way, dizziness, nausea, and gastro-enteritis being conspicuous symptoms. Dimness of vision, often increasing to total blindness, is characteristic of this degree of poisoning. (3) An overwhelming prostration which terminates in coma and death."

The most conspicuous and characteristic feature of wood alcohol poisoning is complete bilateral blindness, appearing sometimes suddenly but in most cases gradually after a period of failing vision. The disturbance of vision will sometimes come after a few hours; in most cases it lasts from one to several days, until a dimness of the sight is noticed. (In our case it took about forty hours.) This progresses until the blindness is absolute. The interval between the ingestion of the poison and the onset of the eye symptoms is very characteristic, and may in some cases, as for instance in ours, hide the real cause of the blindness from the patient. The blindness lasts for a period of several days or even weeks, after which sight returns gradually. The improvement is frequently very considerable, sometimes full restoration takes place; but the improvement is not lasting. After several weeks the vision begins to fail again, and in the great majority of cases this progresses to final and irreparable blindness. Very few cases preserve useful vision; early treatment seems to be favorable to this termination.

Of the objective symptoms the only one constant from the beginning is widely dilated pupils without any reaction whatever. The ophthalmoscopic picture varies. Either it is entirely negative and thus corresponds with the usual assumption of a retrobulbar neuritis, or it shows a papillitis or neuroretinitis of low degree—slight swelling of the nervehead, blurring of the outlines, radiating appearance of the slightly edematous nerve fibres, and congestion of the large bloodvessels, especially the veins. This condition was present in our case in a rather marked degree. A third variety shows pallor of the disc from the outset, with contracted bloodvessels, so that although not so intense it is similar to the appearance in quinine poisoning. But whatever the picture in the beginning, in all cases we ultimately find atrophy of the optic nerve and retina, an extremely pale, bluish or grayish disc with outlines distinct but fuzzy; the large bloodvessels, especially the arteries, contracted, for some distance contoured by a connective-tissue sheath; no smaller bloodvessels or capillaries visible —in a word, the picture of postneuritic atrophy. Nowhere do I find mention made of the presence in the whole macular region, of the yellowish, bright spots described in the above case. I might consider them an accidental circumstance if I had not once seen the same condition in a man whom I treated for alcohol-and-tobacco amblyopia.

The field of vision shows anomalies in all cases. It is nearly always concentrically contracted, and generally there is an absolute or relative central scotoma present. In our case, after six months the right eye showed complete recovery of function (except a moderate diminution of acuteness of vision), probably owing to the small amount of poison ingested and the early institution of treatment. The left eye showed marked although moderate concentric contraction of the field, considerable diminution of central vision, and absence of perception of the green color. A central scotoma for other colors at that time could not be established.

As to the pathology underlying these visual disturbances, opinions are divided, some ascribing it to a retrobulbar neuritis, whereas others believe that the ganglion cells of the retina are the structure primarily affected, followed by ascending—or, rather, descending—atrophy of the optic nerve fibres. The writer is inclined to accept the latter view, although it must be admitted that a number of weighty arguments can be adduced for either of them.

With regard to the course of therapy to be followed in a case of wood alcohol poisoning, sweating by hot bath or pilocarpine, potassium iodide internally, and sufficient diuresis (perhaps by means of a milk diet) suggests itself as rational and has been successful in some cases.

The utmost importance belongs to prophylaxis. The public in

general must be enlightened as to the poisonous nature of this substance, and laws should be enacted forbidding its use in the manufacture of "essences" and proprietary remedies which may be the means of poisoning persons not addicted to the use of intoxicating drinks, and who are entirely ignorant of the danger to which they are exposed.

OBSERVATIONS ON THE THREAD REACTION; ITS OCCURRENCE IN THE HUMAN BODY.

By E. Libman, M.D.,
ADJUNCT VISITING PHYSICIAN, ASSISTANT PATHOLOGIST.

There have been, up to the present time, three forms of specific reactions described—the agglutination reaction, the thread reaction and the "amorphous agglutination reaction." The last named was described by Schmidt during the last year and will not be discussed here.

I wish to speak here on the thread reaction, partly to indicate the necessity for further work on the subject, and partly to put on record an instance of its occurrence in the human body.

The subject was first prominently brought forward by Pfaundler, although other observers had previously noted the phenomenon. Before Pfaundler, Achard showed that the blood of animals (guinea-pigs) acquired agglutinating properties against colon bacilli only with great difficulty. Achard, and Widal and Sicard, demonstrated that the reaction against a colon bacillus which had caused an infection in the human body occurred only exceptionally. Widal had shown that it is difficult to say when an agglutination reaction with a given colon bacillus is specific. Pfaundler investigated eight cases of (non-systemic) infection by colon bacilli (cases of cystitis, peritonitis, etc.). In each of these he obtained a positive reaction with the serum of the case and the respective bacillus at a dilution of at least one to one hundred, if the hanging-drop preparations were observed after twenty-four hours. In the febrile cases he obtained the thread reaction; in the others, a clump reaction. The thread reaction presented the following appearance:

The organisms were arranged in long interwoven threads, the latter being generally coiled in skeins. The spaces between the skeins or threads were clear and none of the bacilli was motile. Very few individual organisms or single groups of bacilli were found in the thread labyrinths. Upon observation with higher powers the organisms in the threads looked granular; some were club-shaped. The bacteria could be demonstrated to be alive. The threads were best seen in the weakest dilution with which it was still possible to obtain a reaction. The threads usually appeared after a few hours. In most cases there was more or less agglutination at first. Pfaundler in his experiments obtained positive reactions only when the patient's blood was tested with the organism causing the infection. He claimed, therefore, that the reaction represented more than a specific reaction, namely, an individualistic one. It is to be noted that the varieties of colon bacilli isolated from the cases differed very widely.

In some unpublished experiments made by the writer in 1898 it was found that the thread reaction was frequently obtained in cases of appendicitis and peritonitis due to the colon bacillus. Only colon bacilli which were closely allied in cultural characteristics were used. Fever was present in all of the cases. The general results of the observations were that the thread reactions occurring in a dilution of one to twenty, if they were complete, seemed to be specific, and no interaction between the various bacilli and a given serum was found. The experiments were too few in number, however, to prove distinctly the absence of any interaction, and in some cases agglutination reactions only were found. (In cases of proteus infection interactions were found.)

Krauss and Loew obtained thread reactions with a number of organisms, with homologous and heterologous sera (that is to say, with the serum from the case from which the organism was isolated, and from other cases) and threw doubt on the claims of Pfaundler. However, their dilutions were in the main very low and the characteristics of the bacilli used in the experiments are not detailed.

Pfaundler in a second paper attempted to show, by means of animal experiments, that the thread reactions obtained with a given serum and bacillus occur only as an individualistic reaction. He states that reaction is practically not as useful as the agglutination reaction, as it is inconstant.

Krauss in a second paper came to the following conclusions:

First.—That the thread reaction is a phenomenon which occurs with certain organisms under the influence of an agglutinating serum.

Second.—Agglutination always precedes it.

Third.—It is not as constant as agglutination.

Fourth.—In general, the same rules that apply practically for agglutination reactions apply for thread reactions, except as regards the bacterium coli.

He bases his conclusions on the occurrence of thread reactions with homologous and heterologous coli sera. He obtained the reaction with normal serum also, and says that it is therefore not specific. He concludes, however, that threads and agglutinations usually occur in specific dilutions and with the use of a homologous serum and a homologous colon bacillus. It is to be noted, however, that a study of Krauss's experiments shows that most of his tests were made with low dilutions. Only once did he obtain a thread reaction at a dilution of one to fifty with a normal horse serum and a heterologous colon bacillus. It is questionable how much value such an experiment has as regards reactions in the human body. It was only with the use of a homologous serum and a homologous colon bacillus that he obtained the thread reaction in a high dilution (one to two hundred).

In the paracolon case described by the writer two years ago, we found that the reaction of the serum with the paracolon bacillus always took the form of a thread reaction, and in that case we found that the reaction was distinctly individualistic. The reactions in that case were of the chain form, which I shall shortly describe. If agglutination reactions alone had been looked for, no specific reactions would have been found.

We found, several years ago, that the same serum with the same organism no longer gave the thread reaction after a number of days if the organism was transplanted daily. The length of time varied for different organisms. It seemed to us that the loss of the reaction was due to the artificial cultivation of the bacillus and not to a loss of power of the conserved serum. Further observations are needed upon this point.

Flexner, Kruse, Duval and Vedder, have noted the occurrence of the thread reaction with an organism more closely allied culturally to the typhoid bacillus than to the colon bacillus, namely, the dysentery bacillus. In their observations, however, the thread reaction was of the same significance as the agglutination reaction.

Recognizing the necessity for further investigation with regard to this subject, we have made observations in this connection whenever possible. We have found that there are two forms of thread reaction. In the first form the bacilli grow out in long, more or less convoluted threads, but still retain their bacillary form. This is the so-called "end to end" reaction. We have found this reaction occur under conditions such that we could be positive that the reaction could not be specific. At any rate, we are prepared to say that such a reaction is even less specific than the agglutination reaction.

In the other form of the thread reaction the organisms assume a coccoid form and on first viewing the hanging-drops one thinks that one is looking at chains of streptococci. This reaction, when complete, in our experience has been specific and individualistic under certain conditions. The reactions are best obtained by making an emulsion in bouillon from a culture of the organism on agar; the suspension must be a very dilute one, just enough of the culture being used to cause a distinct cloudiness. Normal saline solution was used in some of our experiments. Sugar-bouillon cultures should never be used, as in them bacilli of the colon group are apt to take on a coccoid form.

In one case in our observations we found the thread reaction occurring in the human body. The case was one of carcinoma of the duodenum with obstruction of the common bile-duct. (The clinical features of this case are described in full by Dr. Brill in the third volume of the Mt. Sinai Hospital Reports.)

At an exploratory operation made one day before death the gall-bladder was found very much dilated, the wall thickened from chronic inflammation and, on aspirating it, a fluid was obtained which was turned over to the laboratory for examination. The fluid was clear, not bile-stained, and at the bottom of the tube was a small amount of white granular matter. On examining this under the microscope we found what first appeared to be convoluted chains of streptococci. Recognizing the possibility of this really being an instance of the thread reaction occurring in the body, the sediment was stained with the Gram procedure and the organism was found decolorized. A culture made from fluid gave a pure growth of an organism resembling the dysentery bacillus morphologically and culturally. The serum of the patient gave a thread reaction (of the second form described above—the chain reaction) in a dilution of 1 to 1,000. The serum, when tested with colon bacilli, typhoid bacilli and paracolon bacilli, gave no reaction and the sera of a number of other patients suffering from various diseases gave no reaction with the bacillus. On staining the sediment found in the gall-bladder with the Neisser stain, it was found that the bodies which were seen which looked like cocci stained like polar bodies.

It has been shown by a number of authors that the colon bacillus can, under various conditions, assume the coccoid form. Livingood found that when the colon bacillus was inoculated upon media containing unheated liver juice oval forms developed. Rodet found such forms in cultures of the colon bacillus in lactose-bouillon and very often in old cultures of the colon bacillus. He also found the coccoid form in fluid obtained from diseased gall-bladders. Dunbar also noted chain formation of the colon bacillus.

In a very important paper published by Adami, Nicholson and Abbott, a number of very interesting observations on the coccoid form of the colon bacillus are recorded. They succeeded in obtaining coccoid forms of the colon bacillus by the use of acid media, by inoculation into animals, and they describe the occurrence of coccoid forms in bile, ascitic fluid and in the livers of man and a number of animals, both normal and diseased.

Ohlmacher has described a very interesting observation in this connection: In a case of gangrenous cholecystitis with cholangitis due to biliary calculi, the colon bacillus was isolated from the gallbladder, liver and other organs. In the first generation on agar plates very remarkable forms of the organism were found and it was only after three or four transplantations through bouillon that the usual form of the colon bacillus was found. The most marked peculiarities of form were found in the original smears from the gall-bladder and bile-ducts—all gradations from minute coccoid or diplococcoid to long, coarse filamentous forms were observed. Ohlmacher states that they corresponded precisely to those described by Adami, Abbott and Nicholson. Threads were found, some of which were quite thick, others were thin and delicate, some being quite shadowy. Some of the shorter ones showed a row of deeply staining inclusions and others still had clear unstainable spaces or areas with metachromatic staining. "These filaments were often aggregated into groups, several times appearing as a mass of tangled threads." Some of the shorter rods showed short true branches. Some of the filaments or longer rods had median swellings, others among the shorter rods had clubbed ends and many of them were bent at various angles. Ohlmacher was of the opinion that the polymorphism of the bacillus was to be ascribed to certain environmental influences resulting from its abode in the biliary apparatus of the human host.

The observations made in the case which I have described cannot, I believe, be traced to purely accidental influences, nor do I believe that they were due to the icteric condition of the serum, for in the gall-bladder itself the fluid was perfectly clear and not bile-stained, and in the second place the serum did not produce such changes in cultures of other closely related bacillary forms. The reaction must be regarded as a specific one due to the inflammation of the gall-bladder set up by the bacillus in question.

The observations recorded here are of a certain degree of importance because they indicate that we must be very careful in making a diagnosis of streptococci in hanging-drops; we must remember that we may be dealing with the coccoid forms of bacilli. Thus, I have found, in a number of instances, in the urine, long chains of what appeared to be streptococci, but on careful examination these have been found to be the coccoid forms of colon bacilli or other bacilli. In these cases it is probable that the acidity of the urine may have had much to do with the development of the coccoid forms. The difficulty can be avoided, at least to a great extent, by the use of the Gram stain, because up to the present time the thread reaction has been particularly noted with organisms that react negatively to the Gram procedure. In applying the Gram stain to urinary sediments it is important to remember that with very acid urines organisms which are naturally Gram-positive can very easily be decolorized.

LITERATURE.

1. PFAUNDLER: Centralblatt für Bakteriologie. 1898, vol. xxiii.
2. KRAUSS AND LOEW: Wiener klin. Wochenschrift. 1899, p. 95.
3. PFAUNDLER: Ibidem. 1899, p. 342.
4. KRAUSS: Ibidem. 1899, No. 29, p. 761.
5. FLEXNER: Centralblatt für Bakteriologie. Vol. xxx.
6. DUVAL AND VEDDER: Journal of Experimental Medicine. Vol. vi., No. 2.
7. LIBMAN: Journal of Medical Research. Vol. viii., p. 168.
8. LIVINGOOD: Centralblatt für Bakteriologie. Vol. xxiii., p. 980.
9. RODET: Archiv de physiologie norm. et patholog. 1896, p. 968.
10. DUNBAR: Zeitschrift für Hygiene. 1892, p. 485.
11. ADAMI, NICHOLSON AND ABBOTT: Journal of Experimental Medicine. Vol. iv., p. 349.
12. OHLMACHER: Journal of Medical Research. Vol. ii., p. 128.
13. SCHMIDT: Wiener klinische Wochenschrift. 1903, p. 873.
14. McWEENY: British Medical Journal. Sept. 3, 1898, p. 592. A note on the thread reaction with the typhoid bacillus.
15. Of interest in this connection is the paper by ADAMI on Latent Infection. Journal of American Medical Association. Dec. 16, 1899.

NOTES ON THE WIDAL REACTION: (1) THE QUESTION OF DILUTION; (2) THE INFLUENCE OF JAUNDICE.*

By E. Libman, M.D.,
ADJUNCT VISITING PHYSICIAN, ASSISTANT PATHOLOGIST.

The method used in making the tests upon which this paper is based was described in full in the Mt. Sinai Hospital Reports, Vol. I., and in the *Medical News*, March 29, 1902. As a rule, dried blood was used for the tests, but in quite a number of cases the tests were also made with serum. In the larger number of the cases of jaundice to which I shall later refer, serum was used. For the general practitioner the use of the dried blood is undoubtedly much more practical than the use of serum. We have found that the dried blood, if properly sent to the laboratory, gives practically the same results as serum. The drops used are best made a trifle larger than the head of a pin. Should larger drops be used care must be taken that the specimen be dried before the blood coagulates. In a large number of experiments we found that the blood gave a better reaction after three or four hours than when used just after drawing—even after twenty-four hours the dried blood gives good results.

Until the spring of 1902 we were accustomed to make our reactions in the dilution of 1 to 20 only, but as it was claimed by many authorities that reactions ought to be made in the dilution of 1 to 50, we made it a rule at that time to make our reactions in the dilution of 1 to 20 and 1 to 50 (time-limit thirty minutes and one hour respectively).

Previous to the spring of 1902 and since that time, we have examined the blood in 1,500 cases of fever. Of these, 550 were cases of typhoid fever. In the 950 cases which were not typhoid fever, a Widal reaction was never reported positive even in a dilution of 1 to 20. This certainly points to the reliability of a reaction in a dilution of 1 to 20 when interpreted according to the method of considering only complete reactions as being positive.

*From the New York Medical News, January 30, 1904.

We believe that it is advisable, if possible, to make such a standard in the judgment of reactions, that the report of a positive agglutination reaction to the physician should be equivalent to labeling his case as one of typhoid. The practising physician is not interested in a report saying his patient has or has not an agglutination reaction—he wants to know whether his patient has typhoid fever or not.

We will admit for the sake of argument that among the 550 cases of typhoid fever there may have been some cases of paracolon infection, and that the presence of the agglutination reaction in a dilution of 1 to 20 may simply have been a group-agglutination; but, if such a mistake does occur, it is not a serious one, for to the clinician a case of paratyphoid fever is to be considered and handled, at least for the present, as one of typhoid fever.

The question arises, why do we continue making reactions in a dilution of 1 to 50 if we have had such reliable results with a 1 to 20 dilution?

We have been surprised to find, in some instances, a positive result in a dilution of 1 to 50 when the reaction was negative or not clearly positive in a dilution of 1 to 20. There are, we believe, at least two explanations of what seems so anomalous a condition. In some instances, at least, it is due to the fact that in a dilution of 1 to 20 the lytic action of the serum is so marked that one cannot obtain a clear picture. In some cases the explanation lies in the existence of bodies known as proagglutinoids. According to Shiga the proagglutinoids are bodies which are developed from agglutinins through extraneous influences; they possess a greater affinity for the bacilli than the unchanged agglutins; they have lost the group (agglutinophore) which is the carrier of the peculiar agglutinating power, but have retained the other group (haptophore) upon which depends their attachment to the bacteria. Shiga[1] in a very interesting paper on this subject, after referring to the previous observations of Bail, Eisenberg and Falk, gives an account of his own experiments which prove the existence of such bodies. A short account of these experiments will, I think, be of interest here. By heating dysentery immune serum to 60°C. for an hour, or by shaking it with chloroform or exposing it to sunlight for a number of days, he obtained a serum which would agglutinate dysentery bacilli in high dilutions and not in low, whereas previously it had agglutinated in low dilutions as markedly, or even more markedly, than in high dilutions. He applied the term "proagglutinoid zone" to those dilutions in which the reaction disappeared. He not only succeeded in producing a proagglutinoid zone with typhoid immune serum by heating it for four hours at 60°C., but he could, by the prolonged addition of chloroform to dysentery serum, almost completely change the agglutinins into proagglutinoids so that a reaction could not be obtained in any dilution. Further experiments proved that the proagglutinoids were attached to the bacteria and that the proagglutinoid zone could be made to disappear if enough bacteria were added to a mixture of non-agglutinated bacteria and a serum containing proagglutinoids.

Notwithstanding the fact that a 1 to 50 dilution will occasionally give better results than a 1 to 20, it is necessary to make the 1 to 20 dilution, because this is frequently positive before the 1 to 50 dilution becomes positive. Among 165 cases of typhoid fever we found a coincident positive reaction in 1 to 20 and in 1 to 50 in 127 cases. In 12 cases the reaction was positive in a dilution of 1 to 20 two days before it was positive in 1 to 50. In some instances even sixteen days elapsed before the reaction became positive at 1 to 50, and in 8 cases which were positive in a dilution of 1 to 20 there was no reaction in a dilution of 1 to 50 during the time of observation of the patients in the hospital.

From all these data it is evident that it is essential in performing the agglutination test to use dilutions of 1 to 20 and 1 to 50. It is even possible that the 1 to 100 or higher dilutions might be positive when the lower ones are negative. On this point we have thus far had no experience.*

The other point upon which I wish to dwell is the question of whether or not jaundice *per se* can cause a positive Widal reaction. On this subject quite some observations have been made, which we shall detail before we refer to our experiences.

Honl and Eisenberg[2] and Heller[3] found that icteric serum was possessed of a certain amount of agglutinating power. Greenbaum[4]

*Since writing the above we have encountered one case of typhoid fever in which the reaction was absolutely complete in a dilution (approximate) of 1 to 400 in one hour, and negative at all dilutions below and above. After four hours, there was slight clumping at 1 to 200, and stoppage of motility at 1 to 800; 1 to 1,600 was absolutely negative. This case was a typical one in the practice of Dr. Albert Kohn. It would seem necessary, therefore, in cases suspected of being typhoid fever, to make the test in a large number of dilutions.

found a positive reaction in a dilution of 1 to 16 in cases of jaundice. The most extensive observations and experiments, however, were made by Koehler.[5] Koehler used for his experiments sugar-bouillon cultures of the typhoid bacillus; his time-limit was two hours and he considered clumps of four to be significant of the presence of agglutination. In 10 cases of disease of the liver, of which eight were icteric, he found an agglutination reaction present in six. The highest dilution in which he obtained the reaction was 1 to 40; very rarely 1 to 50, and once it was only 1 to 10. His first set of experiments was performed with several varieties of bile. In the bile of dogs in which the common bile-duct had been ligated, he found a decided agglutinating power (even up to 1 to 160). Rabbit's bile was possessed of very slight agglutinating power. Human bile obtained at autopsy occasionally showed a distinct agglutinating power (up to 1 to 80). He had no opportunity of testing bile obtained *intra vitam*. In the bile of typhoid patients post mortem he found no increase in agglutinating power over the bile in other diseases.

In attempting to ascertain what constituent of the bile was responsible for the presence of the agglutinating power, he tested taurochol, glycochol, bilirubin, biliverdin, cholalic acid, glycocholic acid, cholesterin and sodium taurocholate, but found that none of these was possessed of any agglutinating power. Solutions of taurocholic acid, however, gave some positive results (up to 1 to 60). He obtained no result with the serum of rabbits into which he had injected taurocholic acid, but did obtain some positive results in dogs. The reaction generally appeared two or three days after the injection and lasted several days. He obtained results even with some samples of taurocholic acid which in themselves were possessed of no agglutinating power. The serum of dogs in which the bile-ducts had been tied off gave a slight agglutination reaction which disappeared after a communication was established between the gall-bladder and the intestine. On later injecting taurocholic acid into such animals, an agglutination reaction could again be obtained varying in strength from 1 to 40 to 1 to 50. The results in these experiments were not constant.

These experiments of Koehler's are of great interest in showing that taurocholic acid and bile cause a certain amount of agglutination, but they are not significant practically because in making diagnoses by means of the Widal test we deal only with complete reactions. This remark also holds true of his observations on the presence of an agglutinating power in the serum of patients with jaundice. For practical purposes it is inadvisable to use sugar bouillon cultures, a time-limit of two hours is too long, and we shall see that later observations on the whole are contradictory.

Sailer[6] in three cases of intense jaundice obtained no reactions. Zupnik[7] in seven cases of jaundice (two cases of cholelithiasis, one case of cholecystitis and four cases of Weil's disease) found "a more or less positive reaction." In two other cases of Weil's disease the reaction was negative. In one case of carcinoma of the liver without fever he found a positive reaction. He used both macroscopic and microscopic reactions in a dilution of 1 to 40 with a time-limit of eight hours. It is unfortunate that he does not state what he considers to be a positive reaction, and the time-limit is too long.

Eckhardt[8] describes two cases with a clinical picture of Weil's disease of one month's duration in which the reaction was positive at times in a dilution of 1 to 1,000. In these cases the agglutination reaction persisted even after the jaundice had disappeared. In eight cases of jaundice he obtained a positive reaction in a dilution of 1 to 100 in two hours and in one case up to 1 to 1,000. The bile obtained at autopsy and the bile obtained from biliary fistulæ was devoid of agglutinating power. He cites one case of jaundice in which the bile gave no reaction but the blood gave a positive reaction in a dilution of 1 to 100. There was no history of any previous typhoid infection. We will cite a case later which demonstrates that such a condition of affairs can exist in typhoid fever. He also unfortunately does not state what he considers to be a positive reaction. He is of the belief that his cases were probably cases of typhoid fever and bases his belief mainly on the persistence of the reaction after the disappearance of the jaundice. No further bacteriological examinations were made in the cases. We are also inclined to consider that his cases were typhoid fever, but in view of the fact that he obtained positive reactions so often in other cases of jaundice, we believe that less stress should be laid upon the significance of the reactions. In any event, the cases do not prove that jaundice *per se* can cause a positive Widal reaction.

Langstein and Meerwein[9] also made observations in a number of cases of jaundice. Their first case was one of obstruction of the common bile-duct by gall-stones with adhesions about the gall-bladder. The bile was possessed of no agglutinating power. The blood gave a positive reaction in a dilution of 1 to 100 in twelve hours. Later when some bile appeared in the stools they succeeded in obtaining only a partial reaction in a dilution of 1 to 20 in two hours. In two other cases of febrile jaundice, in which the stools were not entirely acholic, the serum did not agglutinate the typhoid bacillus even in a dilution of 1 to 10; and in a fourth case of metastatic carcinoma of the liver there was an entire absence of any agglutination reaction.

Their first case is, however, not conclusive for two reasons. In the first place a time-limit of twelve hours is too long for a reaction in a dilution of 1 to 100, and secondly the question of whether the cholelithiasis could not have been due to typhoid infection is entirely ignored. The conclusion which has been drawn from these two cases, that the serum of an icteric patient with cholangitis gives a positive reaction, whereas that from an icteric patient without cholangitis does not, is hardly warranted.

Joachim[10] describes two cases. The first was a case of febrile jaundice in which at the postmortem examination purulent cholangitis and a thrombosis of the portal vein were found. In this case the blood gave a positive reaction with the typhoid bacillus in a dilution of 1 to 40 in two hours and 1 to 80 in fifteen hours (macroscopic and microscopic tests). From the spleen a paracolon bacillus was cultivated, which was agglutinated by the serum in a dilution of 1 to 40 in two hours. In the second case the jaundice was due to a carcinoma at the papilla of Vater, obstructing the common duct. The blood obtained from the cadaver sixteen hours after death (!) agglutinated the typhoid bacillus in a dilution of 1 to 10 in fifteen hours.

These observations also are of no great significance. In the first place the time-limit was too long for the strength of the reactions. The author does not state what he considers to be a positive reaction; and again, the reaction may have been a group-agglutination reaction. He believed that he was able to confirm the observation of Langstein and Meerwein, that it is particularly in cases of cholangitis with jaundice that the blood gives a positive Widal reaction.

The observations of Koenigstein[11] are, we believe, more conclusive than any of those already mentioned. His reactions were made in a dilution of 1 to 10, 1 to 50 and 1 to 100 and were observed for a period of twenty-four hours. With bile he obtained only false reactions due to mucus, crystals and cellular elements. He could eliminate such reactions by filtering the bile. He examined 21 specimens of bile obtained at autopsy with negative results. The bile of rabbits and oxen also gave negative results. In two dogs in which he had produced jaundice by the subcutaneous injection of a hemolytic poison, he obtained a reaction in only 1 to 10 in one, and no reaction in the other. Among 11 cases of jaundice, seven gave no reaction whatsoever; the other four gave good reactions in a dilution of 1 to 10 and slight reactions in 1 to 50. He believes that in some cases such reactions may be group-agglutinations. He repeated Koehler's experiment with taurocholic acid, but could not substantiate his findings. When one knows that the writer considers an agglutination reaction to consist of agglutination with "incomplete paralysis of the bacteria" his negative results are doubly convincing.

Our own observations consist of tests made with bile and with the serum of jaundiced patients. Ten samples of bile were examined. These specimens were either normal bile or bile from cases of typhoid fever, chronic pancreatitis or cholelithiasis. In no instance could we get a positive Widal reaction. With some there was slight clumping, but in others there was absolutely no effect on the bacilli even in a dilution of 1 to 1. The sera of 35 cases of jaundice (exclusive of four cases to be described later) were tested. These cases included cases of appendicitis, malignant endocarditis, gall-stones with and without cholecystitis, tumors of the liver and duodenum, diseases of the pancreas, a case of Weil's disease, two cases of acute yellow atrophy, a case of general miliary tuberculosis, some cases of catarrhal icterus, hypertrophic cirrhosis, one case of liver abscess with jaundice and cases of jaundice due to septic conditions. In not one of these cases was the serum possessed of any more effect on the bacteria than we often find in normal sera. Not one of them gave a reaction which was at all doubtful.

In only four cases in our experience have we met with a positive Widal reaction in patients with jaundice. The first case was one of paracolon infection reported by the writer in the *Journal of Medical Research* for 1902. In that case the patient had a positive reaction with the paracolon bacillus obtained from the blood in a dilution of 1 to 100 and the typhoid bacillus in a dilution of 1 to 200. At the autopsy healing ulcers were found in the intestine and the question had to remain an open one whether or not the patient suffered from a mixed infection due to the typhoid bacillus and the paracolon bacillus.

The second case was that of a woman who was in the hospital

last year with an attack of typhoid fever complicated by cholecystitis. The Widal reaction was positive in a dilution of 1 to 50. She returned to the hospital yesterday with a severe attack of cholecystitis accompanied by marked jaundice and was operated upon by Dr. Lilienthal. The blood gives a positive Widal reaction in the dilution of 1 to 20. The bile and the markedly icteric urine give no reaction.

The third case was also one of typhoid fever with jaundice due to acute cholecystitis. The Widal reaction was positive in a dilution of 1 to 50 and typhoid bacilli were demonstrated in the fluid in the gall-bladder by Dr. Bernstein of the laboratory staff. The fluid in the gall-bladder in this case was not bile-stained, but consisted of thin seropurulent fluid. This fluid gave a positive Widal reaction in a dilution of 1 to 50.

The fourth case is one of such marked interest that I shall give the history in detail. The patient was a woman, sixty-four years of age, who was in good health up to the age of thirty-four years when she suffered from an attack of jaundice with severe colicky pains and passed gall-stones. There is no history of typhoid fever. One year before admission to the hospital she suffered from severe colicky pains, chills and vomiting; her skin became extremely yellow, the feces very light-colored, the urine very dark and she passed gall-stones. She was well after this attack up to two weeks before admission to the hospital. Then she had a chill, vomited dark green fluid, had severe pain in the upper right quadrant of the abdomen and marked jaundice. She was operated upon by Dr. Lilienthal who found a large purulent exudate around the gall-bladder. The Widal reaction was positive in a dilution of 1 to 50 and typhoid bacilli were isolated by Dr. Bernstein from the pus found at the operation.

It will thus be seen that from our observations there is nothing which convinces us that jaundice *per se* can cause a positive Widal reaction, and have pointed out such deficiencies in the cases cited in the literature, that all we can state is that, while icteric serum may at times be possessed of a certain amount of agglutinating power, there is no definite proof at present that it can produce sufficient agglutination to interfere with our clinical diagnosis.

NOTE.—Since writing this paper, another case of jaundice was found with a positive Widal reaction. The patient was a girl, 23 years of age, in the service of Dr. Brill. She was admitted with a history of jaundice of five years' standing. The liver was enlarged, hard and irregular. The clinical diagnosis wavered between hepatic syphilis and biliary cirrhosis due to calculi. The Widal reaction was positive 1 to 100. On looking up the history, it was found that she had suffered from typhoid fever twelve years before. The autopsy showed a biliary cirrhosis due to calculi in the common duct. In the gall-bladder and in the heart blood typhoid bacilli were found; the interior of the stones showed bacterium coli only.

Of interest is a recent paper (published in May, 1905, by Falta and Noeggerath, in the Deutsches Archiv. fuer klinische Medizin) in which the absence of agglutination in low dilutions when present in high ones in cases of typhoid fever is confirmed. The paper cites similar results published since the appearance of our own by Sahli and Stern. The paper discusses at length the explanation of the phenomenon.

REFERENCES.

[1] SHIGA: Zeitschrift für Hygiene, Vol. xli., p. 261.
[2] Cited by Koenigstein.
[3] Cited by Eckardt.
[4] GREENBAUM: Cited by Eckardt.
[5] KOEHLER: Klinisches Jahrbuch, Vol. viii., Heft I.
[6] SAILOR: Transactions of the Philadelphia Pathological Society, 1902, p. 253.
[7] ZUPNIK: Zeitschrift für Heilkunde, 1901, Vol. ii., p. 334.
[8] ECKARDT: Münchener klin. Wochenschrift, No. 27, 1902.
[9] LANGSTEIN AND MEERWEIN: Wiener Klin., 1903, No. 27.
[10] JOACHIM: Wiener klin. Wochenschrift, 1902, No. 35.
[11] KOENIGSTEIN: Ibid.

A NEW METHOD FOR STAINING THE CAPSULES OF BACTERIA: PRELIMINARY COMMUNICATION.*

By Leo Buerger, M.D.,
PATHOLOGICAL INTERNE.

Although many methods for staining the capsules of bacteria have been devised, the opinion seems to be almost unanimous that they are for the most part very variable in their results. Not this alone, but also the difficulty of differentiating the encapsulated diplococcus, from similar lanceolate organisms, especially of the streptococcus type, led the writer, early in May of this year, to devise a procedure which would enable the bacteriologist to identify the diplococcus lanceolatus with greater ease and precision.

The recognition of the encapsulated organisms in the very first cultures taken from exudates, when for any reason their demonstration in the exudates themselves is impossible, is of prime importance. It is in this particular regard that the method advocated fills a want left by the older procedures.

By it capsules can be obtained not only in exudates but also on certain culture media. The configuration of the capsule of the pneumococcus, when recently isolated, and on certain media, differs from that produced by the methods employed heretofore, and from that of other organisms, in so characteristic a manner that the diagnosis of the organism becomes a comparatively easy matter.

The older stains present the capsule as a diffusely staining, poorly outlined, elliptical band immediately surrounding the diplococcus. With my method it has the following features: There is a refractile, deeply staining, regularly outlined, narrow, elliptical capsule membrane, separated from the diplococcus by a clear area of capsular substance which either remains unstained or takes a faint color. Each of the other encapsulated organisms thus far studied has its own peculiar type of capsule. The bacillus mucosus capsulatus shows a

*Reprinted from The Medical News, December 10, 1904.

broad mucoid envelope with an easily destructible membrane, the "streptococcus mucosus," one of similar nature, and some strains of the pyogenic streptococcus show only a finer linear envelope.

The Method.—The necessary solutions are as follows: (1) Müller's fluid (bichromate of potassium, 2.5 grams; sulphate of sodium, 1.0 gram; water, 100 c.c.) saturated with bichloride of mercury (ordinarily about 5 per cent.). (2) Beef, human or other blood serum diluted with an equal amount of normal salt solution; or ascitic or pleural fluid. (3) 80 to 95 per cent. alcohol. (4) Tincture of iodine, U.S.P. (5) Freshly prepared stain; anilin water gentian violet, made up as follows: Anilin oil 10, water 100, shake, filter and add 5 c.c. saturated alcoholic solution of gentian violet; or, 10 per cent. watery fuchsin (i. e., saturated alcoholic solution of fuchsin 10.0, water 100.0). (6) Two per cent. salt solution in water.

Technic.—The culture is thinly and carefully spread over a perfectly clean cover-slip by means of a drop of diluted serum.* Just as the edges begin to dry the fixing fluid, solution No. 1, is poured on, the cover gently warmed over the flame for about three seconds, rapidly washed in water, flushed once with alcohol, and then treated with iodine for one to two minutes. The iodine is in turn thoroughly washed off with alcohol, and the specimen dried in the air. Staining for two to five seconds, and washing with salt solution, completes the procedure. The specimen is mounted in the salt solution and ringed with vaselin.

Sputum and pus can be stained in a similar manner, the addition of serum being unnecessary, except in very mucoid, stringy purulent exudates.

The method depends, therefore, upon the rapid fixation of the bacteria while still alive and when spread in a medium which prevents dissolution of their capsules. The Müller's fluid, saturated with bichloride of mercury (i.e., Zenker minus acetic acid), which is found ready in every laboratory, has given the best results. However, a simple saturated solution of bichloride of mercury in one-half per cent. salt solution has also been tried, but hitherto has given less distinct pictures. The results obtained by the use of other fixatives will be reported on at a later date.

Thin spreads can be obtained by first emulsifying the culture in a

---

*Hiss: Centralblatt f. Bact., etc., 1902, xxxi., p. 302.

drop of serum on a separate slide. It is of importance to thoroughly rid the specimen of iodine. The preliminary alcohol wash before the iodine steep is not absolutely essential. The whole procedure, taking some two minutes, can be much shortened by reducing the action of the iodine to thirty seconds. This is accomplished by flushing several times with fresh iodine. Thus a good preparation can be finished in about one minute.

As for the stain, watery fuchsin also gives good results. Double staining by means of gentian violet and fuchsin is also feasible. Good permanent balsam mounts can be made from these double stained specimens. Methods for making all mounts permanent are now nearing completion and will be given in detail in a future publication.

The questions of the occurrence and variation of the capsules of different organisms on artificial media, of changes in morphology, and of the differential diagnosis between the pneumococcus and streptococcus by means of this new technic, I will reserve for discussion in a future paper.* The results obtained warrant us in recommending the method to the consideration of the bacteriologist and clinical microscopist.

*Centralblatt fuer Bakteriologie, Bd. 39, Abth. I., Heft 2 and 3.

INVESTIGATIONS IN METABOLISM AND COMPOSITION OF THE URINE IN DISEASE.*

By S. Bookman, M.A., Ph.D., and Edward A. Aronson, M.D.,

1. Typhoid Fever.

In medical literature so little appears in regard to the composition of the urine in various diseases, that this laboratory has taken upon itself to investigate, as carefully as modern methods will admit, the composition of the urine in various diseases, especially as the fevers, on account of their prescribed limitations in affecting primarily but few of the digestive or excretory organs, seem to us a specially fertile field upon which to commence these investigations. On account of the severe emaciation, accompanying the rise in temperature in this disease, suggesting a katabolism of cells and, therefore, proteid matter of the body, we have framed this particular study along the lines of such analyses as would point to the determination of these elements contained in the proteid molecule, viz., N, P, S, and have accordingly determined the total nitrogen and ammonia, the total phosphoric acid, and the free or preformed sulphuric acid and ethereal sulphuric acid. The determination of total solids in their bearing to the inorganic solids is of particular value, since we have consequently before us the relation of organic to inorganic material eliminated.

The total chlorine at the same time gives us the approximate relation of the chlorides to the total solids.

Investigations along these lines are of necessity confined to a hospital laboratory, for in connection with the medical aspect and treatment of the case, the diet, medication and all physical measurements, such as temperature, as well as other bedside observations must be carried on by the medical staff, and the physiological chemist is, therefore, in touch with the physician treating the case, and can then

*From the Physiological Chemical Department of the Pathological Laboratory of Mt. Sinai Hospital.

and then only judge of the particular adaptability of his case, as a pure case of the disease in question, to the subject of his investigations.

These cases can naturally be studied only one or two at a time, and after the collection of sufficient data, then and then only can we arrive at any deductions as to the particular constituent which gives rise to the pathological symptoms noted, or which is itself eliminated by the abnormal process going on in the body. Such investigations as Liebermeister, Leyden, Senator, Traube and others differ upon the essential facts in regard to the temperature in fever. Some of these claim that fever is the result of an increased metabolism, whereas others contend that the increased metabolism is due to the elevated temperature itself. Whatever may be the definite conclusion, only after the most careful and elaborate work upon sufficient numbers of cases, typical for each disease in question, will we be able to draw correct inferences, and it is with this object in view that these researches were begun.

The cases noted below were typical cases of typhoid fever, and besides the diet the temperature changes were noted during each twenty-four hour period in which the urines were collected for these investigations.

Previous work by Hoesslin, Diakonow, Gruzdiev, Gramatchikov and others has shown that the total nitrogen in the feces as compared with the urine was seldom over 10 per cent., and generally below 5 per cent. of the total nitrogen output, and we have, therefore, come to the conclusion that great variations, if present, would be found in the urine and have confined ourselves to the study of this fluid.

On account of the simplicity of milk as a food and the convenience in determining the total nitrogen contents, we have in most instances chosen those cases and confined ourselves to that stage of the disease during which milk formed the principal diet. We have, after careful deliberation, adopted four days as the proper period for these investigations, two and three days being too short for the determination of averages.

We give below our results of investigations upon four cases.

CASE 1.—TYPHOID FEVER.

Date.	July 14-15.	July 15-16.	July 16-17.	July 17-18.	July 25-26.	July 26-27.	July 27-28.	July 28-29.
Amount	1,280 ccm.	1,020 ccm.	1,720 ccm.	1,620 ccm.	1,610 ccm.	850 ccm	1,120 ccm.	420 ccm.
Specific gravity	.1005	.1004	.1003	.1003	.1005	.1007	.1004	.1003
Solids, total	1.648%	1.68%	1.66%	1.48%	2.144%	1.924%	1.17%	0.99%
" , inorganic	21.002	17.085	28.48	24.041	34.518	16.354	13.104	4.158
	0.33%	0.40%	0.35%	0.408%	0.294%	0.634%	0.473%	0.25%
	4.224	4.08	6.02	6.609	4.7334	5.389	5.3088	1.05
Total nitrogen	0.562%	0.54%		0.476%	0.647%	0.605%	0.487%	0.436%
	7.19	5.50		7.711	10.4167	5.1425	5.9414	1.8346
Ammonia	0.04%	0.03%	0.03%	0.034%	0.0595%	0.0578%	0.053%	0.0517
	0.50	0.287	0.585	0.5508	0.9579	0.4913	0.5902	0.2142
Uric acid	0.02%	0.02%	0.016%	0.0075%	0.026%	0.0355%	0.023%	0.0135%
	0.25	0.264	0.275	0.1215	0.4018	0.2167	0.2004	0.0567
Chlorine	0.06%	0.036%	0.10%	0.10%	0.0994%	0.2485%	0.195%	0.0677
	0.77	0.362	1.703	1.604	1.6003	2.1122	2.1868	0.2833
Total phosphates	0.09%	0.33%	0.073%	0.062%	0.065%	0.115%	0.064%	0.015%
	1.15	3.366	1.256	1.004	1.0765	0.9775	0.7168	0.42
Preformed sulphates	0.104%	0.08%	0.53%	0.0646%	0.069%	0.064%	0.0738%	0.0970%
	1.33	0.816	0.998	1.048	1.1259	0.5464	0.8267	0.4099
Ethereal sulphates	0.028%	0.013%	0.17%	0.015%	0.0197%	0.016%	0.0111%	0.008%
	0.36	0.133	0.292	0.243	0.3168	0.1382	0.1244	0.0395
Temperature	102°-102.6°	102.8°-101.6°	101.6°-101.2°	100°-101°	101°-100°	101°-99.6°	98.6°-101°	98.6°-100.6°
Total N in diet			[Full diet given.		Starvation temperature.]			

CASE II.—TYPHOID FEVER.

Date.	July 28-29.	July 29-30.	July 30-31.	July 31-Aug. 1.	August 8-9.	August 9-10.	August 10-11.	August 11-12.	August 23-24.	August 24-25.	August 25-26.	August 26-27.
Amount	430 c.c.	1,200 c.c.	1,280 c.c.	525 c.c.	710 c.c.	680 c.c.	845 c.c.	1,110 c.c.	710 c.c.	975 c.c.	920 c.c.	1,170 c.c.
Specific gravity	1.0143	1.0138	1.0865	1.076	1.0096	1.0096	1.005	1.0058	1.0064	1.0052	1.0069	1.0051
Total solids	3.354%	3.294%	2.108%	2.404%	2.39%	2.586%	1.470%	2.068%	2.02%	1.486%	1.742%	1.232%
	14.422	39.528	26.982	12.631	16.969	17.585	12.472	22.955	14.342	14.489	16.126	14.414
Inorganic solids	0.796%	0.964%	0.658%	0.604%	0.70%	0.712%	0.574%	0.652%	0.546%	0.466%	0.440%	0.262%
	3.423	11.568	8.422	3.171	4.970	4.842	4.85	7.237	3.976	4.544	4.103	3.065
Total nitrogen	1.33%	1.114%	0.952%	0.739%	0.843%	1.054%	0.504%	0.786%	0.604%	0.504%	0.58%	0.472%
	5.719	13.368	12.186	3.88	5.985	7.167	4.259	8.725	4.288	4.914	5.336	5.522
Ammonia NH₃	0.097%	0.078%	0.2975%	0.070%	0.0517%	0.0537%	0.0323%	0.0297%	0.075%	0.128%	0.151%	0.158%
	0.417	0.936	3.808	0.367	0.363	0.360	0.273	0.322	0.533	1.248	1.389	1.849
Uric acid	0.024%	0.032%	0.069%	0.036%	0.0460%	0.0345%	0.0075%	0.0555%	0.033%	0.0188%	0.0263%	0.0263%
	0.103	0.388	0.115	0.189	0.331	0.235	0.063	0.616	0.240	0.188	0.242	0.308
Chlorine	0.131%	0.277%	0.1811%	0.142%	0.135%	0.163%	0.128%	0.114%	0.167%	0.195%	0.142%	0.103%
	0.563	3.284	2.318	0.7455	0.960	1.108	1.082	1.265	1.186	1.901	1.306	1.205
Total phosphoric acid P₂O₅	0.23%	0.215%	0.190%	0.175%	0.175%	0.178%	0.12%	0.171%	0.145%	0.08%	0.115%	0.075%
	0.99	2.58	2.43	0.893	1.242	1.210	1.014	1.898	0.994	0.780	1.058	0.878
Preformed sulphates SO₃	0.239%	0.183%	0.154%	0.141%	0.1340%	0.150%	0.09%	0.1214%	0.105%	0.083%	0.0926%	0.0658%
	1.028	2.196	1.971	0.75	0.956	1.061	0.7605	1.348	0.746	0.809	0.852	0.770
Ethereal sulphates SO₃	0.015%	0.0104%	0.013%	0.009%	0.0143%	0.0125%	0.012%	0.015%	0.0084%	0.007%	0.0116%	0.007%
	0.065	0.125	0.166	0.047	0.101	0.085	0.101	0.166	0.060	0.068	0.107	0.084
Temperature	101.4°	101.4°	102.2°	101.2°	99°-	97.8°-	98°-	98°-	101.6°	102.4°-	103°-	102.4°-
	104°	103.6°	103.8°	104.2°	102.8°	102°	101.6°	101.2°	104°	104.6°	104°	104°
Diet. Total N	19.584	12.556	11.098	10.118	9.792	10.771	10.118	10.445	11.750	12.077	12.730	12.077

Case III.—Typhoid Fever.

Date.	July 31-Aug 1.	August 2-3.	August 3-4.	August 4-5.
Amount	400 ccm.	320 ccm.	620 ccm.	500 ccm.
Specific gravity	.1023	.1019	.1015	1019
Total solids	4.58%	5.11%	3.95%	4.04%
	18 336	16 352	24.49	20.20
Inorganic solids	0.744%	0.67%	0.70%	0.68%
	2.976	2.144	4.34	3 40
Total nitrogen	1.769%	1.867%	1.529%	1.677%
	7.078	5.976	9.48	8.386
Ammonia	0.488%	0.17%	0.105%	0.2703%
	1.951	0.544	0.653	1.3515
Uric acid	0.0037%	0.054%	0.054%	0.0187%
	0.015	0 1752	0.3348	0.0937
Chlorine	0.17%	0 092%	0.089%	0.1065%
	0.6816	0.2953	0.5502	0 5325
Total phosphates	0.43%	0 174%	0.253%	0.22%
	1.72	0.5568	1.5686	1.10
Preformed sulphates	....	0.286%	0.23%	0.288%
	....	0.9174	1.429	4.4392
Ethereal sulphates	....	0 028%	0.02%	0.0178%
	....	0.0917	0.1319	0.089
Temperature	103.4°-104°	103.4°-104°	104°-103°	103°-103.6°
Total N in diet	5.5488	4.4064	4.5696	3.264

Case IV.—Typhoid Fever.

Date.	August 16-17.	August 17-18.	August 18-19.	August 19-20.	August 25-26.	August 26-27.	August 27-28.
Amount	900 c.c.	700 c.c.	1,020 c.c.	1,160 c.c.	1,160 c.c.	770 c.c	1,330 c.c.
Specific gravity	1.016	1.0115	1.010	1.0137	1.011	1.0116	1.005
Total solids	3.27%	3.088%	1.866%	1.85%	2.062%	2.6688%	1.13%
	29.412	21.616	19.233	21.460	23.919	20.544	15.029
Inorganic solids	0.78%	0.592%	0.434%	0.566%	0.634%	0.794%	0.394%
	7.052	4 144	4.427	6.566	7.354	6.114	5.130
Total nitrogen	1.61%	1.414%	1.156%	0.689%	0.84%	0.926%	0.45%
	14.49	9.898	11.790	7.992	9.764	7.130	5.985
Ammonia NH₃	0.277%	0.119%	0.09%	0.417%	0.2646%	0.093%	....
	2.494	0.833	0.918	4.837	3.062	0.716	....
Uric acid	0.01875%	0.0713%	0.051%	0.0075%	0.0038%	0.066%	0.0248%
	0.1667	0.499	0 520	0.088	0.044	0.508	0.330
Chlorine	0.1278%	0.114%	0.085%	0.085%	0.199%	0.234%	0.146%
	1.150	0.798	6.867	0.9860	2.308	1.802	1.939
Total phosphoric acid P₂O₅	0.320%	0.222%	0 202%	0.370%	0.135%	0.145%	0.070%
	2.880	1.554	2.060	4.292	1.566	1.117	0.931
Preformed sulphates SO₃	0.285%	0.238%	0.208%	0.258%	0.132%	0.128%	0.0642%
	2.575	1.656	2.122	2.993	1.532	0.986	0.854
Ethereal sulphates SO₃	0.0137%	0.010%	0.006%	0.0124	0.0048%	0.0134%	0.004%
	0.1233	0.070	0 0612	0.144	0.056	0.103	0.055
Temperature	103°-104°	101.4°-105°	104°-105°	102.4°-104.0°	102.°-104.2°	102°-103°	100.6°-103°
Diet. Total N	8.834	8.16	8.924	7.181	10.118	9.466	9.139

II. Pernicious Anemia.

The only work of value upon the metabolism in diseases of the ductless glands and the blood was performed by Burzhuiski in 1889, Ketche in 1890, and Lepman-Wulf in 1891, in cases of chlorosis, but as this work was rather incomplete and having two typical cases of pernicious anemia at our service, investigations were accordingly commenced along lines similar to the work in typhoid fever above noted.

The increase found in the iron elimination in feces and urine are of particular interest since they show a marked increase over the figures found by Neumann in normal urine, viz., about 0.001 g. per twenty-four hours. These results coincide with figures found by Mayer, Colasanti and Joanguli.

The nature of anemia as regards its relation to metabolism being still obscure, it remains for the further study of more cases of this disease, to draw any conclusions, which the facts at hand at present hardly warrant.

CASE I.—PERNICIOUS ANEMIA. IRON DETERMINATIONS.

Date.	Quantity.	Fe in Urine.	Fe in Feces.
September 29	350 c.c.	0.0039 g	
October 4	1,360 c.c.	0.00685	
October 10	1,625 c.c.	0.0055	
October 16	1,130 c.c.	0.0052	
October 22	1,375 c.c.	0.00385	0.0896
October 29	1,060 c.c	0.01696	0.0241
November 6	1,350 c.c.	0.181	0.0252

CASE II.—PERNICIOUS ANEMIA. IRON DETERMINATIONS.

Date.	Quantity.	Fe in Urine.	Fe in Feces.
October 11	390 c.c.	0.0067	
October 22	360 c.c.	0.0115	0.0414
October 29	660 c.c.	0.0048	0.0442
November 6	980 c.c.	0.0065	0.0392

CASE I.—PERNICIOUS ANEMIA.

Date.	August 28-29.	August 29-30.	August 30-31.	August 31-Sept. 1.	September 3-4.	September 4-5.	September 5-6.	September 6-7.
Amount..................	820 ccm.	660 ccm.	600 ccm.	860 ccm.	1,320 ccm.	980 ccm.	700 ccm.	700 ccm.
Specific gravity.........	.1008	.1012	.1008	.1013	.1007	.1008	.1009	.1011
Solids, total	1.73%	2.08%	2.114%	2.584%	1.774%	1.76%	1.918%	1.637
	14.186	13.754	12.684	22.222	23.4168	17.248	13.426	11.41
Solids, inorganic........	0.75%	0.98%	0.73%	1.25%	0.724%	0.68%	0.638%	0.554%
	6.183	6.494	4.68	10.75	9.557	6.762	4.466	3.878
Sulphates, preformed....	0.116%	0.209%	0.104%	0.30%	0.112%	0.088%	0.1403%	0.1513%
	0.951	1.381	0.625	2.583	1.48	0.967	0.982	1.059
Sulphates, ethereal	0.006%	0.014%	0.077%	0.019%	0.0206%	0.016%	0.0192%	0.0164%
	0.049	0.0909	0.465	0.1598	0.2736	0.158	0.1344	0.1147
Total nitrogen	0.588%	0.649%	0.574%	0.089%	0.563%	0.602%	0.745%	0.702%
	4.822	4.287	3.444	7.7056	7.1289	5.8996	5.2164	4.9196
Ammonia	0.102%	0.314%	0.029%	0.044%	0.143%	0.1615%	0.364%	0.3870%
	0.836	2.0757	0.174	0.3891	1.885	1.5827	2.5466	2.7132
Chlorine................	0.266%	0.287%	0.245%	0.348%	0.266%	0.2378%	0.1633%	0.142%
	2.181	1.898	1.47	2.992	3.5145	2.3309	1.1431	0.994
Phosphates.	0.15%	0.26%	0.15%	0.1655%	0.14%	0.12%	0.243%	0.28%
	1.23	1.716	0.9	1.419	1.848	1.176	1.694	1.96
Uric acid................	0.0075%	0.005%	0.025%	0.025%	0.0225%	0.0277%	0.0075%	0.0045%
	0.0615	0.0346	0.1485	0.2151	0.297	0.2719	0.0525	0.0315

III. Tetanus.

So little has been accomplished in the determination of the metabolism in tetanus, that I feel compelled to add my investigations observed in a case admitted to the wards of the hospital in the service of Dr. Henry Heiman, during the past summer.

Before mentioning my results, I wish to state that the studies were confined only to the urinary excretion—that is, a determination of the solids, both total and inorganic; the total acidity in terms of HCl; the sulphates, both preformed and ethereal; the total nitrogen, ammonia, chlorine, phosphates and uric acid. Only twenty-four hour collections of urine were employed and the work extended over a period of eight days, divided, with an interval of five days, into two series of four days each.

The methods used were as follows: For *solids*, 5 ccm. of unfiltered urine in a platinum vessel, were placed in an oven at 100°C. for three and a half hours and weighed, giving total solids. HNO_3 and H_2SO_4 were added after igniting. Then heated and again weighed, giving inorganic solids as sulphates.

Acidity.—10 ccm. of filtered urine titrated with pheno-phthalein as an indicator and determined in terms of HCl.

Sulphates.—50 ccm. of filtered urine treated with 10 ccm. of acetic acid, heated, and 25 ccm. of barium chloride added, precipitating the sulphates. This was then filtered, ignited and weighed—this gave me the preformed sulphates. To the filtrate, 15 ccm. of HCl were added, boiled until decomposition was complete, filtered, and the precipitate again weighed in a platinum crucible—thus giving the ethereal sulphates.

Total nitrogen.—Five ccm. of unfiltered urine were treated by the Kjeldahl method.

Ammonia.—10 ccm. of filtered urine treated by the Schloesing method.

Chlorine.—10 ccm. of filtered urine were placed in a caserole, $NaCO_3$ and $NaNo_3$ added, and then evaporated. After igniting and taking up with hot water, HNO_3 is added to acidify, $CaCo_3$ to neutralize, and after heating on a water bath, is filtered and washed. The filtrate was then titrated with a 10 $AgNo_3$ solution, using K_2CrO_4 as an indicator.

Phosphates.—50 ccm. of filtered urine, to which 5 ccm. of a solution of sodium acetate and acetic acid are added, are heated and then titrated with a standard solution of uranium acetate.

Uric acid.—To 200 ccm. of filtered urine, Folin's method was applied.

Perhaps it would not be amiss to mention the constituents of a "normal" urine for purposes of comparison later on. Different authorities give different figures, hence there are no arbitrary statistics to be compared with my findings.

Folin,* in a recent publication, gives as the result of an approximately complete and careful analysis of thirty "normal urines" the following figures in a general average:

```
Amount .................................................. 1430 ccm.
Total nitrogen ..........................................   16.9
Urea ....................................................   13.9
Ammonia .................................................    0.85
Kreatinin ...............................................    0.58
Uric acid ...............................................    0.3386
Undetermined nitrogen ...................................    0.6
Total sulphur ...........................................    3.31
Inorganic sulphates .....................................    2.92
Ethereal      "    .......................................    0.22
Neutral sulphur .........................................    0.17
Acidity .................................................  617.
Total phosphates ........................................    3.87
Chlorine ................................................    6.1
```

These figures were obtained while the patients were given the following diet:

```
Milk ................................................... 500 ccm.
Cream (18%—22% fat).................................... 300 ccm.
Eggs (white and yolk).................................. 450 gm.
Horlick's malted milk.................................. 200 gm.
Sugar ..................................................  20 gm.
Salt ...................................................   6 gm.
Water ..............................................up to  2 litres
   "  ..........................................to drink 900 ccm.
```

In looking into the literature of metabolism in tetanus, I found a series of results in five cases, all adults, reported by Vannini,† and I will only mention his conclusions:

First, the patients required considerable quantities of food, which was but poorly absorbed, hence the marked emaciation;

*The American Journal of Physiology, vol. xiii., No. 1.
†Vannini, G. "Contributo allo studio del ricambio materiale uel tetans." Rivista critica di clinica medica, 1902, No. 48-49-50.

Second, increase of albumin metabolism, shown by the marked increase of nitrogen excretion in convalescence;

Third, scant, concentrated and hyperacid urine;

Fourth, urea and ammonia increased, uric acid excretion diminished;

Fifth, often a slight albuminuria with casts;

Sixth, rare or doubtful glycosuria;

Seventh, chlorine diminished, sulphates and phosphates normal.

My case was a child eight years of age and the table on page 411 is given, with the results of the observations.

These studies were made on urine collected after the first twenty-four hours of his stay in the hospital, and for the four succeeding days, during which his temperature never exceeded $100.6°F.$, but marked tetanic symptoms were present all this time. The second series of investigations were begun five days after the last of the preceding series was ended, and during the latter period the symptoms had materially decreased and the condition improved much.

In all metabolism work, one of the most important factors is the determination of the total nitrogen excretion. In accurate observations it is necessary to calculate the total nitrogen in the feces as well as in the urine, for two reasons; first, in ordinary diets a certain proportion of vegetable and animal proteid escapes digestion, and this amount must be estimated and deducted from the total nitrogen intake in order to ascertain what nitrogenous material has actually been used up; second, the secretions of the alimentary canal contain a certain amount of nitrogenous material which represents a genuine excretion and should be included in estimations of the total proteid destruction.

Practical experience has shown that in man about 29 per cent. of the total nitrogen of the feces has this latter origin.

During the first period the boy was fed on a fluid diet of milk, coffee, cocoa and water, but during the second he received a much more nitrogenous diet of soup, milk, egg, cocoa and rice.

It will be seen on closer examination that the table shows no marked increase of nitrogen excretion in the latter period over the former, despite the fact of an increase of nitrogenous food stuffs, signifying that the boy was already convalescing and a probable restoration of the "nitrogen equilibrium."

The solids were diminished throughout; sulphates but slightly

Date.	August 12-13.	August 14-15.	August 15-16.	August 16-17.	August 21-22.	August 22-23.	August 23-24.	August 24-25.
Amount	560 ccm.	440 ccm.	320 ccm.	610 ccm.	600 ccm.	680 ccm.	1,060 ccm.	1,040 ccm.
Specific gravity	1.023	1.027	1.029	1.018	1.019	1.021	1.011	1.011
Acidity	25.9359	35.0108	12.0304	18.9216	Alkaline.	14.892	11.607	15.184
Solids, total	1.15%	6.58%	7.37%	4.22%	2.95%	4.15%	3.06%	2.37%
	23.24	28.97	23.58	27.03	17.70	28.22	32.92	24.606
Solids, inorganic	1.22%	1.04%	0.95%	1.114%	1.71%	1.78%	1.49%	0.986%
	6.832	4.6112	3.0528	7.1296	10.26	12.104	15.815	10.254
Sulphates, preformed	0.32%	0.46%	0.57%	0.203%	0.20%	0.25%	0.14%	0.15%
	1.808	2.034	1.8198	1.297	1.201	1.689	1.52	1.574
Sulphates, ethereal	0.02%	0.02%	0.026%	0.018%	0.013%	0.013%	0.01%	0.01%
	0.1202	0.093	0.0856	0.1172	0.076	0.099	0.1323	0.1106
Total nitrogen	1.86%	2.42%	2.56%	1.389%	0.52%	1.09%	0.85%	0.01%
	10.438	10.6804	8.189	8.8883	3.108	7.4256	8.9634	11.066
Ammonia	0.21%	0.25%	0.23%	0.15%	0.47%	0.06%	0.046%	0.056%
	1.165	1.092	0.729	0.097	2.815	0.366	0.486	0.587
Chlorine	0.61%	0.54%	0.45%	0.74%	0.40%	0.50%	0.34%	0.30%
	3.413	2.374	1.445	4.77	2.385	3.428	3.612	3.14
Phosphates	0.50%	0.48%	0.36%	0.18%	0.34%	0.27%	0.185%	0.20%
	2.805	2.112	1.152	1.152	2.01	1.836	1.961	2.10
Uric acid	0.07%	0.057%	0.094%	0.05%	0.004%	0.06%	0.025%	0.007%
	0.4116	0.2508	0.3008	0.317	0.0295	0.408	0.262	0.0707

diminished, except on the second day, when the patient received some "salts" for catharsis; ammonia varied at times, normal or increased; chlorine diminished; phosphates but little changed; uric acid much diminished.

The urine was at first scant, concentrated and hyperacid, later more copious and less acid. A faint trace of albumin was present only at the first examination, never any casts. Sugar was absent.

The figures from this one case compare favorably in a general way with those observed by Vannini in his five cases.

As yet too few practical clinical deductions can be obtained from the study of the metabolism in tetanus because of the very little that has heretofore been accomplished in this direction, and compels us to trust to the future, with an increase of material and improvement of scientific investigations.

A NEW X-RAY TUBE STAND; A NEW X-RAY TABLE.*

By Walter M. Brickner, M.D.,
RADIOGRAPHIST.

These apparatus were designed to overcome the mechanical defects and the many limitations of the appliances generally in use.

The Tube Stand is made of maple wood. The flat, triangular base, mounted on ball-bearing castors, is light enough to shift easily, yet large enough to prevent tipping over of the stand, even when a heavy tube-shield is placed at the end of the tube arm. The five and one-half foot rectangular upright, graduated in inches, is hollow to accommodate a rectangular lead weight which, by means of a cord moving over a pulley at the top of the stand, accurately balances, and makes easy the movement of, the block that slides up and down on the upright. This block moves upon wooden rollers (fitting into grooves in the upright) and bears also a rubber friction wheel, which not only steadies it in position upon the upright but, by means of an attached wooden handle, also permits fine adjustment of the block at any level. A second rubber friction wheel and handle steady and adjust the graduated horizontal arm that moves back and forth in the block. Two openings in the block, bearing indicators, permit exact readings of the vertical and horizontal scales. Also mounted on the block are two jointed wooden arms, capable of universal adjustment, for the support and separation of the wires running from the coil to the tube. The latter is held on a jointed rod and clamp, articulating on an upright at the end of the horizontal arm. Adjustment of the tube in every plane is very easy.

The manufacturers of this stand have recently modified the sliding block by employing a friction wheel at each side (as described later with the X-ray table). This makes it possible to reverse the horizontal arm (graduated on both sides) and turn the stand so that it can be

*Reprinted from The American Journal of Surgery, April, 1905.

used from either side—right or left—with the adjusting wheels and scales always toward the operator.

The advantages of the stand are that it permits of the adjustment of the tube at any angle and at any level from the floor up to a height of six feet and, therefore, equally well under and over the examining

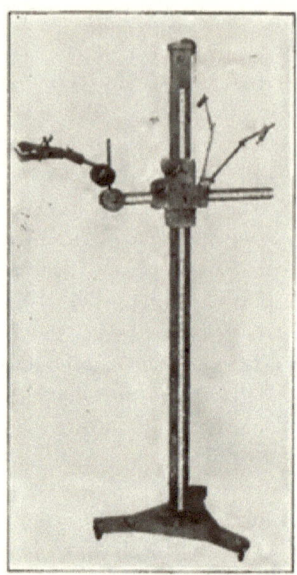

FIG. 1.—X-Ray Tube Stand.

table, that fine adjustment is easy even while the tube is in operation, that it is well adapted to stereoscopic radiography, and that, being of wood, it does not conduct sparks from the wires.

The X-Ray Table is built of a framework of quartered oak, 25 inches wide and 29½ inches high. Including the castors the table has a height from the floor of 32 inches. The top of the table consists of a fixed portion, 42 inches long, and an adjustable portion, 30 inches long. The framework here is 1½ inches wide, thus leaving a space in each portion of the top 22 inches wide for firmly fastened slabs of fibre. This fibre is quite transparent to the X-rays and yet does not yield under the weight of even very heavy patients.

The surface of both the fibre slabs is marked off in small squares by lines corresponding with the inch marks of scales fastened on all four sides of the fibre. Under the larger section of the table top, slides a wooden shelf bearing scales at its sides exactly corresponding with the scales above. The shelf is marked off by crosslines corresponding with those on the fibre, and at each crossing the shelf is perforated by round apertures for the insertion of buttons to hold

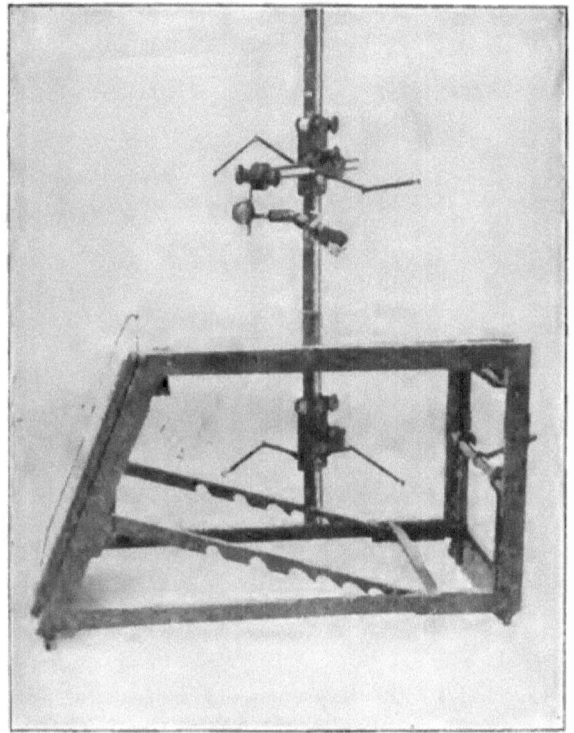

FIG. 2.—X-Ray Table—Closed.

an X-ray plate in position. When the shelf is pushed in and clamped the plate is in direct contact with the under surface of the fibre. By this device a plate can be inserted in just the place under the patient desired, without lifting him, and a second plate can be put in exactly the same position as the first, while the patient remains unmoved, thus fulfilling—with the adjustment of the tube-holder described below—the conditions of stereoscopic radiography. The shelf can be lifted out of the table entirely, and the similar plate shelf under the adjustable portion of the table is hinged so that it can be dropped out of the way—for fluoroscopic examination of a patient with the tube under the table.

It will be seen in the illustrations that ample space for the movement of the tube under the table is provided for by the arrangement of the table legs and their supporting bar, and of the support of the

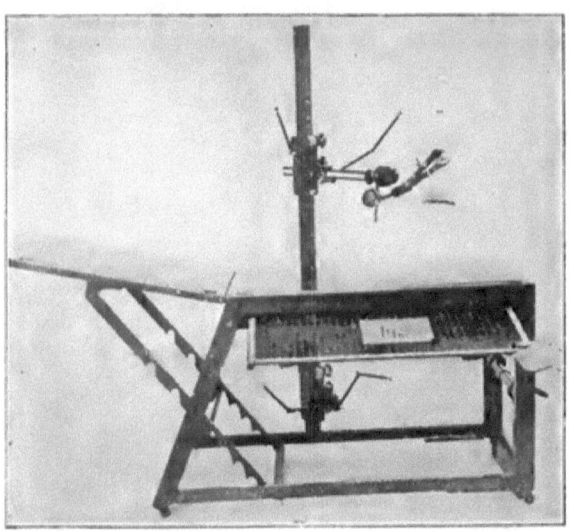

FIG. 3.—X-Ray Table—Opened. Showing plate shelf.

adjustable segment of the table top. This segment is attached to the fixed portion by hinges of fibre so constructed that the movable, directly abuts against the stationary part, in all its adjustments from the lowermost (shown in Fig. 2—table closed) up to the vertical position. This is chiefly of importance, however, when the table is opened out horizontally. In this position the table has a total length of six feet. The length of the adjustable portion is calculated to accommodate comfortably a patient sitting upright, or semi-recumbent, for fluoroscopy of the trunk, etc.

The castors are ball-bearing and the table is easily shifted. At its foot, however, is an arresting device, the width of the table, which, by the movement of a lever, lifts the castors at the foot from the floor and thus prevents the table from rolling. The lever works easily, even with a heavy patient on the table.

Attached to the further side of the table, and movable along its length, is a modification of the tube stand above described. The graduated upright carries two adjustable blocks—one above, and the other below, the level of the table top—and the graduated tube-bearing horizontal arm may be slipped into either block. Two rubber friction

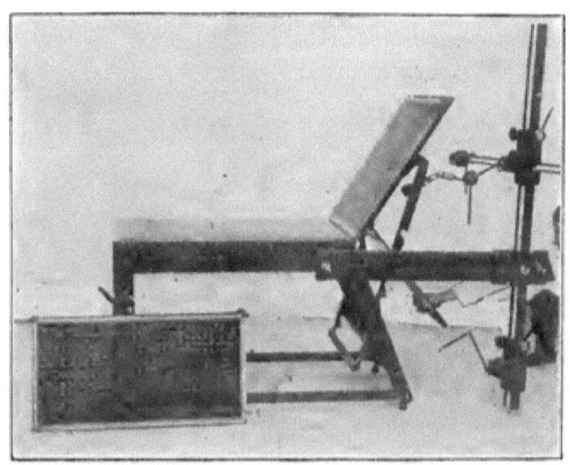

FIG. 4.—X-Ray Table. Arranged for fluoroscopy of chest with patient sitting upright. Plate shelf removed. Tube stand track extended.

wheels on each of these blocks grip the upright, thus dispensing with the counterweight.

The upright revolves, near its middle, in a broad, wide block that can be easily slid on a similarly wide track (near the *top* of the table), consisting of an oak piece the length of the stationary portion of the table, finished on its upper and lower surface with a molded strip of brass. The block bears corresponding brass surfaces. The entire track can be extended to the full length of the opened table, on a wide secondary brass-trimmed track hidden within and fixed to the side of the table. Upon the extended track the tube stand can be rotated behind the adjustable section of the table, when elevated for examination of the chest, neck, etc. Three metal set-screws fasten, respectively, the upright of the tube stand at any angle of rotation in the sliding block, the block at any point along the outer track, and the outer track at any point on the inner track. At no position of the tube holder, or of the table itself, is there any unsteadiness or shaking of one part upon another.

These apparatus are manufactured by the Wappler Electric Controller Co., New York, to whom the writer is indebted for many valuable suggestions in their construction, as well as in the construction of an especially designed X-ray coil and a movable table bearing *all* the switches and adjustments for the coil, and of several other radiographic appliances.

www.ingramcontent.com/pod-product-compliance
Lightning Source LLC
Chambersburg PA
CBHW032143010526
44111CB00035B/993